Biology of Schizophrenia and Affective Disease

Association for Research in Nervous and Mental Disease

NATIONAL UNIVERSITY
LIBRARY ORANGE COUNTY

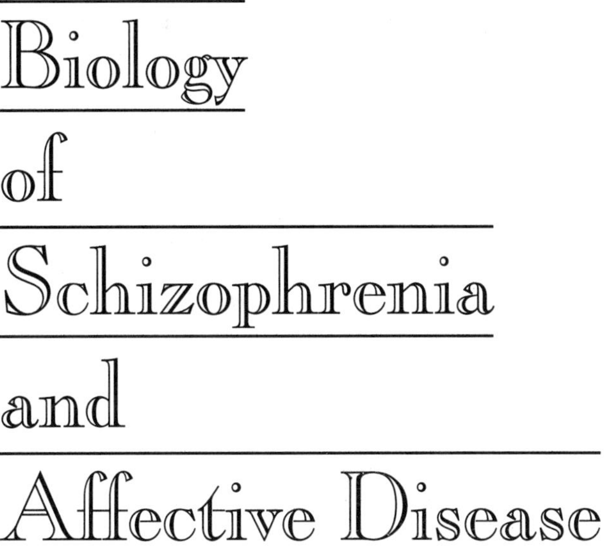

Biology of Schizophrenia and Affective Disease

EDITED BY
Stanley J. Watson, Ph.D., M.D.

Association for Research in Nervous and Mental Disease

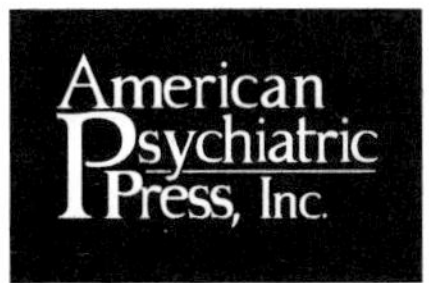

Washington, DC
London, England

NATIONAL UNIVERSITY
LIBRARY ORANGE COUNTY

Note: The authors have worked to ensure that all information in this book concerning drug dosages, schedules, and routes of administration is accurate as of the time of publication and consistent with standards set by the U.S. Food and Drug Administration and the general medical community. As medical research and practice advance, however, therapeutic standards may change. For this reason and because human and mechanical errors sometimes occur, we recommend that readers follow the advice of a physician who is directly involved in their care or the care of a member of their family.

Books published by the American Psychiatric Press, Inc., represent the views and opinions of the individual authors and do not necessarily represent the policies and opinions of the Press or the American Psychiatric Association.

Copyright © 1996 American Psychiatric Press, Inc.
ALL RIGHTS RESERVED
Manufactured in the United States of America on acid-free paper
First Edition
99 98 97 96 4 3 2 1

American Psychiatric Press, Inc.
1400 K Street, N.W., Washington, DC 20005

Library of Congress Cataloging-in-Publication Data
Biology of schizophrenia and affective disease / edited by Stanley J.
Watson. — 1st ed.
p. cm.
Proceedings of the 73rd Meeting of the Association for Research in
Nervous and Mental Disease held Dec. 1993 in New York City.
"Association for Research in Nervous and Mental Disease."
Includes bibliographical references and index.
ISBN 0-88048-746-1
1. Biological psychiatry—Congresses. 2. Schizophrenia—
Physiological aspects—Congresses. 3. Affective disorders—
Physiological aspects—Congresses. 4. Autism—Physiological
aspects—Congresses. I. Watson, Stanley J., 1943– .
II. Association for Research in Nervous and Mental Disease. Meeting
(73rd : 1993 : New York, N.Y.)
[DNLM: 1. Schizophrenia—physiopathology—congresses.
2. Schizophrenia—therapy—congresses. 3. Affective Disorders—
physiopathology—congresses. 4. Affective Disorders—therapy—
congresses. WM 203 B616 1995]
RC327.B55 1995
616.89′82—dc20
DNLM/DLC
for Library of Congress 95-10715
CIP

British Library Cataloguing in Publication Data
A CIP record is available from the British Library.

Contents

Contributors ix

Preface xv

1 Introduction to the 73rd Meeting of the Association for Research in Nervous and Mental Disease 1
Stanley J. Watson, Ph.D., M.D.

2 The Biology of Stress: From Periphery to Brain 15
Huda Akil, Ph.D., and M. Inés Morano, Ph.D.

3 Norepinephrine and Serotonin Transporters: Progress on Molecular Targets of Antidepressants 49
Randy D. Blakely, Ph.D.

4 Excitotoxicity in the Development of Corticolimbic Alterations in Schizophrenic Brain 83
Francine M. Benes, M.D., Ph.D.

5 Dissolution of Cerebral Cortical Mechanisms in Subjects With Schizophrenia 113
Patricia Goldman-Rakic, Ph.D.

6 **Linkage and Molecular Genetics of Infantile Autism 129**
Roland D. Ciaranello, M.D.

7 **Epidemiology and Behavioral Genetics of Schizophrenia 163**
Ming T. Tsuang, M.D., Ph.D., D.Sc., F.R.C.Psych., and Stephen V. Faraone, Ph.D.

8 **Postmortem Studies of Suicide Victims 197**
J. John Mann, M.D., Mark D. Underwood, Ph.D., and Victoria Arango, Ph.D.

9 **Schizophrenia: Postmortem Studies 223**
Joel E. Kleinman, M.D., Ph.D., and Safia Nawroz, M.D.

10 **Brain Circuits and Brain Function: Implications for Psychiatric Diseases 239**
Marcus E. Raichle, M.D., and Wayne C. Drevets, M.D.

11 **Peptides and Affective Disorders 259**
Michael J. Owens, Ph.D., Paul M. Plotsky, Ph.D., and Charles B. Nemeroff, M.D., Ph.D.

12 **Mechanism of Action of Antidepressants: Monoamine Hypotheses and Beyond 295**
Robert M. Berman, M.D., John H. Krystal, M.D., and Dennis S. Charney, M.D.

13 **Dopamine and Schizophrenia Revisited 369**
René S. Kahn, M.D., Ph.D., Michael Davidson, M.D., and Kenneth L. Davis, M.D.

14 **Pathophysiology of Schizophrenia: Insights From Neuroimaging 393**
John Darrell Van Horn, Ph.D., Karen Faith Berman, M.D., and Daniel R. Weinberger, M.D.

15 **Abnormal Frontotemporal Interactions in Patients With Schizophrenia 421**
Karl J. Friston, B.A., M.A., Sigrid Herold, B.M., B.Ch., M.R.C.Psych., P. Fletcher, M.B.B.S., D. Silbersweig, M.D., C. Cahill, B.Sc., R. J. Dolan, M.D., P. F. Liddle, B.M., B.Ch., Ph.D., R. S. J. Frackowiak, M.A., M.D., F.R.C.P., and C. D. Frith, Ph.D.

16 **Mechanism of Action of Atypical Antipsychotic Drugs: An Update 451**
Herbert Y. Meltzer, M.D., Bryan Yamamoto, Ph.D., Martin T. Lowy, Ph.D., and Craig A. Stockmeier, Ph.D.

17 **Overview and Discussion 493**
Steven Matthysse, Ph.D.

Index 505

Contributors

Huda Akil, Ph.D.
Research Scientist and Director of Neurosciences, Mental Health Research Institute, University of Michigan; and Gardner C. Quarton Professor of Neurosciences, Department of Psychiatry, University of Michigan

Victoria Arango, Ph.D.
Assistant Professor, Mental Health Research Center for the Study of Suicidal Behavior and Laboratories of Neuropharmacology, Western Psychiatric Institute and Clinic, University of Pittsburgh School of Medicine

Francine M. Benes, M.D., Ph.D.
Associate Professor, Department of Psychiatry and Program in Neuroscience, Mailman Research Center, McLean Hospital, Belmont, Massachusetts

Karen Faith Berman, M.D.
Chief, Unit on PET, National Institute of Mental Health, Intramural Research Program, Neuroscience Center at St. Elizabeth's

Robert M. Berman, M.D.
Assistant Professor, Department of Psychiatry, Yale University School of Medicine and Psychiatry Service

Randy D. Blakely, Ph.D.
Associate Professor, Anatomy and Cell Biology, Emory University School of Medicine

C. Cahill, B.Sc.
Scientific Officer, MRC Cyclotron Unit, Hammersmith Hospital, London

Dennis S. Charney, M.D.
Professor and Chief, Psychiatry Service, Department of Psychiatry, Yale University School of Medicine and Psychiatry Service

Roland D. Ciaranello, M.D. (deceased)
Professor, Nancy Pritzker Laboratory of Developmental and Molecular Neurobiology, Stanford University School of Medicine

Michael Davidson, M.D.
Associate Professor, Department of Psychiatry, Mount Sinai School of Medicine and Bronx Veterans Affairs Medical Center

Kenneth L. Davis, M.D.
Professor and Chairman, Department of Psychiatry, Mount Sinai School of Medicine and Bronx Veterans Affairs Medical Center

R. J. Dolan, M.D.
Reader in Psychiatry, MRC Cyclotron Unit, Hammersmith Hospital, London

Wayne C. Drevets, M.D.
Department of Psychiatry, Washington University School of Medicine

Stephen V. Faraone, Ph.D.
Associate Professor of Psychology, Department of Psychiatry, Harvard Medical School

P. Fletcher, M.B.B.S.
Research Fellow, MRC Cyclotron Unit, Hammersmith Hospital, London

R. S. J. Frackowiak, M.A., M.D., F.R.C.P.
Professor of Clinical Neurology, MRC Cyclotron Unit, Hammersmith Hospital, London

Karl J. Friston, B.A., M.A.
Senior Clinical Scientist, MRC Cyclotron Unit, Hammersmith Hospital, London

C. D. Frith, Ph.D.
Professor of Neuropsychology, MRC Cyclotron Unit, Hammersmith Hospital, London

Patricia Goldman-Rakic, Ph.D.
Professor of Neuroanatomy, Yale University School of Medicine

Sigrid Herold, B.M., B.Ch., M.R.C.Psych. (deceased)
Senior Registrar in Psychiatry, MRC Cyclotron Unit, Hammersmith Hospital, London

René S. Kahn, M.D., Ph.D.
Assistant Professor, Department of Psychiatry, University Hospital Utrecht, The Netherlands

Joel E. Kleinman, M.D., Ph.D.
Deputy Chief of the Clinical Brain Disorders Branch, Neuroscience Center, National Institute of Mental Health

John H. Krystal, M.D.
Associate Professor, Department of Psychiatry, Yale University School of Medicine and Psychiatry Service

P. F. Liddle, B.M., B.Ch., Ph.D.
Senior Lecturer in Psychological Medicine, MRC Cyclotron Unit, Hammersmith Hospital, London

Martin T. Lowy, Ph.D.
Assistant Professor, Department of Psychiatry, Case Western Reserve University School of Medicine

J. John Mann, M.D.
Professor, Mental Health Research Center for the Study of Suicidal Behavior and Laboratories of Neuropharmacology, Western Psychiatric Institute and Clinic, University of Pittsburgh School of Medicine

Steven Matthysse, Ph.D.
Associate Professor, Mailman Research Center, McLean Hospital, Harvard University

Herbert Y. Meltzer, M.D.
Douglas Bondy Professor, Department of Psychiatry, Case Western Reserve University School of Medicine

M. Inés Morano, Ph.D.
Postdoctoral Candidate, Mental Health Research Institute, University of Michigan

Safia Nawroz, M.D.
Medical Staff Fellow, Neuroscience Center, National Institute of Mental Health

Charles B. Nemeroff, M.D., Ph.D.
Professor and Chairman, Department of Psychiatry and Behavioral Sciences, Emory University School of Medicine

Michael J. Owens, Ph.D.
Assistant Professor, Department of Psychiatry and Behavioral Sciences, Emory University School of Medicine

Paul M. Plotsky, Ph.D.
Professor, Department of Psychiatry and Behavioral Sciences, Emory University School of Medicine

Marcus E. Raichle, M.D.
Professor, Neurology and Radiology, Washington University School of Medicine

D. Silbersweig, M.D.
Assistant Professor, Psychiatry and Neurology, New York Hospital, Cornell Medical Center

Craig A. Stockmeier, Ph.D.
Associate Professor, Department of Psychiatry, Case Western Reserve University School of Medicine

Ming T. Tsuang, M.D., Ph.D., D.Sc., F.R.C.Psych.
Stanley Cobb Professor of Psychiatry, Department of Psychiatry, Harvard Medical School

Mark D. Underwood, Ph.D.
Assistant Professor, Mental Health Research Center for the Study of Suicidal Behavior and Laboratories of Neuropharmacology, Western Psychiatric Institute and Clinic, University of Pittsburgh School of Medicine

John Darrell Van Horn, Ph.D.
Postdoctoral (IRTA) Fellow, National Institute of Mental Health, Intramural Research Program, Neuroscience Center at St. Elizabeth's

Stanley J. Watson, Ph.D., M.D.
Associate Director and Research Scientist, Mental Health Research Institute, University of Michigan; and Associate Chair for Research and Theophile Raphael Professor of Neurosciences, Department of Psychiatry, University of Michigan

Daniel R. Weinberger, M.D.
Chief, Clinical Brain Disorders Branch, National Institute of Mental Health, Intramural Research Program, Neuroscience Center at St. Elizabeth's

Bryan Yamamoto, Ph.D.
Associate Professor, Department of Psychiatry, Case Western Reserve University School of Medicine

Preface

When I was asked to plan the 73rd meeting of the Association for Research in Nervous and Mental Disease (ARNMD) around the topic of the biology of major mental disorders, I realized it was a fine opportunity to showcase the most exciting observations in the field (and the laboratories producing them) for the general practitioner of psychiatry and neurology. After hearing the presentations at the meeting and reading the chapters, I am even more struck by the timeliness of this meeting. The explosive progress in the fields of biochemistry, molecular genetics, neuroscience, and anatomy has synergized with increasing clinical rigor and sophistication to move several steps forward almost every aspect of the biology of the brain and mental illnesses.

We are just now reaping the harvest from major investments made over the last 30 or more years in key basic scientific arenas. Those investments have allowed us to establish linkages between subcellular biology (chemistry, biochemistry, molecular genetics, etc.) and the functioning of neurons. Biological psychiatry and neurology are now able to capitalize on these efforts to begin producing a much more rigorous view of mechanisms of normal and pathological brain function. These points were repeatedly made evident in the presentations at the 73rd meeting of the ARNMD.

At the meeting, I was also struck by the fusion of several types of basic scientific tools and reasoning with clinical areas. The real progress is likely to be made in two domains: the genetics of the several psychoses (although progress to date has been slow and somewhat inconsistent) and the neurobiology and regulatory anatomy of specific brain circuits. Postmortem studies of the brains of individuals with severe mental illness currently involve a very active and exciting integration of biochemistry, molecular genetics, and brain circuit anatomy. Although these studies face considerable technical difficulties, they offer the unprecedented opportunity to evaluate the response of neural circuits to mental illness and its treatment. Furthermore, by combining this direct analysis of the brain's response to illness with contemporary pharmacology and in vivo imaging techniques, we are able to begin to sense the outlines of the scientific future of our field. That future includes the ability to study the responses of particular systems in nervous tissue to specific mental illnesses.

As our understanding of the biology of the brain and its illnesses grows, it should be possible to demonstrate variants of disease and relate them to the genetics, biochemistry, and anatomy of brain circuits. It will also be interesting to see how the appropriate treatments of these illnesses develop. Will these treatments involve pharmacological targeting of circuits of interest? Is it also possible to use gene therapy strategies to correct inherited predispositions for severe brain diseases?

On the other hand, it is ironic that at this moment in scientific history, when we can offer major advances in the understanding and treatment of mental illness, we are faced with a substantial reduction in federal support for research in neurobiology and brain diseases. With the reintegration of the National Institutes of Mental Health, Drug Abuse, and Alcohol back into the National Institutes of Health, they run the risk of losing their identities and therefore their programmatic foci. To add to the confusion, we are facing very low levels of grant funding, in the midst of the Decade of the Brain! We also see national efforts to provide equitable access to health care for all while facing the strange reality of being able to help and/or treat many mental disturbances in a cost-effective way without the financial ability to do so.

If conditions were different, we could reduce pain and suffering and learn more about the bases of mental illness, all at a reasonable cost. Somehow I find myself feeling both very concerned about this state of affairs and very pleased at the dramatic scientific movement in the field of the biology of the brain and its illnesses. Clearly, our ability to see the field of brain biology grow into a field with specific therapeutic approaches for mental illnesses depends on continued research and its funding. Of all the problems besetting humanity, a good proportion is inherent in behavior and therefore in the brain and its genes. We have the opportunity to come to grips with these problems and to substantially improve the mental health and well-being of humanity.

Despite short-term fiscal issues, the future is bright and exciting. It is a pleasure to be a physician and a scientist, and most particularly a neuroscientist, as we see the dawning of a real understanding of the brain in illness and in health.

STANLEY J. WATSON, PH.D., M.D.

CHAPTER

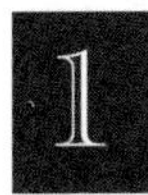

Introduction to the 73rd Meeting of the Association for Research in Nervous and Mental Disease

Stanley J. Watson, Ph.D., M.D.

The 73rd meeting of the Association for Research in Nervous and Mental Disease (ARNMD) was planned in early 1993 with the goal of bringing together some of the most successful lines of work into the causes and biological correlates associated with schizophrenia, mood disorders, and autism. Its theme was the description of the biology of these illnesses, not their clinical manifestations or treatment. The meeting participants attempted to focus on productive, fast-moving areas of research. Although I believe I have succeeded in selecting some of the most forward-thinking groups in this area, I acknowledge that other very

This work was supported in part by program project 42251-06 from the National Institute of Mental Health.

important groups and areas were missed. I can only plead guilty and point to the shortness of the meeting and the fast pace of the field.

The general organizing theme of the meeting was to focus on areas of interface between severe mental illness and the areas of genetics, neurochemistry, pharmacology, and postmortem anatomy and imaging. The speakers were asked to carry out two tasks in their presentations and chapters. The first was an overview of the field and their own work, and the second was their view of future trends in their research field. From the disease perspective, 9 of the 16 presentations were linked to schizophrenia, 6 to mood disorder and suicide, and 2 to autism. Obviously, some basic sessions were relevant to several disease states.

Overview of Mood Disorders, Autism, and Schizophrenia

The clinical syndromes most frequently studied by investigators at this 1993 meeting of the ARNMD were mood disorders (depression and bipolar disease), autism, and schizophrenia. These syndromes are among the most severe in psychiatry. They also represent three of the clearest clinical disease end points for study. The following section is a brief summary of each of these mental illnesses. It is not meant to be a comprehensive clinical presentation but rather an orientation to the key diagnostic issues and characteristics of the natural course of each illness.

Mood Disorders

Mood disorders in psychiatry can be divided into depressive and manic syndromes.

Major depression. Major depression is a severe mood disturbance with a high risk for recurrent depressive episodes throughout life. It affects 4%–7% of individuals at some point during their lifetimes.[1]

The age at onset is usually, but not invariably, after puberty. The mean age at onset is 37 years,[2] and the median patient experiences five to six episodes during his or her lifetime. Untreated, the average episode lasts 6–13 months. There is a predominance of female to male patients with major depression, the ratio being 2:1.

Table 1–1 is a summary of the diagnostic criteria.[3] From the rather dry format of a table it is difficult to get a sense of the disease. If one reads Tables 1–1 and 1–2 carefully, one can discern that life for these depressive patients can be a series of episodes involving severely depressed mood; disinterest in any form of social, sexual, or pleasurable activity; significantly disrupted sleep; agitation; very low energy; strong feelings of guilt; very poor thinking ability; and obsessive thoughts of suicide. Loss of friends, social contacts, marriage, and job are not uncommon. If untreated, an episode may en-

Table 1–1. Summary of DSM-III-R diagnostic criteria for major depression

Five of the following symptoms over the last 2 weeks:

1. Depressed mood
2. Markedly diminished interest in most activities
   (either 1 or 2 must be included)
3. Significant weight loss or gain
4. Daily insomnia or hypersomnia
5. Frequent psychomotor agitation or retardation
6. Daily fatigue or loss of energy
7. Feelings of worthlessness or inappropriate guilt
8. Diminished ability to think or concentrate, or indecisiveness
9. Recurrent thoughts of death, suicidal ideation, or suicide attempts or specific plan

- Should NOT be attributable to organic factors or to death of a loved one
- Should NOT have delusions or hallucinations lasting 2 weeks without prominent mood symptoms
- Should NOT superimpose on schizophrenia, schizophreniform disorder, delusional disorder, or other psychotic disorder not otherwise specified

Source. Adapted from American Psychiatric Association: *Diagnostic and Statistical Manual of Mental Disorders,* 3rd Edition, Revised. Washington, DC, American Psychiatric Association, 1987. Used with permission.

Table 1–2. Summary of DSM-III-R diagnostic criteria for melancholic type of depression

1. Loss of interest in all activities
2. Lack of response to pleasurable stimuli
3. Depression worse in morning
4. Early-morning awakening
5. Psychomotor retardation or agitation
6. Anorexia or weight loss
7. No significant personality disturbance prior to first major depressive episode
8. One or more previous major depressive episode with recovery
9. Previous good response to antidepressant medication

Source. Adapted from American Psychiatric Association: *Diagnostic and Statistical Manual of Mental Disorders,* 3rd Edition, Revised. Washington, DC, American Psychiatric Association, 1987. Used with permission.

tail months of misery before it begins to clear.

Treatment with antidepressants (usually either norepinephrine or serotonin reuptake inhibitors) or electroconvulsive therapy can reduce the recovery time to 2–6 weeks, resulting in complete or almost complete recovery. Some unfortunate individuals experience severe depressive episodes on a regular basis, such as every spring or at times of major stress or life changes.

Bipolar disease. As its name implies, bipolar disease (manic-depressive illness) is characterized by extreme swings of mood from depression to mania and perhaps back. It is diagnosed in 0.6% of the population and is found equally commonly in males and females.[1] The switches between depression and mania can occur quite rapidly, such as within a few hours.

Mania may sound interesting or even pleasant, but it is often severe, highly disruptive, and damaging to the patient's life. Table 1–3 summarizes the DSM-III-R criteria for manic syndrome. It can involve an extended period of sleepless behavior associated with greatly elevated feelings of self-worth or grandiosity, rapid or pressured speech, a flight of ideas, hypersexual behavior, strongly goal-oriented activity, very poor judgment, and finally, impaired social

Table 1–3. Summary of DSM-III-R diagnostic criteria for manic syndrome

A, B, and C

A. A distinct period of occasionally elevated, expansive, or irritable mood

B. Three or more of the following are present and significant:
   1. Inflated self-esteem and grandiosity
   2. Decreased need for sleep
   3. Pressured talking
   4. Flight of ideas or experience of thoughts racing
   5. Easily distracted
   6. Increase in goal-oriented activity or psychomotor agitation
   7. Excessive involvement in pleasurable activities despite potentially painful outcome

C. Severe mood disturbance. Impaired functioning on the job, socially or in relationships, or requires hospitalization to prevent harm to self or others

- NOT experience hallucinations or delusions for 2 weeks without mood disorder
- NOT superimposed on schizophrenia, schizophreniform disorder, delusional disorder, or other psychotic disorder
- NOT related to organic initiating factor

Source. Adapted from American Psychiatric Association: *Diagnostic and Statistical Manual of Mental Disorders,* 3rd Edition, Revised. Washington, DC, American Psychiatric Association, 1987. Used with permission.

relationships and job performance. It is not uncommon for such a patient to lose a great deal of money, to lose a job, or to be divorced.

When a manic patient also experiences severe depression that is temporally linked to mania, the diagnosis of bipolar disease is used. Generally, the onset of disease is in the mid-20s. There is usually a predominance of manic episodes early in life that gradually shift to more depressive episodes in later decades.[4] The average bipolar patient experiences nine ("median") episodes in his or her life. As seen in a classic work by Grof,[5] however, the number of episodes experienced by a patient during a lifetime can vary from 2 to 30. Episodes frequently result in hospitalization.

Treatment for bipolar illness is most effective with lithium chloride and, on occasion, tegretol and valproic acid. Antidepressants and antipsychotic drugs may be used as supplemental therapeutic agents.

Schizophrenia

Schizophrenia is very probably a series of diseases. Its onset is usually in late adolescence to early adulthood, and it usually has a lifelong expression affecting 0.8% of the population.[6] The severity, nature of symptoms, and remitting or unremitting nature of the process have produced several diagnostic subtypes (catatonic, disorganized, paranoid, undifferentiated, and residual).

The exact symptoms of schizophrenia vary rather widely (Table 1–4) but include delusions, hallucinations, very poor logical or associative thinking, catatonic behavior, odd emotional states, and dramatic loss of social contact. Such a patient is intensely internally focused and has a peculiar thinking style and unusual thought content. The disease is very different from depressive withdrawal in that the mood of a depressed patient is most likely the source of the social isolation. In a patient with schizophrenia, thinking processes appear to be fundamentally abnormal, resulting in a distorted view of the world. Once symptoms develop, the patient usually faces a lifetime of disturbances.

Treatments for schizophrenia have largely been in the form of compounds such as haloperidol and, more recently, clozapine. Both are slowly and modestly effective but do not usually result in a return to the level of functioning that was present before the illness.

Autism

Autism is a syndrome, very probably of developmental origin, that is detected in a failure to develop normal early childhood behaviors (Table 1–5). It is diagnosed in 2–4 of every 10,000 children ages 8–10 years.[7] Such children are oblivious to other humans or their feelings. For example, they often will not talk, play, establish friendships, or imitate others. Often the child lacks any mode of communication, or if he or she has speech, it is characterized by abnormal

Table 1–4. Summary of DSM-III-R diagnostic criteria for schizophrenia

A. Presence of 1, 2, or 3 in active phase for 1 week
  1. Two of the following:
    a. Delusions
    b. Prominent hallucination
    c. Incoherence or marked loosening of associations
    d. Catatonic behavior
    e. Flat or grossly inappropriate affect
  2. Bizarre delusions
  3. Prominent hallucinations

B. Dramatic decrease in work, social relations, and self-care

C. Rule out schizoaffective or mood disorder

D. Symptoms 6 months in duration: catatonic, disorganized, paranoid, undifferentiated, and residual

Residual phase

Two of the following:

1. Social isolation or withdrawal
2. Impairment in social roles
3. Marked peculiar behavior
4. Impairment in hygiene
5. Blunted or inappropriate affect
6. Digressive, vague, overelaborate, or circumstantial speech, or poverty of speech or speech content
7. Odd beliefs or marginal thinking
8. Unusual perceptual experiences
9. Lack of initiative, interests or energy

Source. Adapted from American Psychiatric Association: *Diagnostic and Statistical Manual of Mental Disorders,* 3rd Edition, Revised. Washington, DC, American Psychiatric Association, 1987. Used with permission.

content or style. There is often unusual nonverbal communication as well. Autistic children show stereotyped movements, are often strongly bound to routines, and exhibit a narrow range of interests. This lifetime disease undergoes gradual changes so that by adulthood one sees an isolated, poorly socialized, poorly adapted person.

Treatment of autism is generally not successful. It often involves use of antipsychotic compounds, but they are of only very limited value.

Table 1–5. Summary of DSM-III-R diagnostic criteria for autistic disorder

Eight of 16 must be present: 2 from A, 1 from B, and 1 from C

A. Qualitative impairment in reciprocal social interaction (two of the following must be present)
   1. Marked lack of awareness of others or their feelings
   2. No or abnormal seeking of comfort at times of distress
   3. No or impaired imitation
   4. No or abnormal social play
   5. Gross impairment in ability to make peer friendships

B. Qualitative impairment in verbal and nonverbal communications, and in imaginative activity (one of the following must be present)
   1. No mode of communication
   2. Marked abnormal nonverbal communication
   3. Absence of imaginative activity
   4. Marked abnormality in production of speech
   5. Marked abnormality in form or content of speech
   6. Marked impairment in the ability to initiate or sustain conversation with others

C. Markedly restricted repertoire of activities and interests (one of the following must be present)
   1. Stereotyped body movements
   2. Persistent preoccupation with parts of objects
   3. Marked distress over trivial changes in environment
   4. Unreasonable insistence on following precise routines
   5. Markedly restricted range of interests and a preoccupation with one narrow interest

Source. Adapted from American Psychiatric Association: *Diagnostic and Statistical Manual of Mental Disorders,* 3rd Edition, Revised. Washington, DC, American Psychiatric Association, 1987. Used with permission.

General Issues in the Study of Schizophrenia and Mood Disorders

It might theoretically be argued that schizophrenia represents the most complex type of human disease. This syndrome or illness is described only in humans and is characterized by severe but subtle alterations of behavior that involve the highest levels of the human brain. It is clear that the vast majority of physiological functions are perfectly intact in even the most severely schizophrenic patient. Functions ranging from basic regulation of temperature, food intake, and reproduction to basic perceptual functions (color, shape, movement) and even complex interpretations of sensory information (properly interpreting an image on television or understanding a logical argument) are intact and often no different than those seen in individuals with no psychiatric history. Yet such patients may also be quite disturbed across a spectrum of behavioral areas, such as social relationships, sensory events, and affective tone.

Attempts at understanding schizophrenia have forced the hypothesis that the disturbances really involve the most subtle levels of cortical functioning. Schizophrenic patients are very probably not the victims of progressive cortical atrophy similar to that seen in persons with Alzheimer's disease, yet higher components of perception and integration in patients with schizophrenia are prone to profound miscue and distortion. Thus, in a very real sense, the most subtle functions of the most complex structure in the human body are disturbed in a chronic and often unremitting fashion.

In the ARNMD meeting, several bodies of work addressed the general area of cortical organization and functioning in individuals with schizophrenia. Clearly, this is one of the major areas of emphasis in understanding this most complex disease.

In contrast, the disturbances seen in patients with severe affective disease are less "cortical" and more likely to be associated with the basic circuits that regulate drive and mood. There are problems with regulation of core functions, including sleep, sexual activity and even variables such as attention span, endocrine regulation, and reaction times. There is little evidence for persistent perceptual or sensory errors, much less cognitive dysfunction. Furthermore, these "depressed" states are often self-limited, and the patient usually returns to normal functioning. The hypothetical basis for this type of disease is most likely one pointing to a regulatory anomaly in neuronal systems, unlike the cortical structural or developmental hypothesis put forth in schizophrenia. Studies of the stress axis, neuropeptide biology, and monoamine transporters are all related to mood disorders and their etiology and treatment.

The search for the bases of schizophrenia and depression has been a long one but, in my view, one with no real chance of success until only very recently. In clinical research, progress in sharpening the descriptions of the syndromes and clarifying diagnostic schemes has been slow but sure. Much further progress will depend on the integration of biological data with clinical diagnosis.

On the other hand, approaches to basic neurobiology have grown extremely rapidly over the last 20 years and may provide the scientific thrust needed to begin to understand severe mental illness. A large number of scientific areas have flourished in their own right and as they relate to fundamental neurobiology. Among the areas of relevance to the study of severe mental illness, the most important are those that have driven the cellular and molecular approaches to neurobiology. It is not only the growth of specific disciplines themselves, but also their active integration into the study of brain biology, that are likely to drive understanding of mental illness. Table 1–6 lists some of these combinations of scientific areas and the problems or systems they affect, as well as their relationship to the meeting presentations.

Biochemistry of Brain Circuits

As an example of the integration of several scientific areas, the field of biochemical anatomy of the brain has been an extremely rich source of information in both the basic and the clinical arenas. This particular combination of scientific areas (anatomy, biochemistry, pharmacology, and molecular genetics) has dramatically expanded the existing body of knowledge of the brain, its circuits, and the biochemical "machinery" they use. Currently the literature is filled with descriptions of messenger RNA (mRNA) and gene sequences that code for proteins that are critical to the functioning of neurons. Molecules that act as transmitters, enzymes, receptors, transporters, and G proteins, to mention but a few, are increasingly well known at the level of protein, mRNA, and gene. Much of this rapid growth of information can be associated with specific cells and circuits in the brain. It is the ability to move from gene and RNA struc-

Table 1–6. Areas of research in the study of mental illness and neurobiology and their relationship to presentations at the ARNMD meeting

Scientific areas	Areas of study	Speaker	Topic
Pharmacology/imaging	Human brain imaging	K. Friston	Quantitative Imaging in Schizophrenia
		D. Weinberger	Functional Imaging of Schizophrenic Patients
		M. Raichle	Functional Imaging: A Developing Field
Biochemistry/pharmacology	Enzymes, receptors, transporters, transmitters	J. Krystal	Mode of Action of Antidepressants
		R. Blakely	Transporters: Basic and Pharmacological Studies
		C. Nemeroff	Affective Disease and Peptides
		H. Meltzer	Atypical Neuroleptics: How Do They Work?
Development/anatomy/molecular genetics	Formations of and patterns in the central nervous system	P. Goldman-Rakic	Perspectives on Cortical Functioning
		F. Benes	Cortical Changes in Schizophrenia
Biochemistry/molecular genetics/anatomy	Gene and mRNA regulation in neurons/transmitters and circuits/physiology and behavior	H. Akil	Regulation of the Stress Axis and the Hypothalamic-Pituitary-Adrenal Axis in Brain
		P. Goldman-Rakic	Perspectives on Cortical Functioning
		F. Benes	Cortical Changes in Schizophrenia
		J. Kleinman	Schizophrenia: Postmortem Studies
		J. Mann	Postmortem Studies of Suicide Victims
Genetics/clinical	Disease markers	D. Housman	Psychiatric Genetics: New Perspectives
		M. Tsuang	Epidemiology and Behavioral Genetics of Schizophrenia
		R. Ciaranello	Autism Genetics: Clinical and Molecular Approaches
Biochemistry/genetics	Genes causing disease		The Goal

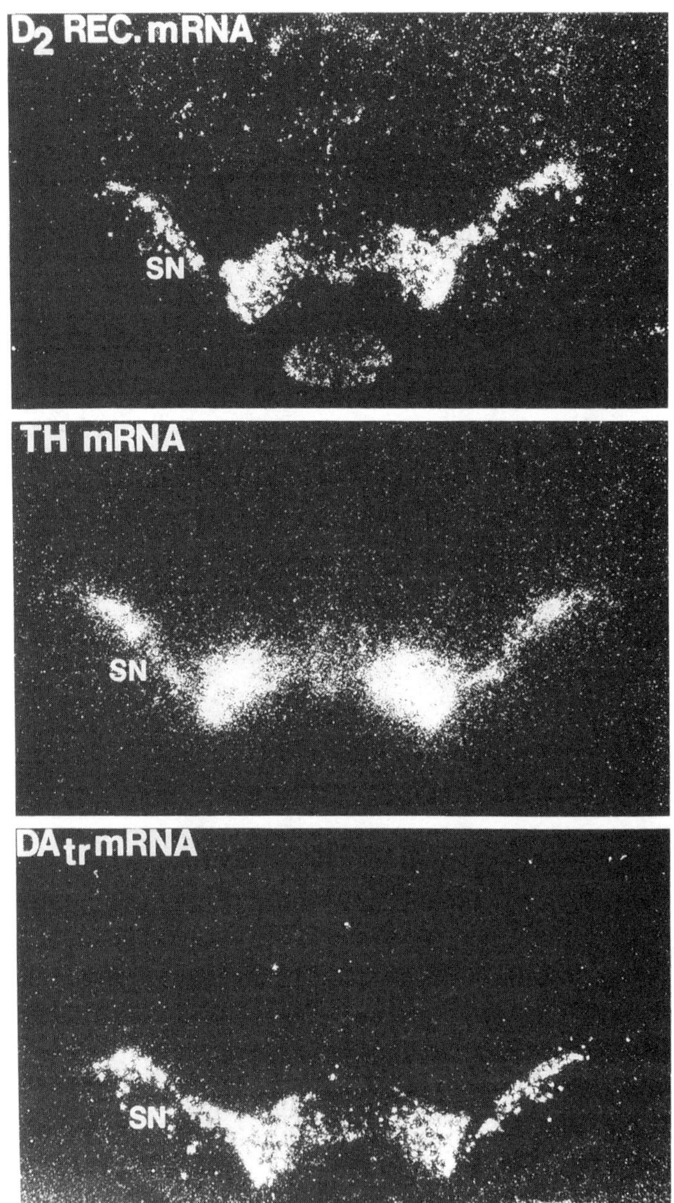

Figure 1–1. In situ hybridization of the mRNAs coding for the D_2 dopamine receptor *(top)*, tyrosine hydroxylase *(middle)*, and the dopamine transporter in the rat substantia nigra (SN) (A_9) and ventral tegmental area (A_{10}) *(bottom)* dopamine-synthesizing cells.

ture to cellular function in specific neurons that allows the cell biology of specific brain circuits to be deduced. The location and connectivity of biochemically known neurons is the basis of modern neuropharmacology and most of current psychiatric and neurological therapeutics.

Currently, the function of a large number of critical proteins can be localized and studied in their neuronal context. In dopamine neurons, for example, the key synthetic enzyme (tyrosine hydroxylase), postsynaptic receptor (dopamine receptors 1–5), autoreceptor (dopamine receptors 2–4), and dopamine reuptake proteins (Figure 1–1) have all been cloned and can be visualized in dopamine-producing cells of the substantia nigra.[8–10] The same general statement can be made for serotonin- and norepinephrine-producing neurons. Studies are very actively under way to learn more about the regulation of these key neuronal proteins and their mRNAs after administration of specific drugs. For example, after administration of antidepressants that block serotonin reuptake back into the serotonin-synthesizing cell, it is possible to detect 100% increases in the mRNA that produces that serotonin transporter.[11] Similar studies on the dopamine reuptake blocker cocaine, as well as studies of receptor and enzyme blockers, are under way in humans. These animal studies have thus led to a mechanistic view of the mode of action of many of the human therapeutics currently used and may help as new compounds are evaluated.

As the cell biology and regulation of neurons become clearer, their response to mental illness may also be quantifiable. Certainly, when causative gene defects for mental diseases are discovered, analysis at the single-neuron and brain circuit level must follow. Once all is said and done, it is the malfunctioning neuron, and therefore its dysfunction in neural circuits, that leads to the disease state.

References

1. Robins LN, Helzer JE, Weissman M, et al: Lifetime prevalence of specific psychiatric disorders in three sites. Arch Gen Psychiatry 41:949–958, 1984

2. Dorzab J, Baker M, Winokur G, Cadoret R: Depressive disease: clinical course. Diseases of the Nervous System 32:269, 1971
3. American Psychiatric Association: Diagnostic and Statistical Manual of Mental Disorders, 3rd Edition, Revised. Washington, DC, American Psychiatric Association, 1987
4. Clayton PJ: The epidemiology of affective disorder. Compr Psychiatry 22:31–43, 1981
5. Grof P, Angst J, Davies T: The clinical course of depression: practical issues, in Classification and Prediction of Outcome in Depression. Edited by Angst J. New York, Symposia Medica, Hoechst FK, Schattauer, Verlag, 1975, pp 141–156
6. Cooper B: Epidemiology, in Schizophrenia: Towards a New Synthesis. Edited by Wing JK. New York, Grune & Stratton, 1978, pp 31–52
7. Lotter V: Epidemiology of autistic conditions in young children, I: prevalence. Soc Psychiatry 1:124–137, 1966
8. Mansour A, Meador-Woodruff JH, Bunzow J, et al: Localization of dopamine D_2 receptor mRNA and D_1 and D_2 receptor binding in the rat brain and pituitary: an in situ hybridization-receptor autoradiographic analysis. J Neurosci 10:2587–2600, 1990
9. Mansour A, Meador-Woodruff JH, Zhou Q-Y, et al: A comparison of D_1 receptor binding and mRNA in rat brain using receptor autoradiographic and in situ hybridization techniques. Neuroscience 45:359–371, 1991
10. Meador-Woodruff JH, Mansour A: Expression of the dopamine D2 receptor gene in brain. Biol Psychiatry 30:985–1007, 1991
11. Lopez JF, Chalmers DT, Vazquez DM, et al: Serotonin transporter mRNA in rat brain is regulated by classical antidepressants. Biol Psychiatry, 35:287–290, 1994

CHAPTER

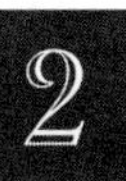

The Biology of Stress: From Periphery to Brain

Huda Akil, Ph.D.
M. Inés Morano, Ph.D.

The concept of "stress" is often invoked as a possible trigger for a number of psychiatric illnesses. Although stress is most commonly associated with various mood disorders (e.g., major depressive, bipolar, and anxiety disorders), there is also evidence that stress can play a role in precipitating psychotic episodes in patients with diseases such as schizophrenia. Typically, an association is made between psychological stress and these illnesses. There is an increasing awareness, however, that physical stress, such as that accompanying viral infections or autoimmune disorders, can also lead to serious psychological sequelae. Indeed, psychologists and neuroscientists attempting to create animal models of depression have typically relied on repeated stressful stimuli in attempting to reproduce the major signs and symptoms of depression.

A key psychological concept that has emerged from both studies in animals and observations in humans is that the stressful nature of any given stimulus resides less in its objective characteristics and more in the organism's ability to cope with it. Thus, the same stimulus can be exceedingly stressful to an animal that cannot control it and relatively nonstressful to an animal that has the ability to terminate it or gain some control over it.

Similarly, unpredictable stressors have more profound consequences than predictable stressors.[1] However, whether stressors are defined on the basis of their physical nature or on the basis of the organism's reaction to them, it is clear that they elicit an array of biological responses that are complex and highly regulated by the brain and that allow both immediate responses and long-term adjustments.

In this chapter, we focus on the basic biology of a key component of the stress system, the limbic-hypothalamic-pituitary-adrenal axis (LHPA). This component represents one of several subsystems that orchestrate the organism's response to stimuli that are conceived of as "stressful," namely, stimuli that disturb the organism's balance or homeostasis and lead to a substantial need for readjustment. Whereas the autonomic nervous system modulates the functions of the visceral organs that it innervates and rapidly alters their functioning through the action of specific neurotransmitters, the LHPA effects its influence via the rapid synthesis of adrenocortical steroids (glucocorticoids), which are released into the peripheral circulation and impinge on numerous target organs. Because glucocorticoids work through a combination of neuronal and genomic mechanisms and the "classical" glucocorticoid receptors alter nuclear events and gene transcription, the consequences of these adrenal steroids can be felt within minutes but can also last long after the stressful event has terminated.

In this chapter, we briefly describe the key features of the LHPA system, focusing on the way in which it orchestrates both its basal tone and its response to stressors. We then describe one natural model of dysregulation of this axis—the aged animal. This model is of interest both because it allows us to examine the dynamics of this system as it readjusts itself in the face of altered conditions and because aging is a critical variable in its expression in several psychiatric illnesses, especially major depression. At the end, we reexamine the concept of stress and LHPA and discuss some avenues for future research.

Basic Biology of the LHPA

Main Elements

Our understanding of the main elements of the LHPA has, generally speaking, proceeded from the more peripheral to the more central. Thus, although a great deal is known about adrenal steroid biology, advances in our understanding of the brain components have been much more recent, and our knowledge of the limbic element is far from complete.

Glucocorticoids are synthesized in the adrenal glands from cholesterol through a series of enzymatic steps. Adrenocortical cells do not contain secretory granules, and there is little storage of glucocorticoids at rest. Rather, synthesis and secretion are closely coupled via activation of the key enzymes and rapid liberation of the highly diffusible corticosteroids. The coupled synthesis-release is activated via the receptor for adrenocorticotropic hormone (ACTH). This receptor, the first to be described as coupled to the activation of adenylyl cyclase,[2] has been recently cloned.[3]

ACTH derives from the pituitary corticotrophs, cells of the anterior pituitary gland that synthesize the hormone and release it in response to stress. Although ACTH had long been identified and sequenced by Li et al.,[4] it was not until the late 1970s that we learned a great deal more about its biosynthetic origin and began to investigate its regulation at the transcriptional and translational levels. Indeed, the precursor for ACTH, a protein called proopiomelanocortin (POMC), was the first mammalian endocrine or neuronal precursor to be cloned,[5] ushering in the revolution in molecular endocrinology and molecular biology that we have witnessed over the last 15 years.

This original cloning coincided with some elegant work on the protein biochemistry of the precursor, confirming and extending it. Thus, basing their work on observations by Lowry et al.,[6] other authors, Mains et al.[7] and Roberts and Herbert,[8] showed that ACTH and the potent opioid peptide beta-endorphin derived from a common protein precursor. The cloning of POMC complementary DNA (cDNA) confirmed these findings and showed the existence of three domains—a carboxy-terminal region containing beta-endorphin, a middle region coding for ACTH, and an N-terminal region of hitherto unknown nature. Beyond the unusual finding that two highly active peptides (ACTH and beta-endorphin) could derive from a common precursor, this work also showed that a single sequence embedded in ACTH (ACTH 4–10) was repeated elsewhere within the parent molecule, once in the midst of beta-melanocyte-stimulating hormone (β-MSH) and a second time, with a slight modification, in the N-terminal domain in a region that was termed γ-MSH. These findings revealed the dramatic complexity of the ACTH precursor and paved the way for extensive studies on the biosynthesis and posttranslational processing of this prohormone.[9] Subsequent information on the gene structure of POMC[10] and its anatomical expression,[11,12] as well as the structure of the processing enzymes involved in its maturation,[13,14] have given the field the full array of tools for the study of the biology and regulation of ACTH at the pituitary level.

It was evident that, for ACTH to be activated by stressors, its secretion had to be stimulated by a hypothalamic-releasing factor or factors. Although arginine-vasopressin (AVP) was known to be an ACTH secretagogue, it was evident to several neuroendocrinologists that another factor, termed *corticotropin-releasing factor* (CRF), must exist. For several years, CRF evaded isolation until Vale et al.[15] determined its structure in 1981 and showed it to be a 41–amino acid peptide highly expressed in the hypothalamus. The cDNA sequence of corticotropin-releasing factor, which was renamed corticotropin-releasing hormone (CRH), was obtained soon thereafter.[16,17] Subsequent anatomical studies[18] revealed that CRH was localized in the medial parvicellular aspect of the paraventricular nucleus of the hypothalamus (mpPVN). AVP is coexpressed in the same neurons, although the vast majority of this peptide is expressed in the neighboring magnocellular elements of the paraventricular nucleus, which also coexpress oxytocin and project to the posterior pituitary. The peptides in the mpPVN, however, project to the external layer of the median eminence and are liberated into the local portal blood system that bathes the anterior pituitary, thereby gaining access to the target corticotrophs. The corticotrophs carry the receptors for both CRH and AVP, both of which are recently cloned members of the superfamily of G-protein coupled receptors.[19,20] It is known that CRH and AVP receptors activate different signal transduction pathways; thus, the two peptides synergize in their actions as secretagogues.[21]

As is the case for ACTH, our understanding of the biology of CRH and AVP has increased dramatically over the last two decades, allowing us the possibility of placing the biology of these elements in the context of the LHPA, understanding how they regulate stress, and how they are in turn regulated by it.

Regulation of the LHPA: Stress Responsiveness

The CRH neuron in the mpPVN appears to be the final common path for brain responses to all stressors. Thus, stressful stimuli converge on these neurons, activating the secretion of CRH and AVP. This in turn causes the release of pituitary ACTH, which is liberated into the general circulation and triggers the synthesis and release of glucocorticoids (corticosterone in rats, cortisol in humans). Although, as mentioned above, these corticosteroids have targets throughout the body, a key set of targets are the pituitary and brain themselves. The effect of corticosteroids on these elements of the LHPA is critical in a series of feedback mechanisms that ensure that stress responses at the brain and pituitary levels are not only initiated promptly but also terminated promptly. Thus, a great deal of the "logic" of this system involves timing of activation and termination. This is probably due to the fact that glucocorticoids are very potent molecules that are capable of exerting long-lasting effects and that constant exposure of the organism to high levels can be deleterious (e.g., can cause immune suppression).

The simplest, though crudest, way to study these negative feedback mechanisms on the pituitary and hypothalamus is to examine the effects of adrenalectomy on POMC, CRH, and AVP. Removal of the adrenal glands, and hence of glucocorticoids, removes the negative feedback effects of these molecules, allowing the observation of the stress axis unchecked by the restraining effects of the steroids. Under these conditions, CRH messenger RNA (mRNA) in the mpPVN is significantly increased and AVP mRNA in those same neurons is dramatically elevated, whereas AVP mRNA in the neighboring magnocellular neurons of the PVN is unaltered, demonstrating the specificity of this negative feedback effect.[22] This increase in gene expression of CRH and AVP is coupled to a significant increase in release, dramatically enhancing the secretion of ACTH from the anterior lobe. POMC mRNA is elevated by 10-fold, paralleling the equally dramatic enhancement in circulating levels of POMC-derived peptides.[23]

This impressive change in pituitary POMC is attributable to both the increased activation by CRH and the loss of direct negative steroid feedback on the pituitary itself. This notion is supported by the observation that the effects of glucocorticoids on the pituitary in vitro are much less dramatic. The consequences of adrenalectomy at both the hypothalamic and the pituitary levels can be shown to be due to glucocorticoid removal, because replacement with exogenous corticosteroids such as dexamethasone can completely reverse the effects of adrenal removal. Furthermore, administration of corticosteroids to intact animals leads to a significant decrease of gene expression and secretion at both the hypothalamic and pituitary levels.

The mechanism of this negative feedback is thought to be genomic, resulting from a steroid receptor–mediated inhibition of transcription of the relevant genes—CRH and POMC. These genomic events are not immediate. Although transcriptional changes can begin immediately after either stress or alteration in steroid levels,[10] the impact of these events on the mRNA pool is a function of the size of the pool; smaller pools exhibit more rapid perturbations. In the case of POMC, for which the mRNA pool is quite large, the steroid-induced changes require hours to days to become fully manifest.[23]

There are, however, more rapid mechanisms of negative feedback that operate in a shorter time frame and are responsible for the moment-to-moment regulation of stress activation and termination. Indeed, release of pituitary peptides after the removal of a stressor is promptly terminated as circulating corticosteroid levels rise. This effect is not due to the depletion of peptide stores, because the fractional release with stress is very small. Furthermore, if the stress-induced rise in corticosteroid levels is prevented, both the magnitude and the duration of the ACTH response will be greatly enhanced, demonstrating the role of these steroids in restraining the response. Keller-Wood and Dallman[24] and Dallman et al.[25] have distinguished multiple times of feedback beyond the genomic, including a fast feedback that appears to be dependent on the rate of rise of the glucocorticoids rather than on their absolute levels. The exact mechanism of such a feedback remains unclear, although neuronal rather than gene regulatory events are likely to be involved.

These feedback loops—genomic versus nongenomic, rapid versus slow—are likely to provide the system with different types of controls. Such nested loops are very intricate but can also be very powerful in regulating the system optimally. (See "The Aged Rat as a Model of a Mildly Dysregulated Stress Axis" in this chapter for an example of the multiple levels of controls.) It is apparent that the genomic control defines the limits of the system, increasing or decreasing its overall capacity through transcriptional changes. Although defining the limits at the level of the CRH neuron may be important because of the small message pool, the physiological significance of altering the limits of POMC gene expression is unclear, given the very large pool available under normal conditions. Indeed, outside of extreme conditions, such as adrenalectomy or very high doses of steroids, the POMC mRNA pool appears to be remarkably stable. Rather, the POMC precursor is capable of altering its biosynthesis at the posttranscriptional and posttranslational levels,[26] possibly via changes in the level or activity of the processing enzymes.

Thus, the most critical mechanisms for steroid-induced negative control of the LHPA remain to be discovered. These mechanisms are likely to be rapid and to include neuronal pathways and circuits that may or may not rely on corticosteroid receptors within the central nervous system.

Regulation of the LHPA: The Circadian Rhythm

So far, we have emphasized the changes induced by stress and the control of these changes by steroid feedback. The basal tone of the entire LHPA, however, is far from static. An essential feature of the stress axis is the fact that it exhibits circadian oscillations whereby glucocorticoid levels are highest upon awakening and lowest at the end of the activity phase. That this rhythm is driven by activity rather than by light can be seen in the difference between humans and nocturnal animals. In humans, the peak levels of glucocorticoids are observed in the morning, around 7:00 A.M. These levels decline steadily throughout the course of the day, reaching their nadir in the late evening hours (e.g., 7:00–12:00 P.M.). They begin to rise again around midnight and peak upon awakening. In contrast, in rats, which are nocturnal animals, the highest levels of glucocorticoids are observed in the evening and the lowest levels are seen in the morning. Circulating levels of ACTH also exhibit parallel, though less marked, rhythms, anticipating the glucocorticoid rhythm by approximately 1–2 hours.[27,28]

Although the suprachiasmatic nucleus, which is classically involved in rhythmic events, plays a role in the control of this cycle, as indicated by lesion studies,[29] it is clearly not the only structure of importance. A major control of the timing of this circadian rhythmicity appears to be food intake. Secretory events in ACTH and adrenal steroids can be observed around mealtimes, not only in response to eating but sometimes in anticipation of it. Altering the timing of meals has been shown to significantly shift the circadian rhythm.[30]

The circadian rhythmicity of the LHPA appears to be driven at the suprapituitary level. Work from our laboratory[27,28] has shown that the expression of CRH mRNA in the parvicellular PVN of rats exhibits a circadian pattern in which the rise in message anticipates the peak of glucocorticoids by several hours, as though in preparation for the increased secretion that takes place at the peak. Thus, the CRH message pool in rats begins to rise in the morning, when glucocorticoid levels are very low, and shows a dramatic drop in late evening as the glucocorticoid levels reach their peak.

Although this may suggest that the pattern is driven by glucocorticoid negative feedback, the CRH mRNA pattern is rather complex in shape and is likely to be controlled by intricate neuronal mechanisms. Indeed, removal of glucocorticoids by adrenalectomy, while dramatically changing the overall level of expression of CRH message, does not lead to a substantial change in the pattern or shape of the CRH mRNA. The only subtle change seen is an alteration in the rate of increase in the message pool during the morning hours, and the normal slope is restored by pelleting the rats to deliver a very low level of glucocorticoids (suggesting mineralocorticoid receptor mediation; see "Receptors Involved in Negative Feedback: Glucocorticoid and Mineralocorticoid Receptors" in this chapter).

The circadian rhythm not only alters basal levels of the hormones along the LHPA axis but is also associated with changes in sensitivity and responsiveness to stressful stimuli. Thus, at the nadir of the rhythm, the organism is exquisitely responsive to stress, showing clear-cut activation responses, and at the same time, the animal is also highly sensitive to negative feedback.[25] Thus, both the initiation of stress responses and their termination appear to be more efficient at the nadir than at the peak of the circadian cycle.

It can be seen from the preceding discussion that the LHPA axis is a highly regulated and well-integrated system that controls many of its features simultaneously. Thus, basal levels oscillate in a circadian fashion; stress responsiveness similarly oscillates across the daily rhythm; and the activation and termination of stress responses is under multiple controls, producing rapid responses that are proportional in amplitude and duration to the severity of the stressor and to its duration but terminating efficiently to return all hormone levels to their appropriate baselines. How does the organism achieve such exquisite control at multiple anatomical levels and in multiple time domains? It appears that the answer lies in the orchestration of a number of mechanisms, some of which are hormonal and some neuronal, affecting almost every level of cellular and integrative control, from gene regulation to neurotransmitter release and electrophysiological events. In the following section we discuss the two major classes of control over the LHPA: hormonal, particularly the glucocorticoid receptors; and neuronal, particularly the pathways of activation and inhibition. We emphasize the role of the brain in orchestrating these phenomena.

Receptors Involved in Negative Feedback: Glucocorticoid and Mineralocorticoid Receptors

Two receptors in the brain recognize the adrenal corticosteroids (cortisol in humans, corticosterone in rats). These receptors had been previously identified on the basis of binding assays and were termed type I and type II by Reul and DeKloet.[31] Whereas type II was found throughout the neuraxis, especially in the hypothalamus and hippocampus, type I was particularly enriched in the hippocampus. After the cloning, expression, and pharmacological characterization of members of the steroid receptor family,[32–34] the type I and type II receptors have been recognized to be the mineralocorticoid receptor (MR) and the glucocorticoid receptor (GR), respectively. Not only did these receptors exhibit the appropriate pharmacological signatures, but they also had the appropriate anatomy as determined by in situ hybridization, with particularly high levels in the pyramidal cells and in the dentate gyrus of the hippocampus.[35,36]

Although it may seem surprising that an MR, which recognizes aldosterone in kidney, would recognize glucocorticoids in brain, MR has, in fact, a better affinity for the natural glucocorticoids than does GR. Thus, the K_d of GR for corticosterone is approximately 5 nM, whereas that of MR for corticosterone is about 0.5 nM. Beyond this difference in affinity, the two receptors have overlapping but distinguishable pharmacological profiles. Most notably, GR recognizes the synthetic glucocorticoid dexamethasone, whereas MR, predictably, has a high affinity for aldosterone. The dual affinity for glucocorticoids and mineralocorticoids could theoretically have been problematic at the level of the kidney, because levels of corticosterone exceed levels of aldosterone. However, it is believed that a specific enzyme exists at the level of the kidney that degrades the glucocorticoids and spares aldosterone, allowing appropriate kidney function.[37]

Both GR and MR are members of a superfamily of receptors that act as ligand-regulating transacting factors. In the case of GR and MR, the protein is thought to reside in the cytoplasm, in a large complex with a number of heat shock proteins that serve to fold it and give it the appropriate configuration for recognizing corticosteroid ligands. Upon binding, these receptors translocate to the nucleus and interact with specific hormone recognition elements on the DNA, thereby effecting changes in transcription rates. The best understood effects are those resulting in an increase in transcription, a phenomenon seen in the regulation of numerous genes by GR. In the LHPA, however, the genomic effects are thought to be primarily inhibitory and are less well understood. The most likely mechanism involves protein-protein interactions in which complexes of transacting factors bind to complex DNA response elements. Some of these interactions would result in the prevention of activation induced by other transacting factors, such as the blockade of the effects of the immediate-early genes c-*fos* and c-*jun*.[38–43] There are a number of complexities in these multiple protein interactions. For example, the exact sequence of events appears to be important in determining whether GR will have stimulatory or inhibitory effects on a target gene; genes previously interacting with c-*fos* and c-*jun* may be suppressed, whereas genes without such interactions may be activated.[44]

Our understanding of gene regulation by MR is considerably more limited than that of GR. MR is often seen as a low-threshold receptor with high affinity but low capacity, and one view of it is that it simply serves as a more sensitive detector, albeit of limited efficacy, of corticosteroid effects. According to this view, GR would take over where MR has left off, effecting much more profound changes in regulating transcription.[33] However, there is also evidence of a more complex interaction whereby MR may be inactive and GR may be active, raising the possibility that MR may act as an antagonist of GR in certain cases.[45,46]

It is evident from the foregoing discussion that a great deal remains to be learned about the interplay between the two corticosteroid receptors at the level of gene regulation and, in particular, about their effects on negatively regulated genes, such as those found in the LHPA (CRH, AVP, POMC).

At the more integrative level, the dual role of MR and GR is equally fascinating. It is clear from a number of studies that MR is important in the control of the circadian rhythm, whereas GR may be more important in modulating the magnitude and duration of stress responses. This is reasonable in view of the differential sensitivity of these two receptors and the fact that at the peak of the daily rhythm a large proportion of MR receptors is expected to be occupied, whereas at the nadir a small proportion is occupied. Yet neither stage of the cycle produces glucocorticoid levels high enough to saturate GR sites, which are then capable of detecting the higher levels of steroids produced by stress.[25,28,47–49]

Beyond circadian rhythmicity, MR and GR are thought to be involved in a number of behavioral functions. Given their high levels of expression in the hippocampus, it is reasonable to investigate their potential role in learning and memory. DeKloet[49] has explored several learning paradigms and has proposed that, at least at the level of the hippocampus, MR and GR may exert opposing effects.

The existence of two receptors with different affinities and capacities, overlapping but distinctive anatomies, and somewhat different genomic effects endows the LHPA with several mechanisms for subtle control, both in terms of basal levels and the circadian rhythm, and in terms of stress responsiveness. A great deal remains to be learned about the subtle interplay between them, especially if we envision them not only at the cellular level but also in the context of the intricate brain circuitry that controls the activation and inhibition of stress responses.

Neuronal Control of the LHPA: Negative Regulatory Circuits

As discussed previously, negative feedback is critical to the termination of the stress response and to the modulation of the overall responsiveness of the axis. This feedback appears to be mediated both directly, at the level of gene regulation, and indirectly, via neuronal circuits that may influence the tone of the CRH neuron at the level of the PVN. The presence of high levels of both GR and MR in the hippocampus has suggested that this structure may play a key role in negative feedback.[49–52] Indeed, hippocampal lesions have been shown to elevate both resting levels of glucocorticoids and stress-induced hormonal responses.[53,54] Three questions remain, however:

1. Is the hippocampus truly the site of negative steroid feedback, or is it primarily a structure that participates in the overall inhibition of the LHPA independently of glucocorticoids?
2. Is this structure primarily involved in controlling basal tone, possibly even the circadian pattern, or is it critical to the control of stress termination?
3. What are the anatomical circuits that may mediate the effect of the hippocampus on the stress system?

Our group embarked on a series of studies addressing these questions at an anatomical and endocrine level. We focused on the circuitry that may be involved in the hippocampal interface with the stress axis. No direct connection had been shown between the hippocampus and the PVN. The possibility remained that a hippocampal-hypothalamic pathway may exist that may be polysynaptic and that may play a role in negative control of the axis. Thus, we needed to achieve two goals in our studies: to establish the existence of anatomical connections between the hippocampus and the PVN, and to relate these connections to a function in controlling the axis.

To achieve these goals, we used lesions as one of our tools and examined CRH and AVP mRNA and ACTH and corticosteroid plasma levels. Our reasoning was as follows: if the hippocampus is indeed critical for inhibiting the overall tone of the LHPA, then its destruction should result in an increase in that tone, and this should result in a chronic increase in circulating stress hormones (ACTH and corticosteroids). Such a finding would support the most basic assumption, namely, that the hippocampus is inhibitory, but would not prove that the hippocampus is involved in steroid feedback. To address the latter question, further measures were required: if, indeed, steroids only have direct effects on CRH/AVP in the PVN and do not depend on hippocampal integrity for their actions, then the high steroid levels resulting from hippocampal lesions should lead to downregulation of the CRH/AVP message. This in turn would decrease ACTH secretion and would eventually restore the homeostasis of the LHPA. Thus, the model of a hippocampus that is generally inhibitory but not critical to steroid feedback would lead us to expect a transient increase in hypothalamic-pituitary-adrenal tone, followed by a return toward normal. If steroid feedback works in part through the hippocampus, however, then inducing lesions at that site should not only increase secretion but also prevent steroid-induced downregulation and actually lead to the unusual condition of increased circulating hormones and increased CRH/AVP.

To date we have studied multiple regions of the hippocampus and have shown that, indeed, hippocampal lesions result in this unusual combination of elevated glucocorticoids and elevated levels of secretagogues.[55,56] This finding suggests that the hippocampus not only plays a role in clamping the tone of the LHPA but that it is also critical to the steroid-mediated control over this basal tone. However, these findings do not allow us to distinguish whether the steroid-mediated feedback is in fact occurring at the level of the hippocampus, at the level of the PVN, or at both. For example, it is possible that negative glucocorticoid feedback at the level of the PVN may somehow require input from the hippocampus in order to be fully effective. Indeed, a recent study suggests that this may be the case, as rats in which the hippocampus was removed did not show negative steroid feedback at the level of the PVN.[57] Thus, our lesion studies establish a role of the hippocampus in controlling basal tone and the importance of this limbic structure in mediating negative steroid feedback on this tone, but they do not directly implicate hippocampal GR and MR in this control. To do so, we would need to selectively block hippocampal GR and demonstrate an effect of this manipulation on the entire axis.

Although several hippocampal sites participate in controlling basal CRH expression, only very discrete regions appear to be involved in the termination of the stress response.[57a] Inducing lesions in the latter sites results in stress response patterns in which activation appears normal but termination appears slow, a pattern seen in aged animals (see "The Aged Rat as a Model of a Mildly Dysregulated Stress Axis" in this chapter). Here again, it is unclear whether GRs within the hippocampus are critical or whether other neurotransmitters and modulators mediate these effects on stress termination.

What are the neural pathways mediating the effects of the hippocampus on both basal tone and termination of the stress response? Extensive anatomical studies in our laboratory have suggested that there are multiple redundant pathways that connect the hippocampus to the PVN through various relays points, including one in the bed nucleus of the stria terminalis (BNST).[58] In some cases, such as in the BNST, the particular site has been linked to PVN control not only anatomically but also functionally (i.e., BNST lesions, like hippocampal lesions, also upregulate CRH mRNA), whereas the role of other sites identified anatomically has not been tested functionally. Thus, these indirect connections between the hippocampus and the PVN may play a role in controlling various aspects of the stress response or may serve other distinct functions.

Taken together, the body of work on the hippocampus suggests that it plays a key role in inhibiting the stress axis, particularly its basal tone, and that it does so at least in part by being permissive for negative steroid feedback that controls the expression of CRH. However, the specific role of hippocampal steroid receptors in these events remains to be determined. The work also suggests that the hippocampus has a role in the control of stress termination, but neither the steroid dependence of this phenomenon nor the role of hippocampal steroid receptors in it have been assessed. Finally, it should be noted that the hippocampal effects, especially on basal tone, may oscillate across the circadian rhythm, having a greater impact at the nadir than at the peak. This may be linked to the possibility that MR may be important in the control of the axis at the nadir and that these receptors reside primarily in the hippocampus.

Neuronal Control of the LHPA: Positive Regulatory Circuits

The neuronal circuits involved in the initiation of the stress response are not well understood. We know that the final common path is in the mpPVN, and we also know that brain stem nuclei are likely to play an important role in stress detection, that is, locus ceruleus and nucleus of the solitary tract. A number of afferent inputs arising from the brain stem have, in fact, been shown to participate in the activation of the hypothalamic-pituitary axis. In particular, noradrenergic and adrenergic neurons of the A2 region in the caudal medulla are known to send direct inputs to the mpPVN,[59] and their modulation alters the tone of the CRH neuron, presumably via a_1 adrenoceptors.[60–65] The nucleus tractus solitarius, which is partly catecholaminergic, has been shown to be critical in inducing ACTH release in response to hypotension.[66] Similarly, serotonergic cell groups (dorsal raphe and raphe magnus) project to parvicellular PVN[67] and appear to be involved in stress responsiveness[68,69] and circadian rhythmicity.[70] Additionally, limbic sites participate in stress responsiveness. The amygdala has been implicated,[71,72] as has the medial BNST.[73] More rostrally, stimulation of the preoptic area and frontal cortex can excite PVN neurons that project to the median eminence.[74]

A major conceptual question remains in the field: Is there a "stress activation pathway," or are stress responses not specifically tied to a unique anatomy but rather to a common endpoint, namely, activation of the PVN? Different types of stressors, for example, physical or psychological, painful or nonpainful, are likely to engage the system from different starting points. But at what level do they converge? Is it only at the level of the CRH/AVP neuron in the parvicellular PVN? Or do they do so more proximally, for example, in limbic sites that need to be activated for a stimulus to be labeled "stressful" by the organism? If we draw an analogy to sensory motor organization, the sensations and perceptions of the stimuli—for example, pain, severe heat or cold, homeostatic imbalance, an immune insult, or a fear-provoking stimulus—would constitute the sensory component. The secretion of CRH/ACTH/corticosteroids would constitute the output, or motor component. But what are the circuits that link the two and simultaneously encode this wide array of stimuli as "stressful"? These circuits may be important to our understanding not only of the integration of stress responses but also of the biology of many illnesses, especially mood disorders.

A major stumbling block in the identification of these circuits has been the need for a strategy for detecting stress activation at the level of the central nervous system, as opposed to relying only on peripheral endocrine indices. This is a prerequisite to carrying out lesion studies in order to disrupt the circuit(s) and begin to delineate the key elements. One must have the ability to reliably monitor central nervous system correlates of acute activation by various stressors in order to discern the existence of unique pathways as well as common components. The measure must be rapid enough to detect the activation before negative feedback mechanisms (steroid and nonsteroid) dampen or even reverse the response.

In an effort to map brain regions activated by various stressors, several recent studies have been undertaken using immediate-early genes such as c-*fos*, c-*jun*, and *zif-268* as markers for early neuronal activity.[75–77] To date the Watson laboratory has examined and compared immediate-early gene responses after restraint stress and swim stress.[78] The results suggest that, in addition to activation of the mpPVN, a widespread number of cortical and subcortical limbic brain areas are activated in response to both stressors, as are certain brain stem nuclei (e.g., catecholaminergic cell groups) implicated in activation of the hypothalamic-pituitary axis. Although both stressors, despite their differences, appear to activate common sites, it is premature to suggest that these sites represent the stress activation circuit. Indeed, the activation of *fos* mRNA by both stressors is so widespread that it is rather difficult to ascertain whether it is revealing specific circuitry or a nonspecific generalized response of the central nervous system to a powerful input. Clearly, more work needs to be carried out in this area, relying not only on immediate-early genes but also on other strategies for detecting rapid activation in an anatomical context.

The Aged Rat as a Model of a Mildly Dysregulated Stress Axis

A naturalistic model of a disrupted LHPA offers the opportunity to better understand the system by uncovering the problem at the root of the disturbance and evaluating its consequences on stress control. The aged rat offers such a model. Sapolsky et al.[79–81] first described an abnormal pattern of response to some stressors in aged rats: the amplitude of the response to restraint stress was similar to that of young animals, but the turnoff pattern was aberrant and corticosterone levels remained elevated for a long period in aged animals, suggesting aberrant negative feedback. These workers then examined steroid receptors in brain and found them to be low in the hippocampus, probably due to loss of hippocampal pyramidal cells in the aged rats. This correlation suggests, but does not prove, that the hippocampal deficiency may be responsible for the aberrant turnoff of the stress response.

A number of studies have examined various aspects of the LHPA in aged rats, resulting in a number of controversies. There are several reports of increased basal levels of corticosterone in older rats[79,82–88] although a number of other investigators, including those in our own laboratory, have seen no such elevation.[89–98] Similarly, not all stressors result in an increase in responsiveness in aged rats.[79] There is general agreement (including our own work) that, in aged rats, hippocampal adrenal steroid receptors are lower than those in young control subjects after short-term adrenalectomy (to remove circulating corticoids).[79,85,99] These "missing receptors" are thought to be on pyramidal hippocampal neurons, and the loss is presumably due to neuronal death.[83,100,101] A related notion is that the death of the pyramidal cell is the result of the toxic effects of elevated corticosterone.[51] Thus, a positive feedback loop of dysregulation may be established—elevated steroids lead to the death of neurons involved in inhibition of stress responsiveness, and this in turn results in decreased inhibition of the CRH/AVP neuron, leading to enhanced secretion, further steroid rises, and further neuronal death.

This hypothesis is elegantly attractive, but it has not been proven. Indeed, a number of observations suggest that the situation may be more complex. For example, as discussed previously, not all investigators agree that circulating glucocorticoids are basally elevated in aged animals. We found completely superimposable steroid levels across the circadian rhythm in old versus young Fisher rats. Yet the same aged rats exhibited an aberrant response to restraint stress, replicating the pattern reported by others.[79] This finding suggests that basal levels and stress responsiveness of steroids can be dissociated in aged animals. In addition, the abnormal response to stressors is observed only after some, but not all, stressors,[79] indicating another level of complexity. Finally, the issue of differences in the sex[90] and the strain of rats should be considered. Thus, in contrast to Fisher, Long Evans, and Wistar rats, Brown Norway rats display a decrease of MR, but not GR, in the hippocampus.[98]

The picture that emerges suggests an uneven pattern of dysregulation of the LHPA with age. It is conceivable that earlier stages, or animals with certain histories or genetic propensities, first show the aberrant negative feedback with certain stressors and the concomitant hippocampal degeneration. A continuous dysregulation of even basal levels may appear only in more "advanced" cases. Such a heterogeneity has been suggested by Issa et al.,[102] who demonstrated that only 30% of aged rats (23–27 months) showed memory impairment, and that this subgroup showed more profound aberrations in hippocampal receptor binding and in circulating corticosterone levels than their non–memory-impaired counterparts.

Even the finding of altered steroid binding in the hippocampus is not without complications, many of which are due to the intrinsic difficulties of quantitating type I and type II receptors. Both types of steroid receptors do not readily dissociate their ligands and are highly sensitive to circulating steroids. In addition, not only are they occupied when steroid levels are high, but they become translocated to the nucleus, thus changing cellular compartments.

In order to quantitate cytoplasmic steroid receptors, it is customary to perform adrenalectomy on rats and allow a brief period of recovery (12–36 hours), allowing circulating steroids to disappear. An assumption made in all such binding studies is that the treatment does not alter the amount of receptor protein or the receptor affinity but merely removes the steroids. It is known, however, that a longer period without circulating glucocorticoids does lead to significant upregulation of steroid receptor binding[103] and of steroid receptor mRNA.[55]

If the sensitivity to adrenalectomy is different in aged animals, this could confound the results. Indeed, recent work by Eldridge et al.[104] suggests that the decreased level of glucocorticoid binding in the hippocampus of aged animals may occur in adrenalectomized but not in intact rats. Thus, Eldridge et al.[105] proposed that aged rats start with binding sites comparable to those of young rats but do not upregulate after adrenalectomy, leading to the lowered measured levels after adrenalectomy. This group proposes that the major difference seen in aging is a change in GR affinity to the ligand[106] and in GR sensitivity to steroid-induced up- and downregulation.[104,105]

On the basis of these difficulties, we felt it would be advantageous to look at GR and MR mRNA in the hippocampus of aged and young rats, because mRNA measurements are not subject to the complexities associated with steroid receptor binding. We simultaneously examined binding and mRNA levels and looked at the effects 36 hours after adrenalectomy on both parameters, mRNA levels and steroid receptor binding. To quantitate receptor binding in intact rats, we used the method of Eldridge et al.[105] In addition, we examined GR and MR dissociation constants in adrenalectomized rats.

The results were revealing. As reported by others, we found type I and type II binding in the hippocampus of aged male Fisher rats (26–27 months) to be significantly lower than that in young rats (5–6 months). Pituitary binding was unaltered with age. Unlike Eldridge's group, we found that this difference in hippocampal receptor binding could be seen even without adrenalectomy, with more than a 50% decrease in both types of receptors. Neither receptor showed a change in association/dissociation constants. The cell nuclei of intact aged rats also contained less corticosterone per milligram of protein, consistent with the presence of fewer receptors.

In the intact aged rats, both GR and MR mRNAs exhibited a 30% decrease in level ($P < .01$ for both), consistent with the 50% decrement in binding. This supports the notion of a selective loss of receptor and/or cells bearing the receptors within the hippocampus. Thirty-six hours after adrenalectomy, however, the aged rats exhibited a rise in mRNA levels, whereas the young control rats did not. This elevation brought the levels of steroid receptor mRNAs in the aged rats to the same as those seen in young animals (intact or adrenalectomized). It should be recalled, however, that at this point, binding is significantly decreased in aged rats. This suggests that the adrenalectomy-induced mRNA elevation did not translate into a change in protein synthesis. Indeed, the ratio of receptor maximal binding capacity to mRNA in adrenalectomized aged rats is approximately half that seen in young rats.[107]

Because prior evidence from our laboratory had indicated that hippocampal lesions result in induction of CRH and AVP mRNA in the mpPVN,[55,56] it was of interest to examine the aged rat as a model of a "mildly lesioned" hippocampus. We found, however, that CRH mRNA content and peptide contents were similar in the PVN of young and old animals. Interestingly, the CRH content in the median eminence was decreased by nearly 70% in the aged group, suggesting a higher release of CRH in the portal blood of aged rats.

We then studied the in vitro CRH release in total hypothalami from young and old rats. Although the basal CRH release was not significantly different in these conditions, the CRH release after stimulation with 10 nM norepinephrine was higher in the aged group. On the other hand, the AVP content in the two groups was not significantly different in the median eminence of the same animals. Moreover, in the hypothalamus incubation experiment, we did not see differences in the basal or stimulated AVP release in the two groups.

This work suggested that aging may result in a selective activation of the release of CRH, but not of AVP, and that this elevation is not necessarily accompanied by an induction of CRH mRNA levels, at least at this stage of aging. This observation is consistent with our more recent lesion results showing that limited hippocampal lesions produce limited or undetectable elevation in CRH message in the PVN. Taken together, the data lead to the notion that changes in the releasability of secretagogues represent an earlier stage of dysregulation, whereas changes in mRNA levels may represent the extreme case of full loss of hippocampal input.

These changes in CRH levels and releasability appear to result in altered sensitivity at the level of the pituitary. We have studied the control of ACTH secretion of young and old corticotroph cells in vitro, using a perifusion system where cells from a pool of young and old pituitary anterior lobes were stimulated with different doses of CRH or AVP or both. The dose-response curves of AVP-induced ACTH secretion in young and old corticotrophs were completely superimposable, consistent with the absence of a hypothalamic change in

AVP. However, in response to each dose of CRH, the old corticotrophs secreted 50% less ACTH than the young ones, suggesting a profound downregulation. Moreover, the combination of CRH and AVP produced less potentiation in the aged rats. Taken together, these results suggest that aged animals show a selective increase in CRH release and releasability, which is compensated for by a downregulation of pituitary CRH receptors.

Finally, there are multiple other changes at the level of the pituitary and adrenal, which are beyond the scope of this chapter. Suffice it to say, however, that every change appears to be compensated for by a secondary change at the next step, leading to a new but still fairly effective homeostasis. Thus, as mentioned previously, we were unable to detect any change in the resting levels of plasma corticosterone of the aged rats; the circadian rhythms of plasma corticosterone and corticosterone-binding capacity were superimposable in the two groups of rats.

In conclusion, our data demonstrate that, although exhibiting several changes at different levels of the LHPA, Fisher rats at this stage of aging were able to compensate through the interplay of multiple levels of control (e.g., increased CRH release coupled with downregulation of CRH receptors), resulting in normal circulating levels of corticosterone under resting conditions. However, under stress conditions (restraint), these same aged rats showed a delayed recovery to basal corticosterone levels even hours after the termination of the stressor. This model underscores the complexities of studying a closed, highly regulated system such as the LHPA and the need for using multiple probes to uncover a change in the individual elements of the axis.

The Stress Concept Revisited

So far, we have outlined both the molecular and the neuronal elements of the LHPA and have described its checks and balances in the context of the mild dysregulation seen in aging. Although the phenomenology is fairly well understood in the field, there are several conceptual issues that we have touched upon along the way but that may be worth reconsidering here in an effort to place this whole system in a context of relevance to mental health and mental illness. The following section is clearly speculative but represents our current conceptualization of the brain aspects of the stress axis based on anatomical, behavioral, and clinical considerations.

It may be relatively easy to imagine a fairly hard-wired set of connections that monitor physiological functions such as respiration, glucose levels, or blood pressure and transduce any deviations from homeostasis into neuronal and endocrine responses. However, stress is also typically defined as the body's response to stimuli that are external and evoke responses of "fight or flight," that is, more psychological stimuli. The central conceptual issue is: How is a psychological stimulus defined as stressful? How is this definition arrived at neuronally?

Psychologists agree that the perception of psychological stress is closely tied to the notion of control and of coping. Thus, the same stimulus presented to different individuals will be perceived differently, as a function of their past experience and their ability to face the stressor, to control it, or even to use it as a challenge. This being the case, we have to conceive of the neuronal underpinning of this process not only in terms of a throughput system that carries information to the PVN but as a comparator system that monitors the external and internal environment of the organism, compares it with past experience, and imparts valence to it. This idea of assigning valence is important not only in allowing the organism to focus on the correct stimulus but also in discounting irrelevant stimuli and to terminate responses when the stimuli cease to be important. Put in this context, we need to broaden our view of this monitoring system to encompass the detection not only of negative events but also of positive events that require the organism's full attention and take precedence over other ongoing stimuli (such events can, in fact, be associated with glucocorticoid secretion). Viewed in this manner, the stress system becomes an active monitoring system that is constantly matching current events to past experience, interpreting their importance and relevance (salience) to the survival of the organism, assigning to them a degree of valence (positive or negative), and determining the organism's ability to cope with them while recruiting several physiological, endocrine, and motor mechanisms to respond as needed.

Such a conceptualization would require us to include a number of key neuronal elements in this axis that may not be obvious if we had a more hard-wired view of stress responsiveness. Thus, beyond the primary detectors of a deviation from homeostasis, such as the nucleus tractus solitarius, we would invoke higher structures involved in coding emotions (e.g., the amygdala), interpreting the stimuli (e.g., cortex), or comparing current stimuli to past events, requiring learning and memory (e.g., hippocampus and cortex).

In this context, the role of the hippocampus, discussed previously, can be reinterpreted. In this ongoing monitoring process, the hippocampus may be critical in assigning salience (a function in which it has been implicated) and in participating in the comparator function, given its proposed role in mediating short-term memory and spatial learning. The hippocampus would not only influence our perception of stressors but would also in turn need to monitor the current stress status of the organism as it codes information into memory. Thus, the role of the glucocorticoid receptors within the hippocampus may have little to do with steroid feedback onto the stress axis, but rather may serve a role of keeping the hippocampus apprised of stress conditions as it codes novel information.

What would happen if this highly complex system involving the interplay of several circuits becomes disrupted? One might imagine that stress responses may be initiated in response to the "wrong" stimuli, that is, that stimuli may be coded as stressful that may not be perceived as such by most individuals or by the given individual at other times. One might also imagine that appropriate stress responses may not be terminated in a timely manner and that basic functions (eating, sexual activity) that are often superseded by stress responses become dysregulated. Many of these phenomena are observed in individuals with major mood disorders. Although it is clear from a large body of work that mood disorders, particularly major depression, can lead to chronic dysregulation of the LHPA, it is also possible to see how a disruption in the limbic and cortical aspects of the LHPA can participate in precipitating and/or maintaining depressive episodes. Thus, a more thorough understanding of the neuronal systems underlying stress biology and psychology should prove essential to an understanding of the biology of depression and of several other psychiatric disorders.

References

1. Henn FA, Edwards E, Muneyyirci J: Animal models of Depression. Clinical Neuroscience 1:152–156, 1993
2. Haynes RC, Berthet L: Studies on the mechanism of action of the adrenocorticotropic hormone. J Biol Chem 225:115–124, 1957
3. Mountjoy KG, Robbins LS, Mortrud MT, et al: The cloning of a family of genes that encode the melanocortin receptors. Science 257:1248–1251, 1992
4. Li CH, Evans H, Simpson ME: Adrenocorticotropic hormone. J Biol Chem 149:413–414, 1943
5. Nakanishi S, Inoue A, Kita T, et al: Nucleotide sequence of cloned cDNA for bovine corticotropin-β-lipotropin precursor. Nature 278:423–427, 1979
6. Lowry PJ, Hope J, Silman RE: The evolution of corticotropin, melanotropin and lipotropin, in Proceedings of the Fifth International Congress of Endocrinology, Vol 1. Edited by James VHY. Amsterdam, Excerpta Medica, 1976, pp 71–76
7. Mains RE, Eipper BE, Ling N: Common precursor to corticotropins and endorphins. Proc Natl Acad Sci U S A 74:3014–3018, 1977
8. Roberts JL, Herbert E: Characterization of a common precursor to corticotropin and β-lipotropin: cell-free synthesis of the precursor and identification of corticotropin peptides in the molecule. Proc Natl Acad Sci U S A 74:4826–4830, 1977
9. Akil H, Watson SJ, Young EA, et al: Endogenous opioids: biology and function. Annu Rev Neurosci 7:223–255, 1984
10. Roberts JL, Lundbland JR, Eberwine JH, et al: Hormonal regulation of POMC expression in pituitary. Ann N Y Acad Sci

512:275–285, 1987

11. Bloom FE, Battenberg E, Rossier J, et al: Endorphins are located in the intermediate and anterior lobes of the pituitary gland, not in the neurohypophysis. Life Sci 20:43–48, 1977
12. Watson SJ, Akil H, Richard CW, et al: Evidence for two separate opiate peptide neuronal systems and the coexistence of beta-LPH, beta-endorphin and ACTH immunoreactivities in the same hypothalamic neurons. Nature 275:226–228, 1978
13. Seidah NG, Gaspar L, Mion P, et al: cDNA sequence of two distinct pituitary proteins homologous to Kex2 and furin gene products: tissue-specific mRNAs encoding candidates for prohormone processing proteinases. DNA Cell Biol 9:415–424, 1990
14. Smeekens SP, Steiner DF: Identification of a human insulinoma cDNA encoding a novel mammalian protein structurally related to the yeast dibasic processing protease Kex2. J Biol Chem 265:2997–3000, 1990
15. Vale W, Spiess J, Rivier C, et al: Characterization of a 41-residue ovine hypothalamic peptide that stimulates secretion of corticotropin and β-endorphin. Science 213:1394–1397, 1981
16. Furutani Y, Morimoto Y, Shibahara S, et al: Cloning and sequence analysis of cDNA for ovine corticotropin-releasing factor precursor. Nature 301:537–540, 1983
17. Thompson RC, Seasholtz AF, Herbert E: Rat corticotropin-releasing hormone gene: sequence and tissue-specific expression. Mol Endocrinol 1:363–370, 1987
18. Swanson LW, Sawchenko PE, Lind RW, et al: The CRH motoneuron: differential peptide regulation in neurons with possible synaptic, paracrine and endocrine outputs. Ann N Y Acad Sci 512:12–23, 1988
19. Chen R, Lewis KA, Perrin MH, et al: Expression cloning of a human corticotropin-releasing factor receptor. Proc Natl Acad Sci U S A 90:8967–8970, 1993
20. Morel A, Lolait SJ, Brownstein MJ: Molecular cloning and expression of V1a and V2 arginine vasopressin receptors. Regul Pept 45:53–59, 1993
21. Antoni FA: Hypothalamic control of adrenocorticotropin secre-

tion: advances since the discovery of 41-residue CRF. Endocr Rev 7:351–378, 1986

22. Sawchenko PR: Adrenalectomy-induced enhancement of CRF and vasopressin immunoreactivity in parvicellular neurosecretory neurons: anatomic, peptide, and steroid specificity. J Neurosci 7:1093–1106, 1987
23. Birnberg N, Lissitsky J, Hinman M: Glucocorticoids regulate pro-opiomelanocortin gene expression at the level of transcription and secretion. Proc Natl Acad Sci U S A 80:6982–6986, 1983
24. Keller-Wood ME, Dallman MF: Corticosteroid inhibition of ACTH secretion. Endocr Rev 5:1–24, 1984
25. Dallman MF, Akana SF, Scribner KA, et al: Stress, feedback and facilitation in the hypothalamo-pituitary-adrenal axis. J Neuroendocrinol 4:517–526, 1991
26. Shiomi H, Watson SJ, Kelsey JE, et al: Pretranslational and posttranslational mechanisms for regulating β-endorphin-adrenocorticotropin of the anterior pituitary lobe. Endocrinology 119: 1793–1799, 1986
27. Kwak SP, Young EA, Morano MI, et al: Diurnal corticotropin-releasing hormone mRNA variation in the hypothalamus exhibits a rhythm distinct from that of plasma corticosterone. Neuroendocrinology 55:74–83, 1992
28. Kwak SP, Morano MI, Young EA, et al: Diurnal CRH mRNA in the hypothalamus: decreased expression in the evening is not dependent on endogenous glucocorticoids. Neuroendocrinology 57:96–105, 1993
29. Szafarczyk A, Izart G, Malaval F, et al: Effects of lesions of the suprachiasmatic nuclei and of p-chlorophenylalanine on the circadian rhythms of adrenocorticotrophic hormone and corticosterone in the plasma, and on locomotor activity of rats. J Endocrinol 83:1–16, 1979
30. Krieger DT, Hauser H: Comparison of synchronization of circadian corticosteroid rhythms by photoperiod and food. Proc Natl Acad Sci U S A 75:1577–1588, 1978
31. Reul JM, DeKloet R: Anatomical resolution of two types of corticosterone receptor sites in rat brain with in vitro autoradiog-

raphy and computerized image analysis. Journal of Steroid Biochemistry 24:269–272, 1986
32. Hollenberg SM, Weinberger C, Ong ES, et al: Primary structure and expression of a functional human glucocorticoid receptor cDNA. Nature 318:635–641, 1985
33. Ariza JL, Weinberger C, Cerelli G, et al: Cloning of the human mineralocorticoid receptor complementary DNA: structural and functional kinship with the glucocorticoid receptor. Science 237:268–275, 1987
34. Patel PD, Sherman TG, Goldman DJ, et al: Molecular cloning of a mineralocorticoid receptor cDNA from rat hippocampus. Mol Endocrinol 3:1877–1885, 1989
35. Herman JP, Patel PD, Akil H, et al: Localization and regulation of glucocorticoid and mineralocorticoid receptor messenger RNAs in the hippocampal formation of the rat. Mol Endocrinol 3:1886–1894, 1989
36. Swanson LW, Simmons DM: Differential steroid hormone and neural influences on peptide mRNA levels in CRH cells of the paraventricular nucleus: a hybridization histochemical study in the rat. J Comp Neurol 285:413–435, 1989
37. Funder JW, Pearce PT, Smith R, et al: Mineralocorticoid action: target tissue specificity is enzyme, not receptor, mediated. Science 242:583–585, 1988
38. Dalman FC, Scherrer LC, Taylor LP, et al: Direct evidence that the glucocorticoid receptor binds to hsp90 at or near the termination of receptor translation in vitro. J Biol Chem 264:19815–19821, 1991
39. Caamaño CA, Morano MI, Patel PD, et al: Bacterially expressed mineralocorticoid receptor is associated in vitro with the 90-kDa heat shock protein and shows typical hormone- and DNA-binding characteristics. Biochemistry 32:8589–8595, 1993
40. Sakai D, Feldman S: Effects of neural stimuli on paraventricular nucleus neurons. Brain Res Bull 14:401–407, 1985
41. Drouin J, Trifiro MA, Plante RK, et al: Glucocorticoid receptor binding to a specific DNA sequence is required for hormone-dependent repression of proopiomelanocortin gene transcription. Mol Cell Biol 9:5305–5314, 1989

42. Schule R, Rangarajan P, Kliewer S, et al: Functional antagonism between oncoprotein c-Jun and the glucocorticoid receptor. Cell 62:1217–1226, 1990
43. Yang-Yen HF, Chambard JC, Sun YL, et al: Transcriptional interference between c-Jun and the glucocorticoid receptor: mutual inhibition of DNA binding due to direct protein-protein interaction. Cell 62:1205–1215, 1990
44. Diamond MI, Miner JN, Yoshinaga SK, et al: Transcription factor interactions: selectors of positive or negative regulation from a single DNA element. Science 249:1266–1272, 1990
45. Pearce D, Yamamoto KR: Mineralocorticoid and glucocorticoid receptor activities distinguished by nonreceptor factors at a composite response element. Science 259:1161–1165, 1993
46. Funder JW: Mineralocorticoids, glucocorticoids, receptors, and response elements. Science 259:1132–1133, 1993
47. Reul JM, DeKloet ER: Two receptor systems for corticosterone receptors in rat brain: microdistribution and differential occupation. Endocrinology 117:2505–2511, 1985
48. Herman JP, Watson SJ, Chao HM, et al: Diurnal regulation of glucocorticoid receptor and mineralocorticoid receptor mRNAs in rat hippocampus. Molecular and Cellular Neurosciences 4:181–190, 1993
49. DeKloet ER: Brain, corticosteroid receptor balance and homeostatic control. Front Neuroendocrinol 12:95–164, 1991
50. Dallman MF, Akana SF, Cascio CS, et al: Regulation of ACTH secretion: variations on a theme of B. Recent Prog Horm Res 43:113–171, 1987
51. Jacobson L, Sapolsky R: The role of the hippocampus in feedback regulation of the hypothalamic-pituitary-adrenocortical axis. Endocr Rev 12:118–134, 1991
52. McEwen BS, Weiss JJM, Schwartz LS: Selective retention of corticosterone by limbic structures in rat brain. Nature 220:911–912, 1986
53. Feldman S, Conforti N: Participation of the dorsal hippocampus in glucocorticoid negative feedback effect on adrenocortical activity. Neuroendocrinology 30:52–55, 1980
54. Fischette CT, Komisaruk BR, Edinger HM: Differential fornix ab-

lations and the circadian rhythmicity of adrenal corticosteroid secretion. Brain Res 195:373–387, 1980

55. Herman JP, Schafer MK-H, Young EA, et al: Evidence for hippocampal regulation of neuroendocrine neurons of the hypothalamo-pituitary-adrenocortical axis. J Neurosci 9:3072–3082, 1989
56. Herman JP, Cullinan WE, Young EA, et al: Selective forebrain fiber-tract lesions implicate ventral hippocampal structures in tonic regulation of paraventricular nucleus CRH and AVP mRNA expression. Brain Res 592:228–238, 1992
57. Feldman S, Weidenfeld J: The dorsal hippocampus modifies the negative feedback effect of glucocorticoids on the adrenocortical and median eminence CRF-41 responses to photic stimulation. Brain Res 614:227–232, 1993

57a. Herman JP, Cillinan WE, Morano MI, et al: Contribution of the ventral subiculum to inhibitory regulation of the hypothalamo-pituitary-adrenocortical axis. J Neuroendocrinol, in press

58. Cullinan WE, Herman JP, Watson SJ: Ventral subicular interaction with the hypothalamic paraventricular nucleus: evidence for a relay in the bed nucleus of the stria terminalis. J Comp Neurol 332:L1–L20, 1993
59. Cunningham ETJ, Bohn MC, Sawchenko PE: Organization of adrenergic inputs to the paraventricular and supraoptic nuclei of the hypothalamus in the rat. J Comp Neurol 292:651–657, 1990
60. Alonso G, Szafarczyk A, Balmefrezol M: Immunocytochemical evidence for stimulatory control by the ventral noradrenergic bundle of parvicellular neurons of the paraventricular nucleus secreting corticotropin releasing hormone and vasopressin in rats. Brain Res 3967:297–307, 1986
61. Gibson A, Hart SL, Paterl S: Effects of 6-hydroxydopamine-induced lesions of the paraventricular nucleus, and prazosin, on the corticosterone response to restraint in rats. Neuropharmacology 25:257–260, 1986
62. Mezey E, Kiss JZ, Skirboll LR: Increase of corticotropin-releasing factor staining in rat paraventricular nucleus neurons by depletion of hypothalamic adrenaline. Nature 310:140–141, 1984
63. Plostky PM, Otto S, Sutton S: Neurotransmitter modulation of

corticotropin releasing factor secretion into the hypophysial-portal circulation. Life Sci 41:1311–1317, 1987

64. Szafarczyk A, Malaval F, Laurent A: Further evidence for a central stimulatory action of catecholamines on adrenocorticotropin release in the rat. Endocrinology 121:883–892, 1987
65. Szafarczyk A, Guillaume V, Conte-Devolx B: Central catecholaminergic system stimulates secretion of CRH at different sites. Am J Physiol 255:E463–E468, 1988
66. Darlington DN, Shinsako J, Dallman MF: Medullary lesions eliminate ACTH responses to hypotensive hemorrhage. Am J Physiol 251:R106–R115, 1986
67. Sawchenko PE, Swanson LW, Steinbusch HWM: The distribution and cells of origin of serotonin inputs to the paraventricular and supraoptic nuclei of the rat. Brain Res 277:355–360, 1983
68. Feldman S: Neural pathways mediating adrenocortical responses. Federation Proceedings 44:169–175, 1985
69. Feldman S, Conforti N: Modifications of adrenocortical responses following frontal cortex stimulation in rats with hypothalamic deafferentations and medial forebrain bundle lesions. Neuroscience 15:1045–1047, 1985
70. Szafarczyk A, Hery M, Laplante E: Temporal relationships between the circadian rhythmicity in plasma levels of pituitary hormones and in hypothalamic concentrations of releasing factors. Neuroendocrinology 30:369–376, 1980
71. Alexopoulos GS, Young RC, Kocsis JH, et al: Dexamethasone suppression test in geriatric depression: effect of age and sex on cortisol and beta-endorphin. Biol Psychiatry 33:73–85, 1993
72. Beaulieu S, DiPaolo T, Barden N: Control of ACTH secretion by the central nucleus of the amygdala: implications of the serotonergic system and its relevance to the glucocorticoid delayed negative feedback mechanism. Neuroendocrinology 44:247–254, 1986
73. Dunn JD, Whitener J: Plasma corticosterone responses to electrical stimulation of the amygdaloid complex: cytoarchitectonic specificity. Neuroendocrinology 42:211–217, 1986
74. Saphier D, Feldman S: Effects of neural stimuli on paraventricular nucleus neurons. Brain Res Bull 14:401–407, 1985

75. Hoffman GE, Smith MS, Verbalis JG: c-Fos and related immediate early gene products as markers of activity in neuroendocrine systems. Front Neuroendocrinol 14:173–214, 1993
76. Schreiber SS, Tocco G, Shors TJ, et al: Activation of immediate early genes after acute stress. Neuroreport 2:17–20, 1991
77. Imaki T, Shibasaki T, Hotta M, et al: Intracerebroventricular administration of corticotropin-releasing factor induces c-fos mRNA expression in brain regions related to stress responses: comparison with pattern of c-fos mRNA induction after stress. Brain Res 616:114–125, 1993
78. Cullinan WE, Herman JP, Battaglia DF, et al: Pattern and time course of immediate early gene expression in rat following acute stress. Neuroscience, in press
79. Sapolsky RM, Krey LC, McEwen BS: The adrenocortical stress-response in the aged male rat: impairment of recovery from stress. Exp Gerontol 18:55–64, 1983
80. Sapolsky RM, Krey LC, McEwen BS: The adrenocortical axis in the aged rat: impaired sensitivity to both fast and delayed feedback inhibition. Neurobiol Aging 7:331–336, 1986
81. Sapolsky RM, Krey LC, McEwen BS: The neuroendocrinology of stress and aging: the glucocorticoid cascade hypothesis. Endocr Rev 7:284–301, 1986
82. Chiueh CC, Nespor SM, Rapoport SI: Cardiovascular, sympathetic and adrenal cortical responsiveness of aged Fisher-344 rats to stress. Neurobiol Aging 1:157–163, 1980
83. DeKlotsky S, Scheff S, Cotman C: Elevated corticosterone levels: a possible cause of reduced axon sprouting in aged animals. Neuroendocrinology 38:33–38, 1984
84. Meaney MJ, Aitken DH, Bhatnagar S, et al: Postnatal handling attenuates neuroendocrine, anatomical and cognitive impairments related to the aged hippocampus. Science 238:766–768, 1988
85. Meaney MJ, Viau V, Aitken D, et al: Stress-induced occupancy and translocation of hippocampal glucocorticoid receptors. Brain Res 514:37–48, 1988
86. Meaney MJ, Aitken DH, Sharma S, et al: Basal ACTH, corticosterone and corticosterone-binding globulin levels over the di-

urnal cycle, and age related changes in hippocampal type I and type II corticosteroid receptor binding capacity in young and aged, handled and nonhandled rats. Neuroendocrinology 55: 204–213, 1992
87. Sapolsky RM, Krey LC, McEwen BS: Corticosterone receptors decline in a site-specific manner in the aged rat. Brain Res 289:235–240, 1983
88. Steward J, Meaney MJ, Aitken D, et al: The effects of acute and life-long food restriction on basal and stress-induced serum corticosterone in young and aged rats. Endocrinology 123:1934–1941, 1988
89. Algieri S, Calderini G, Lomuscio G, et al: Changes with age in rat central monoaminergic system responses to cold stress. Neurobiol Aging 3:237–242, 1982
90. Brett LP, Chong GS, Coyle S, et al: The pituitary-adrenal response to novel stimulation and ether stress in young adult and aged rats. Neurobiol Aging 4:133–138, 1983
91. Brodish A, Odio M: Age-dependent effects of chronic stress on ACTH and corticosterone responses to an acute novel stress. Neuroendocrinology 49:496–501, 1989
92. Goya RG, Castro MG, Sosa YE: Diminished diurnal secretion of corticosterone in aging female but not male rats. Gerontology 35:181–187, 1989
93. Hess GD, Riegle GC: Adrenalcortical responsiveness to stress and ACTH in aging rats. J Gerontology 25:354–358, 1970
94. Hylka VW, Sonntag WE, Meites J: Reduced ability of old male rats to release ACTH and corticosterone in response to CRF administration. Proc Soc Exp Biol Med 175:1–4, 1984
95. Odio M, Brodish A: Age-related adaptation of pituitary-adrenocortical responses to stress. Neuroendocrinology 49:382–388, 1989
96. Sonntag WE, Golieszek AG, Brodish A, et al: Diminished diurnal secretion of adrenocorticotropin (ACTH) but not corticosterone in old male rats: possible relation to increased adrenal sensitivity to ACTH in vivo. Endocrinology 119:1793–1799, 1986
97. Tang F, Phillips JG: Some age-related changes in pituitary-adrenal function in the male laboratory rat. J Gerontol 33:377–382,

1978

98. vanEekelen JAM, Rots NY, Sutanto W, et al: The effect of aging on stress responsiveness and central corticosteroid receptors in the Brown Norway rat. Neurobiol Aging 13:159–170, 1989
99. Reul JM, Tonnaer J, DeKloet ER: Neurotropic ACTH analog promotes plasticity of type I corticosteroid receptors in brain of senescent male rats. Neurobiol Aging 9:253–257, 1988
100. Landfield P, Waymire J, Lynch G: Hippocampal aging and adrenocorticoids: quantitative correlations. Science 202:1098–1102, 1978
101. Sapolsky RM, Krey LC, McEwen BS: Prolonged glucocorticoid exposure reduces hippocampal neuron number: implications for aging. J Neurosci 5:1222–1227, 1985
102. Issa AM, Rowe W, Gauthier S, et al: Hypothalamic-pituitary-adrenal activity in aged, cognitively impaired and cognitively unimpaired rats. J Neurosci 10:3247–3254, 1990
103. Reul JM, VanDebosch FR, DeKloet ER: Differential response of type I and type II corticosteroid receptors to changes in plasma steroid level and circadian rhythmicity. Neuroendocrinology 45:407–412, 1987
104. Eldridge JC, Brodish A, Kute TE, et al: Apparent age-related resistance of type II hippocampal corticosteroid receptors to down-regulation during chronic escape training. J Neurosci 9:3237–3242, 1989
105. Eldridge JC, Fleenor DG, Kerr DS, et al: Impaired up-regulation of type II corticosteroid receptors in hippocampus of aged rats. Brain Res 478:248–256, 1989
106. Landfield PW, Eldridge JC: Increased affinity of type II corticosteroid binding in aged rat hippocampus. Exp Neurol 106:110–113, 1989
107. Morano MI, Akil H: Age-related changes in the POMC stress axis in the rat, in New Leads in Opioid Research. Edited by VanRee JM, Mulder AH, Wiegant VM, et al. Amsterdam, Excerpta Medica, 1990, pp 9–11

CHAPTER

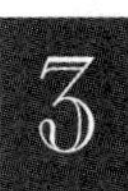

Norepinephrine and Serotonin Transporters: Progress on Molecular Targets of Antidepressants

Randy D. Blakely, Ph.D.

One of the underlying tenets of molecular psychiatry is that the elucidation of the structure and regulation of genes required for neuronal synapse formation and function will provide insights into disease processes and offer prospects for novel biochemical therapeutics. Indeed, it is safe to say that our present abilities to provide pharmacologic interventions in life-threatening psychoses and affective disorders derives largely from the manipulation of an ever-expanding list of molecular targets localized to specific brain synapses.

Surprisingly, neurotransmitter transporters, the principal targets for the most widely prescribed agents in psychiatry, the antidepressants, have resisted molecular scrutiny for nearly three decades.

Support for R. D. Blakely was provided by Grant DA 07390 from the National Institutes of Health and by the Mallinckrodt Foundation.

In the late 1950s and early 1960s, it became clear[1,2] that the fate of secreted monoamines, particularly norepinephrine (NE), was to be efficiently sequestered back into sympathetic neuronal terminals by transport activities (Figure 3–1), a process inhibited by both cocaine and tricyclic antidepressants.[3,4] Although enzymatic mechanisms capably degrade intracellular and circulating catecholamines, the acute effects on sympathetic transmission of enzymatic inhibition were minimal compared with the profound changes after transport blockade. The presence of transport activities in presynaptic terminals (and, in some cases, glia) reflects a requirement for tightly controlled temporal and spatial chemical signaling and an opportunity for biosynthetic economy in the repackaging and rerelease of previously utilized transmitter. Pharmacologic blockade of transport activities, therefore, leads quickly to an increase in synaptic transmitter availability and the opportunity for neurotransmitter to "spill over" to extrasynaptic sites, both of which in the long term may correct chemical signaling abnormalities underlying neuropsychiatric disorders.

The revelation that serotonin (5-hydroxytryptamine [5-HT]) was also subject to antidepressant-sensitive "reuptake";[2,5] that both NE and 5-HT were synthesized in terminals of widespread brain stem projections to limbic, cortical, and subcortical structures, where they could regulate mood, appetite, sleep, and aggression;[6] and that manipulation of monoamine biosynthesis and storage induced characteristic behavioral disturbances led to a formulation of a biogenic amine hypothesis of affective disorders.[7,8] Since that time, evidence for altered transport in affective disorders has been gathered, focused largely on measurements of 5-HT transport due to readily accessible platelet serotonin transporters.

Such findings invariably led to tests for proper structure or regulatory control of the transporters themselves in disease states, an effort that requires a knowledge of monoamine transporter structure and of the genes that encode each protein. Only within the past few years has the latter goal become reality, with the molecular cloning of biogenic amine transporter genes and gene products[9–13] within the GAT/NET gene family.[14] In this chapter, I review these advances with an eye to how increased understanding of neurotrans-

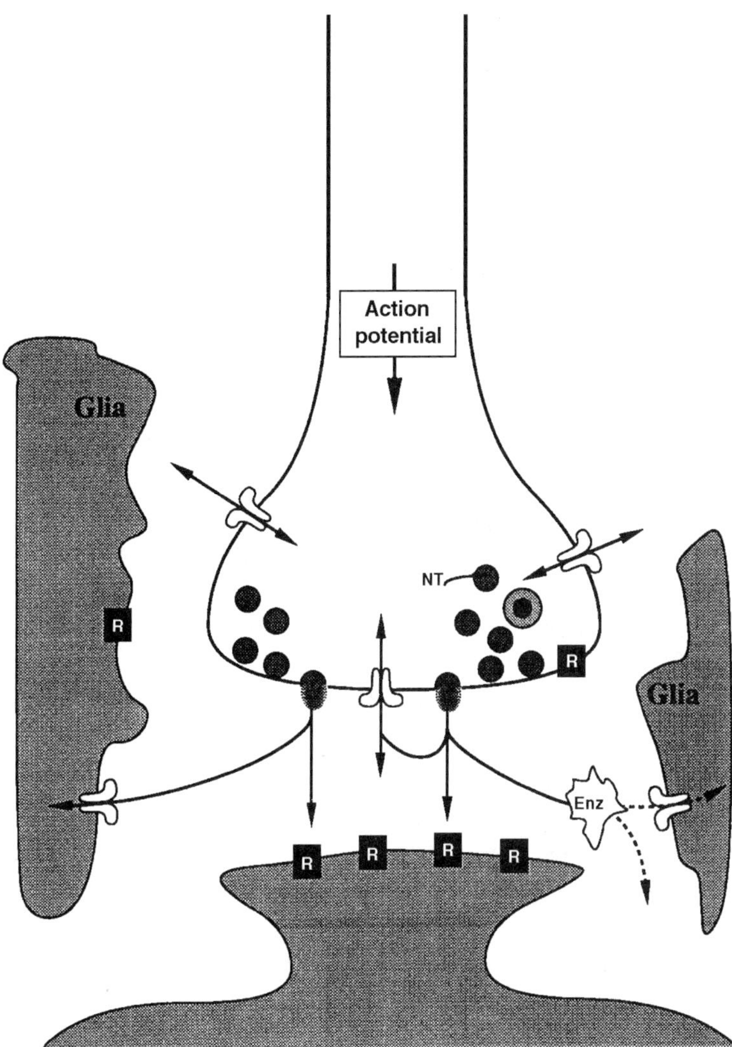

Figure 3–1. Schematic illustration of a typical neuronal synapse depicting vesicular release of neurotransmitters following depolarization and the subsequent clearance of transmitter by presynaptic and/or glial transporters. Transmitter vesicles within the presynaptic cytoplasm are shown co-localized with large dense core secretory granules containing neuropeptides. Transporters are given bidirectional arrows to indicate a capacity for both influx and efflux depending on transmembrane ion gradients and voltage. NT = neurotransmitter being packaged into synaptic vesicles for release. R = receptors on presynaptic and postsynaptic membranes. Enz = enzyme.

mitter transporter structure and regulation may contribute to future insights in human psychiatric illness.

Norepinephrine Transporter: Molecular Basis of Uptake 1

Due to the low-affinity, high-capacity accumulation of catecholamines by target tissues, Iversen[2] introduced the terms *uptake 1* and *uptake 2* to discriminate between the neuronal and nonneuronal absorptive processes, respectively. Although a certain degree of specificity is present in the uptake 2 process, this activity remains poorly defined and lacks the ion dependence and antagonist sensitivity of uptake 1. Uptake 1 is defined as a neuronal NE transport activity dependent on extracellular Na^+ and Cl^-, believed to reflect the cotransport of these ions with the positively charged catecholamine[15] (Figure 3–2). Each transport cycle appears to move the three substrates in a 1:1:1 stoichiometry.[15,16] Intracellular K^+ may also participate in the uptake of extracellular substrates,[16] although the exact role for this ion has yet to be precisely defined. The imposition of a negative membrane potential on resealed membrane vesicles accelerates NE influx, suggesting that net charge moves each transport cycle, compatible with the aforementioned stoichiometry.[15,16] Uptake 1 actually prefers dopamine (DA) to NE as a substrate for influx,[2] although it is unlikely that significant extracellular DA ever presents itself at adrenergic synapses.

Other phenylethylamines, including amphetamine and tyramine, are substrates for uptake 1, capable of not only blocking NE uptake but also of entering the presynaptic neuronal cytoplasm, where they can deplete vesicular NE storage pools and augment nonvesicular NE release. Secondary amine antidepressants, such as desipramine and nortriptyline, are more uptake 1-selective antagonists than are their tertiary amine derivatives imipramine and amitriptyline; the latter compounds display greater potency in the inhibition of 5-HT uptake. Other agents, including cocaine, mazindol, nomifensine, and nisoxetine, potently inhibit uptake 1 in both

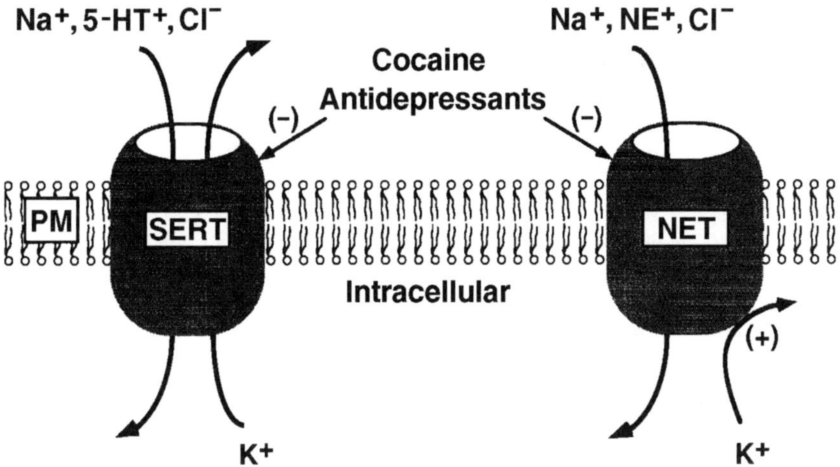

Figure 3–2. Ion-coupled norepinephrine (NE) and 5-hydroxytryptamine (5-HT) uptake. At left is the proposed mechanism for the 5-HT transporter (SERT), whereby uptake of 5-HT is dependent on cotransport of Na^+ and Cl^- and countertransport of K^+. This model predicts no net charge movement per complete cycle and is hence termed *electroneutral*. At right is the NE transporter (NET) model showing Na^+- and Cl^--dependent NE uptake, where intracellular K^+ stimulates NE uptake but may not directly cross the plasma membrane. This model predicts the inward movement of a single positive charge in each transport cycle and is termed *electrogenic*. PM = plasma membrane.

peripheral and central nervous system (CNS) preparations.

Protein-directed strategies achieved only limited success in the elucidation of neurotransmitter transporter structure, and particularly so for the NE transporter (NET). Howard et al.[17] labeled a 54-kilodalton (kDa) species in PC12 cells with the alkylating agent xylamine in a cocaine-dependent manner; the correspondence of this protein to NET, however, could not be further ascribed to the carrier itself. To circumvent traditional biochemical purification strategies and clone NET complementary DNAs (cDNAs) in the absence of protein-derived sequence information, Pacholczyk et al.[9] turned to expression cloning in COS cells, where uptake 1 activity induced by cDNA clones could be efficiently screened. The outline for the technique is shown in Figure 3–3.

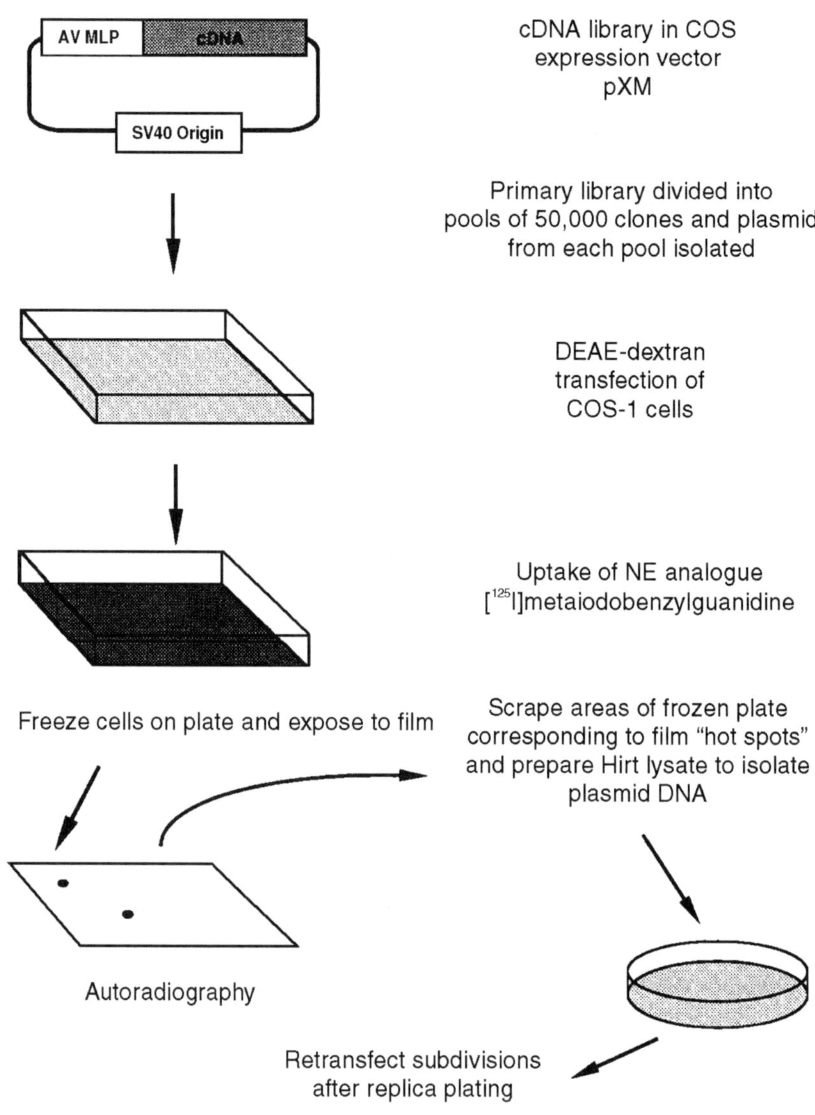

Figure 3–3. Expression cloning strategy for the identification of the norepinephrine transporter. AV MLP = adenovirus major late promoter. cDNA = complementary DNA. DEAE = diethylaminoethyl. NE = norepinephrine.

cDNA libraries were first prepared from the human, uptake 1-expressing neuroblastoma SK-N-SH.[18] Screening for cDNA-induced transport activity relied on the use of [^{125}I]metaiodobenzylguanidine (MIBG) as a surrogate substrate for positively transfected COS cells. The accumulation of [^{125}I]MIBG in transfected cells could be imaged autoradiographically, and transporter-expressing cells could then be isolated and plasmid DNA extracted to identify the clones responsible for inducing transport, leading to the eventual identification of a single human NET (hNET) cDNA. Subsequent NET expression studies made use of the vaccinia-T7 expression system, a remarkably efficient tool for the expression of cloned transport proteins.[19]

Because the NET activity conferred by the identified cDNA was sensitive to blockade by tricyclic antidepressants, amphetamine, and cocaine, the cloning of an hNET cDNA both defined the transporter's primary structure and established a single protein as the site of both drug recognition and transport activity. Still lacking is a knowledge of the native stoichiometry of NET expression, that is, how many NET monomers form the functional complex and whether accessory proteins are organized with hNET in the active unit. Expression of pharmacologically appropriate uptake 1 in nonneuronal host cells suggests, however, that if such accessory proteins exist, they are likely to be modulatory rather than essential to function and widely expressed outside the nervous system. With regard to the latter point, it must be borne in mind that the gene family within which NET resides[14] now contains transporters unrelated to synaptic neurotransmitter uptake, and thus almost every cell may express one or more family member.

The primary sequence of the hNET cDNA[9] predicts a highly hydrophobic, 617–amino acid polypeptide of 67 kDa with 12 potential transmembrane domains (TMDs), following algorithms of the type first proposed by Kyte and Doolittle[20] (Figure 3–4). The NH2 terminus lacks the hydrophobicity that is characteristic of a signal sequence for membrane insertion and bears no asparagine-linked glycosylation sites; thus, as for many other transport proteins, the NH2 terminus is predicted to reside in the cytoplasm. An even number of TMDs following the NH2 terminus places the COOH terminus

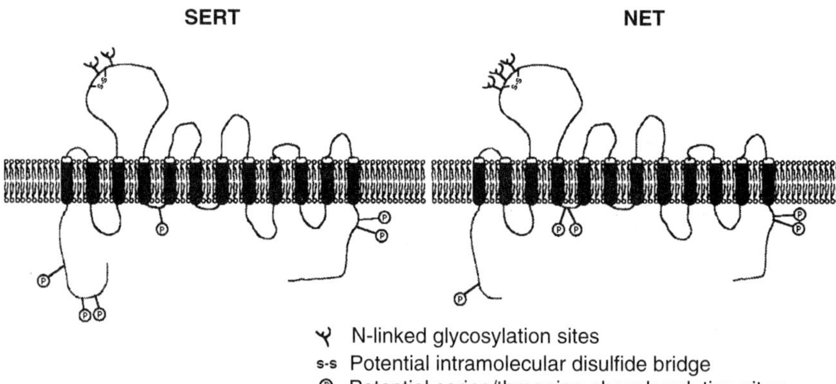

Figure 3–4. Proposed transmembrane topology and structural features of serotonin transporter (SERT) and norepinephrine transporter (NET) as derived from cloned complementary deoxyribonucleic acids. Note the 12 proposed transmembrane domains (TMDs), the large extracellular loop between TMD3 and TMD4 bearing multiple N-linked glycosylation sites, cytoplasmic -NH2 and -COOH tails, and sites for potential inter- or intramolecular disulfide bridge formation and cytoplasmic transporter phosphorylation.

also in the cytoplasm. Following TMD3, hNET contains a large hydrophilic loop with three canonical asparagine-linked glycosylation sites, suggesting an extracellular localization of this domain.

Consistent with these predictions, Melikian et al.[21] have found 80-kDa hNETs expressed in transfected cells to exhibit a sizeable electrophoretic mobility shift (to 46 kDa) after complete enzymatic deglycosylation. The difference between the estimated 46 kDa and the 67 kDa predicted from the primary sequence[9] probably represents the increased mobility of highly hydrophobic membrane proteins on the sodium dodecyl sulfate–polyacrylamide gels used for hNET mass estimation. Glycosylation of membrane proteins can contribute to their folding, stability, trafficking, or ligand recognition. In the case of hNET, stepwise glycosylation appears to be required for normal protein stability and cell surface expression[21] rather than contributing defining characteristics of ligand recognition. The fact that NET bears no other sites for N-linked glycosylation except on the large loop between TMDs 3 and 4 strongly favors an extracellular localization of this domain, as predicted by the initial model. Further support for the topological correctness of the model arises from detergent dependence of antibody recognition[21] when the NET antibody is directed at a predicted intracellular loop that may require membrane permeabilization for antibody access.

Protein phosphorylation at serine, threonine, and tyrosine residues is involved in the acute regulation of many ion channels and cell surface receptors. The putative cytoplasmic domains of hNET contain multiple, canonical sites for serine-threonine phosphorylation (Figure 3–4), and acute regulation of NET activity by exogenous hormones, which in other systems elevate protein kinase regulatory second messengers, has been reported (see below). To date, validation of the phosphorylation of any of these sites has not been achieved, and efforts to do so have been limited largely by an absence of hNET purification methods that are suitable for phosphoprotein analysis. Metabolically labeled NET proteins can now be efficiently immunoprecipitated from transfected cells,[21] providing new opportunities for accelerated progress on NET phosphorylation or other common membrane protein posttranslational modifications (e.g., acylation).

Comparison of the hNET primary amino acid sequence with that of a cloned γ-aminobutyric acid transporter (GAT1)[22] revealed 46% absolute identity, establishing the existence of an Na^+/Cl^- cotransporter gene family likely to contain additional neurotransmitter transporter proteins.[14] This supposition has been amply validated with the identification of additional GAT/NET homologues encoding DA, 5-HT, glycine, taurine, proline, creatine, and betaine transporters, among others. Estimates from genomic hybridization studies suggest that there are as many as 30 members within the GAT/NET gene family; indeed, additional GAT/NET homologues have been cloned by several laboratories that, at present, lack defined substrates.[23] Na^+/L-glutamate and Na^+/glucose cotransporters, which lack a requirement for extracellular Cl^- for substrate influx, reside in distinct gene families unrelated to the GAT/NET group.[24] Approximately 40% identity is detected in 2 × 2 comparisons of hNET with other GAT/NET homologues; NE, DA, and 5-HT transporters are most closely related to each other, defining a small subdivision united by both sequence and pharmacology (Figure 3–5). Approximately 20% of hNET residues are absolutely conserved across all GAT/NET family members. Interestingly, this sequence

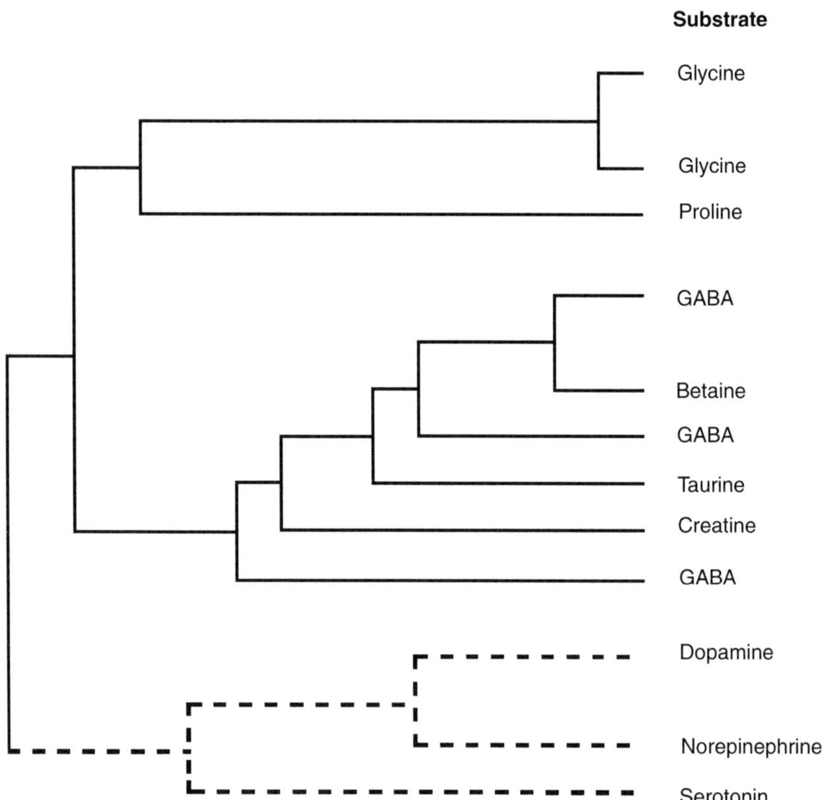

Figure 3–5. GAT/NET gene family relationships. Transporters are identified by their most likely endogenous substrate. Multiple species variants of the transporters presented are not included, nor are additional gene products with yet unidentified substrates. The GAT/NET subdivision containing cocaine- and antidepressant-sensitive transporters is highlighted with dashed lines. The distance of horizontal lines connecting each transporter to a branch point is inversely proportional to sequence similarity. Thus, dopamine and norepinephrine transporters are more closely related to each other than to the serotonin transporter, although these three as a group are more similar to each other than they are related to other GAT/NET homologues. GABA = γ-aminobutyric acid.

identity is distributed nonuniformly, with particularly high conservation evident in TMDs 1–2 and 5–8. These residues are most likely to represent sites involved in shared tasks such as Na^+ and Cl^- binding or, alternatively, they outline the global architecture required for the conformational changes required for transporter function. Regions devoid of sequence conservation may contribute to transporter-specific ligand recognition, cell trafficking, or regulation.

One feature that separates the NE, 5-HT, and DA transporters (DATs) from other GAT/NET homologues is high-affinity recognition of the psychoactive agents cocaine and amphetamine; NETs and the 5-HT transporters (SERTs) also share recognition of tricyclic antidepressants. Could individual human differences in primary transporter sequence thus lead to enhanced or reduced drug sensitivity and predispose some to addiction and others to a regimen of ineffective pharmacotherapy? Although the sites of antagonist recognition have yet to be directly established, the expression of cloned and mutant NETs, SERTs, and DATs in transfected cells is rapidly illuminating functional properties of shared structural features. Sequence comparisons show the NH2 and COOH termini to be poorly conserved and thus potentially involved in unique attributes of each carrier. However, chimera studies in which these domains were swapped between NETs and SERTs revealed no alteration in substrate or antagonist selectivity;[25] in addition, direct digestion or removal by mutagenesis of GAT1 tails fails to alter transport properties,[26,27] suggesting that NH2 and COOH termini are inconsequential for ligand recognition. Attempts to form functional chimeras between NETs and SERTs in which more than the NH2 or COOH terminal tails are transferred have not proven successful despite clear evidence of chimeric protein synthesis[28] consistent with an involvement of multiple TMDs in surface expression or formation of the ligand-binding pocket.

The simple structure of catecholamine substrates for NET invites comparisons between modes of catecholamine recognition by receptors and transporters. Perhaps a common strategy has been arrived at by evolutionarily unrelated proteins due to the rather limited number of contact sites on the catecholamine molecule.[29] In adrenergic receptors, the protonated NH2 group on NE is believed to ion-pair with an intramembrane aspartate residue, whereas catechol OH groups are tethered by hydrogen bonds of serine residues on a nearby TMD.[30] Likewise, structural features of catecholamines required for high-affinity recognition by NETs confirm the importance of ring hydroxyl groups and a protonated, unsubstituted NH2 group.[2] In addition, TMD aspartate and serine residues are among the handful of monoamine transporter–specific residues, raising the possibility of convergent development of catecholamine contact points in transporters and adrenergic receptors.

Site-directed mutagenesis of the TMD1 aspartate residue in NET[31] and the DAT[29] markedly alters substrate and antagonist recognition. For DAT, retention of low-affinity cocaine binding and substrate recognition suggests a selective alteration in the ligand binding pocket by the aspartate mutation rather than a gross destabilization of transporter protein. Antibody studies reveal no difference between wild-type and TMD1 aspartate-mutant NET proteins,[31] consistent with a direct alteration at the binding site rather than a global modification of protein stability. However, the idea that the TMD1 aspartate residue coordinates the catecholamine NH2 group via salt-bridge formation is problematic in light of the fact that other GAT/NET proteins, bearing an uncharged glycine residue in the position occupied by the NET, DAT, and SERT aspartate, also bind substrates with protonated NH2 groups. Moreover, what is unique about NE, DA, and 5-HT as GAT/NET substrates is not the presence of a protonated NH2 group to possibly bind the TMD1 aspartate but the absence of an acidic side chain linked to each substrate's α-carbon. One or more of the residues shared by NET, SERT, and DAT, but not by other GAT/NET homologues, such as the TMD1 aspartate, may represent a binding site for catecholamine and indoleamine substrates at regions of the substrate occupied by the acidic carboxyl moiety in other substrates.

Disregarding species variations, are all NETs identical to the transporter expressed by SK-N-SH cells? Similar transport activities could arise from more than one gene product, as found in numerous examples of receptor heterogeneity. Two distinct genes are known to encode CNS and adrenal vesicular transporters responsible for NE packaging for release.[32] Multiple genes also encode several pharmacologically distinct GABA transporter isoforms[33] (Figure 3–5). Tissue-specific differences in ligand recognition by NETs have been reported,[2] although these discrepancies may reflect assay differences more than the properties of NET structural variants.

To date, only a single human genomic locus for NETs has been identified,[34] spanning a locus of least 10 kilobases (kb) on chromosome 16q12.2 with multiple introns evident. Multiple messenger RNAs (mRNAs) are revealed by hNET cDNA probes in SK-N-SH and PC-12 cells, as well as in primary tissues.[9,16] In SK-N-SH cells, this heterogeneity appears to derive from 3′ noncoding variants providing different polyadenylation sites,[35] the functional importance of which remains unexplored. Coding region variants could be derived from the single hNET gene, as occurs with the cell-specific alternative splicing of RNAs derived from a single glycine transporter gene (GLYT1 and GLYT2; see Figure 3–5) that results in two transporters with different NH2 termini.[36] Differences in posttranslational modifications (e.g., glycosylation) of NETs expressed in CNS and periphery may also contribute regional variations in structure, as appears to be the case for CNS DATs.[37]

The powerful impact of exogenous transporter blockers raises the question as to what endogenous mechanisms ensure the proper level and localization of transporter expression and whether these mechanisms are compromised in individuals with brain disorders. Catecholamine biosynthesis and release in noradrenergic neurons is modulated by electrical activity and presynaptic receptor stimulation, raising the question as to whether NETs also possess the capacity for acute regulation. Disturbances in NET regulation might lead to inappropriate spatial and temporal actions of released NE, chronically altering the properties of target cells by feedback mechanisms of noradrenergic neurons themselves. Obeying Michaelis-Menten–type saturation kinetics, synaptic NET activity is expected to increase as the concentration of extracellular NE increases until NETs reach maximal velocity at saturating NE concentrations. The kinetic properties of NETs in native and transfected cells demonstrate a Michaelis constant (K_m) of approximately 0.5 μM,[9] indicating transporter saturation at low micromolar concentrations.

Synaptic concentrations of NE at peripheral synapses, which generally have wide synaptic spaces, may reach high micromolar levels, and even higher concentrations may be reached transiently in the more confined synaptic spaces in the CNS. At saturation, NETs must be either converted to a more active state or joined by other NETs previously held in intracellular compartments; otherwise, synaptic recovery will not keep pace with release, NE may spill over to extrasynaptic sites, and less NE will be recovered for repackaging. Alternatively, an alteration in the activity or number of NETs at noradrenergic synapses could be utilized to alter the level and lifetime of synaptic NE independent of control mechanisms regulating release.

Gillis[38] first demonstrated a rapid increase in the retention of NE by cat atrium after stimulation of the heart's sympathetic innervation. Rorie et al.,[39] utilizing electrical stimulation of adrenergic fibers in the dog saphenous vein and measurement of both NE overflow and metabolite production, detected enhanced NE transport paralleling the increase in impulse flow. Similar findings have been reported by Eisenhofer et al.,[40] using pharmacologic manipulation of peripheral sympathetic neurons in unanesthetized rabbits in vivo.

These studies indicate that NE uptake increases in parallel with increased firing rate and release. Whether the increased NET activity reflects the increased velocity of a fixed number of NETs expected as extracellular substrate levels rise or involves an alteration in NET density or turnover capacity is unclear. Sustained elevation of intracellular Ca^{2+} after repetitive terminal depolarization could provide an intrinsic signal to move transporters from subcellular sites to the terminal membrane.

NE release is altered by a number of endogenous agents that act on presynaptic terminals; likewise, acute hormonal regulation of NET activity has been reported. Beginning with the studies of Palaic and Khairallah,[41] multiple groups of investigators[42,43] have found NETs in CNS and peripheral nervous system to be sensitive to angiotensin II or III. Angiotensin peptides typically reduce transport and increase release, although acute stimulation of transport has been reported for rat brain stem neuronal cultures.[42] Interestingly, captopril, an angiotensin-converting enzyme inhibitor, has been reported to improve cardiac function in mild heart failure by increasing NE uptake.[44]

Atrial natriuretic peptide has been reported to acutely elevate NET activity in brain stem and adrenal slice preparations, reversing the inhibitory effects of angiotensin II and III at dosages subthreshold for its own response.[45,46] Insulin produces a rapid (within 1 minute), dose-dependent reduction in NE uptake in rat brain synaptosomes and PC12 cells.[47,48] In synaptosomes, insulin reduces NET maximal velocity (V_{max}) with no effect on K_m, consistent with either a reduction in surface pools of NETs or an alteration in capacity of a fixed number of transporters.[48] Insulin's effects are observed in PC12 cells despite reserpine depletion of vesicular catecholamine stores and are thus not likely to arise from alterations in DA or NE release.[47]

Although the intracellular effectors of these responses are not known, direct treatment of bovine adrenal chromaffin cells in vitro with agents that elevate or mimic intracellular cyclic adenosine monophosphate (cAMP) also alters NE uptake.[49] Clearly, the presence of serine/threonine phosphorylation sites on hNET (Figure 3–4) raises the question as to whether any of these effects are mediated by protein phosphorylation. Unfortunately, only a few studies report a kinetic basis for hormone-altered transport, and the presence of an NE release pathway, often modulated in parallel, confounds analysis. Use of purified NET proteins and heterologous expression systems should help clarify these effects and permit a direct evaluation of NET phosphorylation. The availability of NET-specific antibodies[21] should allow regulatory modifications of NET proteins, if they exist, to be identified biochemically in parallel with activity or hormone-induced changes in NET activity.

Hormones may also modulate NE uptake capacity by altering NET gene expression. For example, Figlewicz et al.[50] have shown that chronic intraventricular administration of insulin to rats in vivo significantly reduces steady-state levels of NET mRNA in the locus ceruleus. In vitro, chronic insulin treatment reduces NE uptake and levels of desmethylimipramine (DMI)-labeled NETs in PC12 cells.[47] Pertussis toxin treatment of chromaffin cells also appears to modulate NET expression in a delayed fashion that is most compatible with reduced gene expression.[49] These studies indicate that expression levels of NETs can be modulated by external hormonal influences, a finding of potential clinical relevance particularly where endocrine dysfunction is suspected. Indeed, sympathetic NETs have been reported to be upregulated in human diabetic cardiomyopathy[51] as well as in rodents, where insulin-secreting β cells have been destroyed with streptozocin.[52]

It has also been reported that NETs can be regulated in parallel with tissue NE concentrations; depletion of brain NE with reserpine causes a decrease in uptake sites, whereas conversely, increased synaptic NE availability due to monoamine oxidase inhibitors induces an increase in sites as labeled by [^{3}H]DMI.[53] An inability of the NET gene to respond to hormonal cues in CNS neurons could result in inappropriate levels of synaptic NE clearance and improper receptor stimulation, precipitating behavioral disturbances. Although this idea is clearly speculative, DNA and antibody probes are now available to examine hNET protein and gene regulation in the context of human neuropsychiatric disorders.

Serotonin Transporters: Platelet and Brain Targets for Antidepressants

Like the NETs, SERTs are believed to be responsible for removing neurotransmitter (5-HT) from synapses in the CNS and the enteric nervous system. In addition to neuronal expression, pharmacologically identical 5-HT uptake occurs in platelets, placenta, pulmonary endothelium, and mast cells.[54] In the lung, 5-HT transporters efficiently clear plasma-borne 5-HT and, with platelets, keep blood levels of free 5-HT low. Placental SERTs may protect the heavily vascularized tissue from premature constriction arising from maternal 5-HT.

Platelet SERTs have played an important role as a readily accessible peripheral index of CNS serotonergic gene expression, particularly in depression.[8,55] Extrapolation from data on platelet SERT to disturbances in CNS SERT levels or function assumes common SERTs in the CNS and periphery, relies on the specificity of SERT ligands, and presumes a parallel responsiveness of CNS and platelet SERT gene expression or protein modifications to genetic and environmental insults. SERT sites have been historically characterized through the binding of [^{3}H]imipramine, which bears a moderately higher affinity for human SERTs than for hNETs. Due to the high nonspecific binding of [^{3}H]imipramine in brain preparations, most recent investigations have adopted more selective ligands, such as [^{3}H]paroxetine, [^{3}H]citalopram, and [^{3}H]nitroquipazine. Autoradiographic studies using [^{3}H]citalopram and [^{3}H]imipramine[56] have identified the amygdala, thalamus, hypothalamus, CA3 region of the hippocampus, substantia nigra, locus ceruleus, and the raphe nuclei of the midbrain as the rat and human brain regions with the highest levels of uptake sites. Similarly, immunocytochemistry with SERT-specific antibodies demonstrates heavy innervation of these nuclei by SERT-immunoreactive fibers.[56a] Toxin-induced lesions of serotonergic neurons in rat brain reduce antidepressant binding sites in raphe projection areas, consistent with a presynaptic origin of SERTs in vivo.[56]

The cloning of the first brain SERT cDNA provides a clear example of the power inherent in a combination of molecular biological and anatomical techniques. Blakely et al.[12] synthesized degenerate oligonucleotide probes capable of recognizing both GAT1 and NET sequences and, presumably, many other transporter molecules. Use of these oligonucleotides in polymerase chain reaction amplifications of rat and human cDNAs resulted in the identification of a large number of novel transporter-like sequences. Each of these new partial clones could then be converted into RNA probes for in situ hybridization to identify sites of endogenous gene expression. One clone hybridized exclusively with neurons of the substantia nigra/ventral tegmental area, suggesting that it encoded a segment of the DAT. This suspicion was verified with the cloning of functional rodent DATs[10,11] by a similar approach, with DAT sequences matching that of our partial clone in overlapping regions. A second partial clone hybridized exclusively with mRNA expressed in brain stem and midbrain neurons of the serotonergic raphe complex (Figure 3–6)

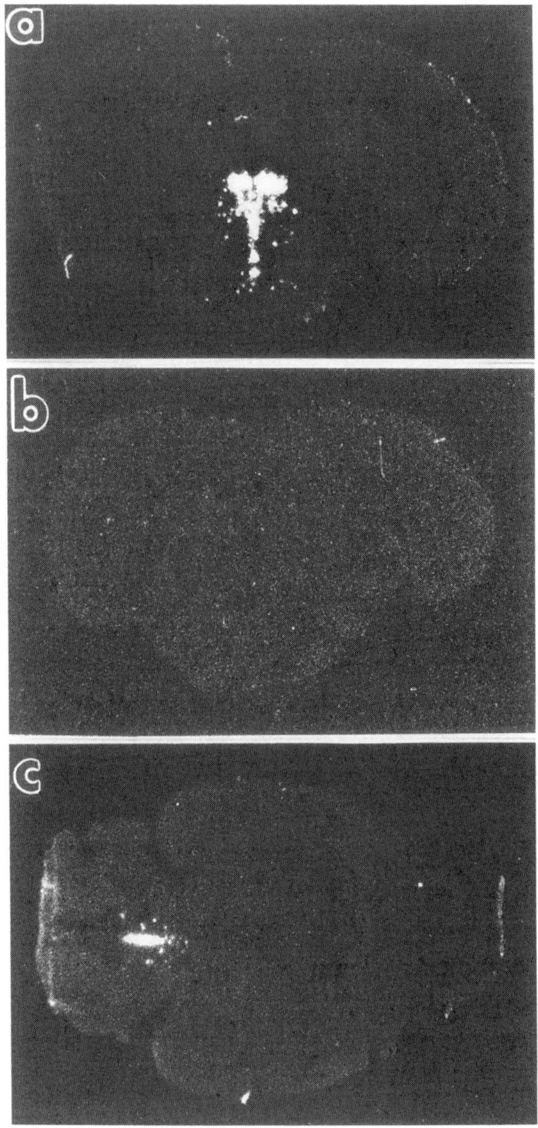

Figure 3–6. In situ hybridization of serotonin transporter (SERT) messenger ribonucleic acid expression in rat brain. *A:* Coronal section of rat brain at the level of the dorsal and median raphe nuclei probed with SERT antisense ribonucleotide probe. *B:* Same level as in panel A but probed with a control SERT sense ribonucleotide probe. *C:* Horizontal rat brain section incubated with SERT probes as in panel A depicting the anterior-posterior organization of brain stem raphe nuclei.

and in subsequent efforts led to the identification of a functional SERT cDNA.[12]

Similar efforts also resulted in the identification of a SERT cDNA from RBL cells, a cognate mast cell line.[13] Despite sequence differences in the original reports, both brain and RBL cDNAs are now known to encode a GAT/NET homologue of 630 amino acids with a predicted size of 68 kDa and greatest similarity to NET and DAT within the GAT/NET gene family (Figure 3–5). The size of the polypeptide predicted from SERT cDNAs is in good agreement with purification[57] and antibody[58] studies of endogenous SERTs that reveal 80-kDa proteins. Like the hNET, hydrophobicity analysis of SERTs suggests a structure of 12 TMDs (Figure 3–4), a large extracellular loop between TMD3 and TMD4 containing consensus sequences for asparagine-linked glycosylation, with both the NH2 and COOH termini located intracellularly. Like all members of the GAT/NET gene family, SERT has two cysteine residues located within this large extracellular loop, providing for potential intramolecular (or intermolecular) disulfide bridge formation.

The primary sequence identity of the rat SERT from brain and RBL cells provides strong support for identical peripheral and CNS transporters, which is particularly important in light of the frequent use of platelets as model 5-HT neurons for studies of human depression. Because these findings were from rodent studies, human SERTs could arise from distinct proteins. Due to limited availability of human midbrain tissue for mRNA isolation, we turned to a placental cDNA library to clone a functional human SERT cDNA, the sequence of which, like the rat transporter, predicts a 630–amino acid polypeptide with 92% sequence homology with the rat SERT. Recently, Lesch et al.[59] have amplified SERT cDNAs from human platelet and brain mRNAs, obtaining identical sequences to that reported for the placental carrier and validating cross-tissue inferences from rodent studies. Whereas a single RNA species hybridizes to SERT cDNA probes on Northern blots of rodent tissues, at least three SERT mRNAs are detected on blots of human tissues and cell lines.[60,61]

The significance of these multiple human SERT RNA bands is presently unknown, but like the hNET gene, the human SERT gene, located on chromosome 17q11.1–17q12, possesses multiple exons.[61] Whether the observed multiple SERT transcripts reflect noncoding SERT variants, as suggested for hNET, or encode novel coding region splice variants is under investigation. The human SERT genomic locus has been cloned and is presently being examined for evidence of structural variants.[62]

Mouse[63] and *Drosophila*[64] SERT cDNAs have recently been identified, offering prospects for studies of SERT genes in these developmentally and genetically well-characterized organisms. What would be the phenotype of a "SERT-less" animal or of one given to unregulated SERT overexpression? Would this be a lethal phenotype, or could the organism accommodate by altering release and receptor mechanisms, with a phenotype informative of human disorders? Can human SERT alleles be identified that result in altered but not absent SERTs? Might it be possible to engineer a mouse model of compromised SERT expression as an animal model of neuropsychiatric illness? With the cloning of SERT genes and gene products, it has become possible to test these and other questions.

Transfection of single rodent and human SERT cDNAs into mammalian cells confers high-affinity, Na^+- and Cl^--dependent 5-HT transport that is inhibited by the 5-HT-selective uptake antagonists paroxetine, fluoxetine, citalopram, and others. Consistent with in vivo studies, cocaine and the neurotoxic amphetamines also block 5-HT uptake in these transfected cells, whereas SERT only weakly recognizes NE and DA. Single SERT cDNAs confer 5-HT transport and antagonist sensitivity; however, like NET, it remains to be established whether protein monomers alone are competent for all functions or whether monomers are actually subunits of a larger, homomultimeric complex. Endogenous human SERTs, sized by gel filtration, are much larger than the size of a single SERT monomer;[65] however, the contribution of detergent and lipid to these estimates cannot be completely discounted.

As with NET, the structural features of SERT responsible for the many characteristics governing transport are still unidentified. The critical TMD1 aspartate residue required for NET and DAT function is conserved in SERTs. In preliminary studies, site-directed mutagenesis of this residue reveals a need for a charged amino acid at this position for high-affinity substrate and antagonist recognition.[57] Substitution with a smaller but equivalently charged glutamate residue results in an increased 5-HT K_m and reduced affinity for cocaine and imipramine.

We have also identified other residues that uniquely alter antidepressant recognition, leaving cocaine and 5-HT recognition unaffected. Could endogenous human genetic variations, mimicking those we have induced in SERT cDNAs in vitro, contribute to poor performance of some patients on antidepressant regimens? The cocaine analogue 3β-(4-[^{125}I]iodophenyl)tropane-2β-carboxylic acid methyl ester ([^{125}I]RTI-55) labels SERTs in platelet and transfected cell membranes in a largely Na^+-dependent manner.[66] In contrast to other ligands, including 5-HT, [^{125}I]RTI-55 binding is independent of Cl^- and displays a distinct pH dependence, suggesting that cocaine and its congeners interact with SERT in a manner distinct from substrates and antidepressants and perhaps reflecting contact sites outside of the substrate-binding pocket. Future studies should be capable of directly identifying exactly where and how molecularly distinct antidepressants and cocaine block SERTs from moving 5-HT across the plasma membrane.

Although further experiments based on GAT/NET sequence conservation are warranted, species differences in antagonist potency may help direct studies addressing ligand-binding sites. Binding sites for ligands on 5-HT receptors have recently been elucidated by tracing species-specific drug discrimination to the interactions of key residues on cloned proteins.[67] In this regard, tricyclic antidepressants show greater potency (approximately an order of magnitude) for endogenous and cloned human SERTs than for rodent homologues. Other ligands, including cocaine and heterocyclic antidepressants, fail to demonstrate this species bias. Sequence comparison between rat and human SERT identify only 16 amino acid differences within the putative TMDs, the regions we suspect may contribute to ligand binding and antagonist recognition. Human and rat SERT chimeras allow the contribution of structural differences to pharmacologic properties to be tracked,[67a] with divergent residues within TMD12 dictating human-specific tricyclic potency.

Like NE transport, SERT activity is dependent on extracellular

Na^+ and Cl^-, which is thought to represent the ion-cotransport function of these proteins (Figure 3–2). A model for this multisubstrate process has been proposed in which one Na^+, one Cl^-, and a single protonated 5-HT molecule bind to the transporter, forming a quaternary complex that then undergoes a conformational change to release 5-HT and the ions into the cytoplasm.[68] Intracellular K^+ then associates with the transporter and is released into the external medium, making the transporter available for another transport cycle. Na^+ and Cl^- ions not only contribute the driving force for the transport process but also increase the transporter's affinity for the substrate 5-HT.[69] Data from kinetic analyses of 5-HT uptake in humans and rats are consistent with a stoichiometry of one Na^+ ion for both binding and transport of one 5-HT molecule.[70,71]

A conflicting study reports that two Na^+ ions are required for 5-HT transport in membrane vesicles from mouse cerebral cortex.[72] Extracellular Cl^- sensitivity of 5-HT transport is also hyperbolic, suggesting a 1:1 Cl^- to 5-HT^+ stoichiometry.[69,70] Intracellular K^+, which can be substituted for experimentally by H^+, accelerates 5-HT influx, perhaps by facilitating a conformational change required for external exposure of unoccupied 5-HT binding sites.[68] Surprisingly, SERT and NET appear to differ on the role of intracellular K^+ in transport (Figure 3–2). Although intracellular K^+ stimulates both NET and SERT activity,[15,69] only SERT has been predicted to translocate K^+ as part of the transport cycle. Because the homologous transporter GAT1 appears to lack sensitivity for intracellular K^+ altogether,[68] structural variations among GAT/NET family members may reflect important mechanistic distinctions acquired in the evolutionary divergence from a common ancestral transporter.

The model for ion-coupled 5-HT uptake also predicts that the SERT transport cycle is electrically neutral; however, some studies show increased SERT activity by membrane hyperpolarization.[73] As previously noted for NET, flux studies provide insights into ionic requirements of transport but may be misleading if interpreted literally as indicative of cumulative charge movement. Indeed, Risso et al.,[74] using sensitive, whole-cell voltage clamp techniques, recently observed 5-HT–dependent transport currents in cells transfected with human SERT cDNA. These findings suggest that additional ions unaccounted for in radiotracer flux studies transit the membrane through SERT in each transport cycle.

Such studies also underscore the importance of identifying transporter cDNAs that are capable of expression in novel contexts. Without cloned transporters overexpressed in heterologous expression systems, the behavior of SERTs (or NETs) as a function of membrane potential would remain indirect, because the small size of neuronal NE and 5-HT terminals precludes direct recordings of transporter currents in situ. Kinetic analysis of SERT activity in platelet membrane vesicles indicates a flux rate for 5-HT of 8 per second, which is slightly greater than that found for NET.[75] To date, the speed of clearance of 5-HT from mammalian synapses by SERTs has not been determined, although elegant work on leech serotonergic synapses formed in vitro[76] provides convincing support for the ability of rapid SERT action to dictate the kinetics of postsynaptic 5-HT responses.

Analysis of the amino acid sequences of the cloned human SERT reveals six potential sites of phosphorylation by protein kinase A and protein kinase C;[61] five of these recognition sites also are conserved in rat SERT. Acute and chronic regulation of SERT by protein kinase C and cAMP have been reported, possibly involving one or more of these potential phosphorylation sites. Activation of protein kinase C with phorbol esters causes a dose-dependent inhibition of SERT activity in bovine pulmonary endothelial cells, platelets, and RBL cells that is blocked by protein kinase C inhibitors.[77–79] SERT activity can also be acutely upregulated by adenosine agonists.[78] After treatment with cholera toxin and forskolin, human placental choriocarcinoma (JAR) cells displayed enhanced SERT activity; however, the delayed nature of this effect compared with the rapid rise in intracellular cAMP levels suggested an effect on steady-state mRNA stability or gene transcription.[80] Consistent with this idea, increases in the levels of SERT mRNA have recently been found to coincide with increased cell surface density of SERTs after cholera toxin treatment.[81]

Although it is unclear whether the placental JAR model system faithfully depicts gene regulation exhibited in brain serotonergic neurons, SERTs, like NETs, clearly exhibit a capacity for chronic second-messenger–based regulation. These studies are important steps in understanding the susceptibility of SERT genes to aberrant modulation, because an inability to establish the appropriate level of transporter expression could render monoamine synapses susceptible to use-dependent disturbances in cell-cell information processing and ultimately lead to behavioral disturbances.

Blockade of 5-HT uptake is an immediate effect of the antidepressant 5-HT uptake inhibitors, whereas the therapeutic effects of these drugs are observed only after 2–3 weeks of treatment. Therefore, the adaptive responses in SERT expression associated with chronic antidepressant treatment are of much interest. Several studies in both humans and rats have shown decreases in [^{3}H]imipramine-binding sites after chronic administration of antidepressants; other reports have failed to corroborate these findings,[8] and the questionable specificity of [^{3}H]imipramine as a SERT ligand has limited the certainty of these findings. Long-term treatment with selective SERT antagonists, but not with monoamine oxidase inhibitors, induces a decrease in the steady-state levels of SERT mRNA,[82] which is consistent with differential effects of these agents on SERT sites measured with radioligand binding.[83]

Although still a matter of controversy, SERT activity and density have been reported to be significantly diminished in platelets from drug-free depressed patients and in human brains after suicide.[8] However, other studies have found no alterations in 5-HT transport in these conditions, possibly due to heterogeneous origins of such disorders. In addition to depression, SERT inhibitors have found clinical usefulness in the treatment of obsessive-compulsive disorder, panic disorder, eating disorders, alcoholism, and premenstrual syndrome,[84] although none of these disorders has yet been directly linked to altered SERT gene expression. The identification of the human genetic locus for SERT and the isolation of human SERT genomic clones should assist in evaluating possible hereditary SERT variations that might underlie a predisposition to psychiatric disease. In addition, greater inspection of SERT expression in humans in vivo should be feasible due to the combination of advanced brain imaging techniques with potent and selective SERT ligands.[85]

Conclusions

NETs and SERTs have long figured prominently in experimental and clinical neuroscience but also have long evaded a molecular description that could lead to new insights linking alterations in transporter structure and regulation to mental illness. The cloning of NET and SERT cDNAs has generated an initial set of transporter structural predictions and provided the necessary tools and expression systems to more directly examine transporter genes and proteins in vivo.

Are there additional transporters related to NETs and SERTs, perhaps specific for histamine or octopamine or as yet unknown chemical messengers? We still know little about how substrates bind to the transporters and are thereby shuttled across the plasma membrane, or about how antagonists bind. Could such information contribute to an understanding of inherited variations in transporter sequence? As integral membrane proteins, neurotransmitter transporters have a formal capacity to be regulated in situ not only by extracellular drugs but also by cytoplasmic effectors. Could knowledge of cellular regulatory mechanisms offer guidance in the design of novel therapeutics or direct a search for aberrant regulatory steps in disease?

The role of protein phosphorylation or other posttranslational modifications in regulating transporter function is only beginning to be evaluated. Antibodies specific for each carrier, suited to an estimation of transporter abundance, turnover, and modulation, are likely to be far superior to radioligands as informative protein probes. But are the most relevant regulatory events for transporters acutely or chronically maintained, or are both levels of regulation involved in setting the proper absorptive capacity of brain synapses? Hints of altered NET and SERT gene regulation after hormonal stimulation suggest significant gains to be acquired from systematic analysis of genomic regulatory elements that control transporter expression. Chronic or hereditary disturbances in regulatory cascades leading to altered transporter expression may underlie reports of transporter loss in psychiatric disease, particularly depression, a hypothesis that can now be approached directly. Thus, for many impressed with the abilities of transporter proteins to alter synaptic signaling and the behavioral effects of transporter-blocking drugs, a new era has dawned. The focus has shifted from the establishment of the primary structures of neurotransmitter transporters like NETs and SERTs to exploiting transporter nucleic acid and antibody probes for a determination of just how alterations in transporter behavior may contribute to altered human behavior.

References

1. Axelrod J: Noradrenaline: Fate and control of its biosynthesis. Science 173:598–173, 1971
2. Iversen LL: Uptake processes for biogenic amines, in Handbook of Psychopharmacology. Edited by Iversen LL, Iversen SD, Snyder SH. New York, Plenum, 1975, pp 381–442
3. Axelrod J, Whitby LG, Hertting G: Effect of psychotropic drugs on the uptake of H^3-norepinephrine uptake by tissues. Science 133:383–384, 1961
4. Furchgott RF, Kirkepar SM, Rieker M, et al: Actions and interactions of norepinephrine, tyramine, and cocaine on aortic strips of rabbit and left atria of guinea pig and cat. J Pharmacol Exp Ther 142:39–58, 1963
5. Ross SB, Renyi AL: Accumulation of tritiated 5-hydroxytryptamine in brain slices. Life Sci 6:1407–1415, 1967
6. Carpenter MB, Sutin J: Human Neuroanatomy. Baltimore, MD, Williams & Wilkins, 1983
7. Siever LJ: Role of noradrenergic mechanisms in the etiology of the affective disorders, in Psychopharmacology: The Third Generation of Progress. Edited by Meltzer HY. New York, Raven, 1987, pp 493–504
8. Meltzer HY, Lowy MT: The serotonin hypothesis of depression, in Psychopharmacology: The Third Generation of Progress. Edited by Meltzer HY. New York, Raven, 1987, pp 513–526
9. Pacholczyk T, Blakely RD, Amara SG: Expression cloning of a

cocaine and antidepressant-sensitive human noradrenaline transporter. Nature 350:350–354, 1991

10. Shimada S, Kitayama S, Lin C-L, et al: Cloning and expression of a cocaine-sensitive dopamine transporter complementary DNA. Science 254:576–578, 1991
11. Kilty J, Lorang D, Amara SG: Cloning and expression of a cocaine-sensitive rat dopamine transporter. Science 254:78–79, 1991
12. Blakely RD, Berson HE, Fremeau RTJ, et al: Cloning and expression of a functional serotonin transporter from rat brain. Nature 354:66–70, 1
13. Hoffman BJ, Mezey E, Brownstein MJ: Cloning of a serotonin transporter affected by antidepressants. Science 254:579–580, 1991
14. Amara SG, Kuhar MJ: Neurotransmitter transporters: recent progress. Annu Rev Neurosci 16:73–93, 1993
15. Harder R, Bönisch H: Effects of monovalent ions on the transport of noradrenaline across the plasma membrane of neuronal cells (PC-12 cells). J Neurochem 45:1154–1162, 1985
16. Ramamoorthy S, Prasad PD, Kulanthaivel P, et al: Expression of a cocaine-sensitive norepinephrine transporter in the human placental syncytiotrophoblast. Biochemistry 32:1346–1353, 1993
17. Howard BD, Cho AK, Zhang MB, et al: Covalent labeling of the cocaine-sensitive catecholamine transporter. J Neurosci Res 26:149–158, 1990
18. Richards ML, Sadee W: Human neuroblastoma cell lines as models of catechol uptake. Brain Res 384:132–137, 1986
19. Blakely RD, Clark J, Rudnick G, et al: Vaccinia-virus T7 polymerase transient expression system: evaluation for the expression cloning of plasma membrane transporters. Anal Biochem 194:302–308, 1991
20. Kyte J, Doolittle RF: A simple method for displaying the hydropathic character of a protein. J Mol Biol 157:105–132, 1982
21. Melikian HE, MacDonald JK, Gu H, et al: Human norepinephrine transporter: biosynthetic studies using a site-directed polyclonal antibody. J Biol Chem 269:12290–12297, 1994

22. Guastella J, Nelson N, Nelson H, et al: Cloning and expression of a rat brain GABA transporter. Science 249:1303–1306, 1990
23. Uhl GR, Kitayama S, Gregor P, et al: Neurotransmitter transporter family cDNAs in a rat midbrain library: "orphan transporters" suggest sizeable structural variations. Brain Res Mol Brain Res 16:353–359, 1992
24. Amara SG: A tale of two families. Nature 360:420–421, 1992
25. Blakely RD, Moore KR, Qian Y: Tails of serotonin and norepinephrine transporters: deletions and chimeras retain function, in Molecular Biology and Function of Carrier Proteins. Edited by Reuss L, Russell JM, Jennings ML. New York, Rockefeller University Press, 1993, pp 283–300
26. Bendahan A, Kanner BI: Identification of domains of a cloned rat brain GABA transporter which are not required for its functional expression. FEBS Lett 318:41–44, 1993
27. Mabjeesh NJ, Kanner BI: Neither amino nor carboxyl termini are required for function of the sodium- and chloride-coupled g-aminobutyric acid transporter from rat brain. J Biol Chem 267:2563–2568, 1992
28. Moore KM, Blakely RD: Restriction site independent formation and expression of chimeras from homologous genes. Biotechniques 17:130–136, 1994
29. Kitayama S, Shimada S, Xu H, et al: Dopamine transporter site-directed mutations differentially alter substrate transport and cocaine binding. Proc Natl Acad Sci U S A 89:7782–7785, 1992
30. Strader CD, Sigal IS, Dixon RAF: Structural basis of β-adrenergic receptor function. FASEB J 3:1825–1832, 1989
31. Blakely RD, Melikian HE, McDonald JK, et al: Characterization of the human norepinephrine transporter with an anti-peptide antibody. Society for Neuroscience Abstracts 19:206.2, 1993
32. Edwards RH: The transport of neurotransmitters into synaptic vesicles. Curr Opin Neurobiol 2:594–596, 1992
33. Borden LA, Smith KE, Hartig PR, et al: Molecular heterogeneity of the γ-aminobutyric acid (GABA) transport system. J Biol Chem 267:21098–21104, 1992
34. Brüss M, Kunz J, Lingen B, et al: Chromosomal mapping of the human gene for the tricyclic antidepressant-sensitive noradren-

aline transporter. Hum Genet 91:278–280, 1993
35. Pacholczyk T: Expression cloning of a cocaine- and antidepressant-sensitive human noradrenaline transporter (doctoral thesis). New Haven, CT, Yale University School of Medicine, 1992
36. Borowsky B, Mezey E, Hoffman BJ: Two glycine transporter variants with distinct localization in the CNS and peripheral tissues are encoded by a common gene. Neuron 10:851–863, 1993
37. Lew R, Patel A, Vaughn RZ, et al: Microheterogeneity of dopamine transporters in rat striatum and nucleus accumbens. Brain Res 584:266–271, 1992
38. Gillis CN: Increased retention of exogenous norepinephrine by cat atria after electrical stimulation of the cardioaccelerator nerves. Biochem Pharmacol 12:593–595, 1963
39. Rorie DK, Hunter LW, Tyce GM: Dihydroxyphenylglycol as an index of neuronal uptake in dog saphenous vein. Am J Physiol 257:H1945–H1951, 1989
40. Eisenhofer G, Cox HS, Esler MD: Parallel increases in noradrenaline reuptake and release into plasma during activation. Naunyn Schmiedebergs Arch Pharmacol 341:192–199, 1990
41. Palaic D, Khairallah PA: Effect of angiotensin on uptake and release of norepinephrine by brain. Biochem Pharmacol 16:2291–2298, 1967
42. Sumners C, Raizada MK: Angiotensin II stimulates norepinephrine uptake in hypothalamus-brain stem neuronal cultures. Am J Physiol 250:C236–C244, 1986
43. Vatta MS, Bianciotti LG, Locatelli AS, et al: Monophasic and biphasic effects of angiotensin II and III on norepinephrine uptake and release in rat adrenal medulla. Can J Physiol Pharmacol 70:821–825, 1992
44. Agostini D, Merlet P, Dubois-Rande JL, et al: Improvement of cardiac uptake 1 function induced by captopril in mild heart failure. Circulation 82:1516, 1990
45. Vatta MS, Bianciotti LG, Fernandez BE: Influence of atrial natriuretic factor on uptake, intracellular distribution, and release of norepinephrine in rat adrenal medulla. Can J Physiol Pharmacol 71:195–200, 1993
46. Vatta MS, Bianciotti LG, Papouchada ML, et al: Effects of atrial

natriuretic peptide and angiotensin III on the uptake and intracellular distribution of norepinephrine in medulla oblongata of the rat. Comp Biochem Physiol 99C:293–297, 1991

47. Figlewicz DP, Bentson K, Ocrant I: The effect of insulin on norepinephrine uptake by PC12 cells. Brain Res Bull 32:425–431, 1993
48. Raizada MK, Shemer J, Judkins JH, et al: Insulin receptors in the brain: structural and physiological characterization. Neurochem Res 13:297–303, 1988
49. Bunn SJ, O'Brien KJ, Boyd TL, et al: Pertussis toxin inhibits noradrenaline accumulation by bovine adrenal medullary chromaffin cells. Naunyn Schmiedebergs Arch Pharmacol 346:649–656, 1992
50. Figlewicz DP, Szot P, Israel PA, et al: Insulin reduces norepinephrine transporter mRNA in vivo in rat locus ceruleus. Brain Res 602:161–164, 1993
51. Ganguly PK, Dhalla KS, Innes IR, et al: Altered norepinephrine turnover and metabolism in diabetic cardiomyopathy. Circulation Res 59:684–693, 1986
52. Fushimi H, Inoue T, Kishino B, et al: Abnormalities in plasma catecholamine response and tissue catecholamine accumulation in streptozotocin diabetic rats: a possible role for diabetic autonomic neuropathy. Life Sci 35:1077–1081, 1984
53. Lee CM, Javitch JA, Snyder SH: Recognition sites for neurotransmitter uptake: regulation by neurotransmitter. Science 220:626–629, 1983
54. Fozard J (ed): Peripheral Actions of 5-Hydroxytryptamine. New York, Oxford University Press, 1989
55. Langer SZ, Galzin AM: Studies on the serotonin transporter in platelets. Experientia 44:127–130, 1988
56. Duncan GE, Little KY, Kirkman JA, et al: Autoradiographic characterization of imipramine and citalopram binding in rat and human brain: species differences and relationships to serotonin innervation patterns. Brain Res 591:181–197, 1992

56a. Qian Y, Melikian HE, Rye DB, et al: Identification and characterization of antidepressant-sensitive serotonin transporter proteins using site-spcific antibodies. J Neurosci 15:1261–1274, 1995

57. Launay JM, Geoffroy C, Mutel V, et al: One-step purification of the serotonin transporter located at the human platelet plasma membrane. J Biol Chem 267:11344–11351, 1992
58. Melikian H, Moore KR, Qian Y, et al: Structure and function of plasma membrane serotonin transporters. Society for Neuroscience Abstracts 19:206.1, 1993
59. Lesch KP, Wolozin BL, Murphy DL, et al: Primary structure of the human platelet serotonin uptake site: identity with the brain serotonin transporter. J Neurochem 60:2319–2322, 1993
60. Austin MC, Bradley CC, Mann JJ, et al: Expression of serotonin transporter mRNA in the human brain. J Neurochem 62:2362–2367, 1994
61. Ramamoorthy S, Bauman AL, Moore KR, et al: Antidepressant- and cocaine-sensitive human serotonin transporter: molecular cloning, expression, and chromosomal localization. Proc Natl Acad Sci U S A 90:2542–2546, 1993
62. Ramamoorthy S, Bradley CC, Bauman AL, et al: Human serotonin transporter: molecular cloning, genomic organization, and mRNA regulation. Society for Neuroscience Abstracts 19:7.5, 1993
63. Chang AS, Chang SM, Starnes DM, et al: Cloning and expression of the mouse serotonin transporter. Brain Res Mol Brain Res, in press
64. Demchyshyn LL, Pristupa ZB, Sugamori KS, et al: Cloning, expression, and localization of a chloride-facilitated, cocaine-sensitive serotonin transporter from *Drosophila melanogaster*. Proc Natl Acad Sci U S A 91:5158–5162, 1994
65. Ramamoorthy S, Leibach FH, Mahesh VB, et al: Partial purification and characterization of the human placental serotonin transporter. Placenta 14:449–461, 1993
66. Wall SC, Innis RB, Rudnick G. Binding of the cocaine analog 2β-carbomethoxy-3β-(4- [^{125}I]iodophenyl)tropane to serotonin and dopamine transporters: different ionic requirements for substrate and 2β-carbomethoxy-3β-(4-[^{125}I]iodophenyl)tropane binding. Mol Pharmacol 43:264–270, 1993
67. Oksenberg D, Marsters SA, O'Dowd BF, et al: A single amino-acid difference confers major pharmacological variation between human and rodent 5-HT1b receptors. Nature 360:161–163, 1992

67a. Barker EL, Kimmel HL, Blakely RD: Chimeric human and rat serotonin transporters reveal domains involved in recognition of transporter ligands. Mol Pharmacol 46:799–807, 1994
68. Kanner BI, Schuldiner S: Mechanism of transport and storage of neurotransmitters. CRC Critical Reviews in Biochemistry 22:1–38, 1987
69. Humphreys CJ, Beidler D, Rudnick G: Substrate and inhibitor binding and translocation by the platelet plasma membrane serotonin transporter. Biochem Soc Trans 19:95–98, 1991
70. Cool DR, Leibach FH, Ganapathy V: Modulation of serotonin uptake kinetics by ions and ion gradients in human placental brush-border membrane vesicles. Biochemistry 29:1818–1822, 1990
71. Mann CD, Hrdina PD: Sodium dependence of [^{3}H]paroxetine binding and 5-[^{3}H]hydroxytryptamine uptake in rat diencephalon. J Neurochem 59:1856–1861, 1992
72. O'Reilly CA, Reith ME: Uptake of serotonin into plasma membrane vesicles from mouse cerebral cortex. J Biol Chem 263:6115–6121, 1988
73. Kanner BI, Bendahan A: Transport of 5-hydroxytryptamine in membrane vesicles from rat basophilic leukemia cells. Biochim Biophys Acta 816:403–410, 1985
74. Risso S, DeFelice LJ, Duke BJ, et al: Electrogenic serotonin transport in stably transfected HEK-293 cells. Submitted for publication to Biophysical Society Abstract, 1993
75. Talvenheimo J, Nelson PJ, Rudnick G: Mechanism of imipramine inhibition of platelet 5-hydroxytryptamine transport. J Biol Chem 254:4631–4635, 1979
76. Bruns D, Engert F, Lux HD: A fast activating presynaptic reuptake current during serotonergic transmission in identified neurons of *hirudo*. Neuron 10:559–572, 1993
77. Anderson GM, Horne WC: Activators of protein kinase C decrease serotonin transport in human platelets. Biochim Biophys Acta 1137:331–337, 1992
78. Miller KJ, Hoffman BJ: Regulation of the serotonin transporter by PKC and adenosine receptor activation. Society for Neuroscience Abstracts 19:95.9, 1993

79. Myers CL, Lazo JS, Pitt BR: Translocation of protein kinase C is associated with inhibition of 5-HT uptake by cultured endothelial cells. Am J Physiol 257:L253–L258, 1989
80. Cool DR, Leibach FH, Bhalla VK, et al: Expression and cyclic AMP-dependent regulation of a high affinity serotonin transporter in the human placental choriocarcinoma cell line (JAR). J Biol Chem 266:15750–15757, 1991
81. Ramamoorthy S, Cool DR, Mahesh VB, et al: Regulation of the human serotonin transporter: cholera toxin-induced stimulation of serotonin uptake in human placental choriocarcinoma cells is accompanied by increased serotonin transporter mRNA levels and serotonin transporter-specific ligand binding. J Biol Chem 268:21626–21631, 1993
82. Lesch KP, Aulakh CS, Wolozin BL, et al: Regional brain expression of serotonin transporter mRNA and its regulation by reuptake inhibiting antidepressants. Brain Res Mol Brain Res 17:31–35, 1993
83. Graham D, Tahraoui L, Langer SZ: Effect of chronic treatment with selective monoamine oxidase inhibitors and specific 5-hydroxytryptamine uptake inhibitors on [^{3}H]paroxetine binding to cerebral cortical membranes of the rat. Neuropharmacology 26:1087–1092, 1987
84. Fuller RW, Wong DT: Serotonin uptake and serotonin uptake inhibition. Ann N Y Acad Sci 600:68–78, 1990
85. Laruelle M, Baldwin RM, Malison RT, et al: SPECT imaging of dopamine and serotonin transporters with b-CIT: pharmacological characterization of brain uptake in nonhuman primates. Synapse 13:295–309, 1993

CHAPTER

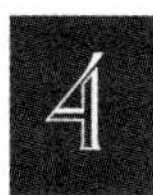

Excitotoxicity in the Development of Corticolimbic Alterations in Schizophrenic Brain

Francine M. Benes, M.D., Ph.D.

For more than a century, there have been discussions as to whether schizophrenia is a neurodegenerative disorder.[1–5] The idea that neuronal death might play a role in chronic psychosis has emanated from the clinical observation that many schizophrenic patients show a progressive deterioration in mental functioning in the early stages of their illness.

Over the past 20 years, studies in which computerized axial tomography and, later, magnetic resonance imaging have been used

---

I thank the staff in the Laboratory of Structural Neuroscience for the fortitude that has made these studies possible and Mrs. Patti Fitzpatrick for her expert assistance in preparing this manuscript.

have reported ventricular enlargement and cortical sulcal widening in schizophrenic subjects.[6] Although these changes are often thought to be the result of neuronal degeneration, findings of this type are nonspecific in nature and, in some instances, may even be reversible.[7] Over the past decade, however, histopathologic investigations have reported volume loss,[8,9] reduced numbers of neurons,[10–15] and altered arrangements of neurons[16–18] in several corticolimbic brain regions of subjects with schizophrenia. It is noteworthy that no studies in which quantitative techniques have been used have found evidence of gliosis,[10,13,19,20] and the absence of increased numbers of astroglial cells has been used to argue against a typical adult degenerative process, like that seen in Alzheimer's disease or Huntington's chorea, accounting for the reduced neuronal numbers observed in patients with schizophrenia.[7]

Although some negative results have been reported,[21–23] the majority of postmortem studies are providing support for the viewpoint that a nondegenerative process may cause a loss of neurons in the corticolimbic system of some individuals with schizophrenia.

The challenge now being faced by investigators who study schizophrenia is to define the mechanism(s) that may account for the loss of neurons observed in some subjects with schizophrenia. Alternative processes that have been proposed include a genetically determined cytoarchitectural variant,[10,24] a prenatal or perinatal disturbance of normal ontogeny,[10,16,17,25,26] and an excitotoxic injury.[27,28] In the following discussion, the possibility that excitotoxicity might account for the reduction in the numbers of neurons observed in postmortem brains from schizophrenic subjects is considered. Toward this end, evidence for an increase in glutamatergic transmission occurring alone or in combination with diminished γ-aminobutyric acid (GABA)-ergic activity is discussed with respect to the potential vulnerability of schizophrenic individuals to excitotoxic injury. The possibility that there may be a neurodevelopmental time frame for the induction of such vulnerability in individuals "at risk" for schizophrenia is also discussed. Finally, a working system model is used to consider how an excitotoxic injury might arise through the interaction of key corticolimbic brain regions, each with discrete alterations of intrinsic neural circuits.

Evidence for Glutamatergic Dysfunction in Subjects With Schizophrenia

Anatomical Findings

In an attempt to gain some insight into how the reduced number of neurons may have been induced in schizophrenic subjects, a novel stereomorphometric analysis was developed and applied to this problem.[18] The data obtained with this method suggested that schizophrenic individuals might have neuronal clusters in layer II of the anterior cingulate region that are smaller in size and separated by wider distances.[18] On the basis of the known organization of the cortex,[29] it was postulated that the cell-free zones lying between the neuronal clusters might contain increased numbers of associative afferent axons projecting to layer I.[18]

To test this hypothesis, polyclonal antibodies against phosphorylated epitopes of the NFP200K cytoskeletal subunit were used to visualize axons in human postmortem cortex.[30] When this method was blindly applied to a cohort of control subjects and schizophrenic patients, an increased density of vertical, but not of horizontal, axons was observed in superficial laminae of the cingulate region in the patient group.[31] A subsequent replicative study indicated that the increased density of vertical axons was present in the anterior cingulate, but not the prefrontal, cortex of schizophrenic subjects.[32] Because the immunolocalization of cytoskeletal protein allows visualization of many different types of axons, regardless of their region of origin or their neurotransmitter system, it was necessary to find an alternative strategy that could be used to localize associative fibers in the upper layers of the cingulate cortex so that this potentially important finding could be replicated and extended.

Suspecting that the vertical fibers that were increased in number in schizophrenic patients might be incoming associative axons, I employed monoclonal antibodies against glutamate because such inputs are believed to use this amino acid as a transmitter.[33] The method developed yielded an extensive visualization of vertical fibers in superficial layers of human cortex[34] (Figure 4–1). When this method was blindly applied to a cohort of postmortem tissues, an increased density of glutamate-immunoreactive vertical fibers with a small caliber similar to that of cortical axons was found in layer II and upper portions of layer IIIa of the anterior cingulate region of schizophrenic subjects (Figure 4–2).

These data were not only a replication of earlier findings of the previously mentioned studies in which the immunolocalization of NFP200K subunits was used but also provided support for the idea that the vertical fibers that are increased in schizophrenic subjects might employ glutamate as a neurotransmitter. This region, however, also receives glutamatergic afferent inputs to superficial laminae from the amygdala[35] and the thalamus.[36] In the case of the amygdala, a reduced volume of this region has been observed in schizophrenic subjects,[8] although quantitative estimates of neuronal numbers have not yet been performed. With regard to the thalamus, no difference in the number of neurons has been observed in anterior nuclei, but a substantial reduction in neuronal density has been observed in the dorsomedial nucleus.[15,37] Although it seems less likely that the amygdala and thalamus are the sources for the increased vertical fibers in superficial layers of the anterior cingulate cortex, these regions cannot yet be definitively excluded as candidate regions.

Another possible source of these fibers are pyramidal neurons in deeper laminae of the cingulate region. For example, pyramidal neurons in layer V[38] and Martinotti cells found in both layers V and VI[39] project axons in a vertical direction toward layer I and could contribute to the increased fibers observed in layer II of schizophrenic subjects. Although the neurotransmitter employed by Martinotti cells is not yet known, that for pyramidal neurons is thought to be glutamate.[33,40] Nevertheless, pyramidal neurons in layer V of the anterior cingulate region itself do not appear to be a likely source of vertical axons increased in layer II of schizophrenic subjects, because two previous postmortem analyses revealed a reduction in the density of pyramidal cells in layer V in schizophrenic subjects.[10,20] In the prefrontal area, however, an unexpected increase in the density of pyramidal neurons has been observed.[20] Although most associative

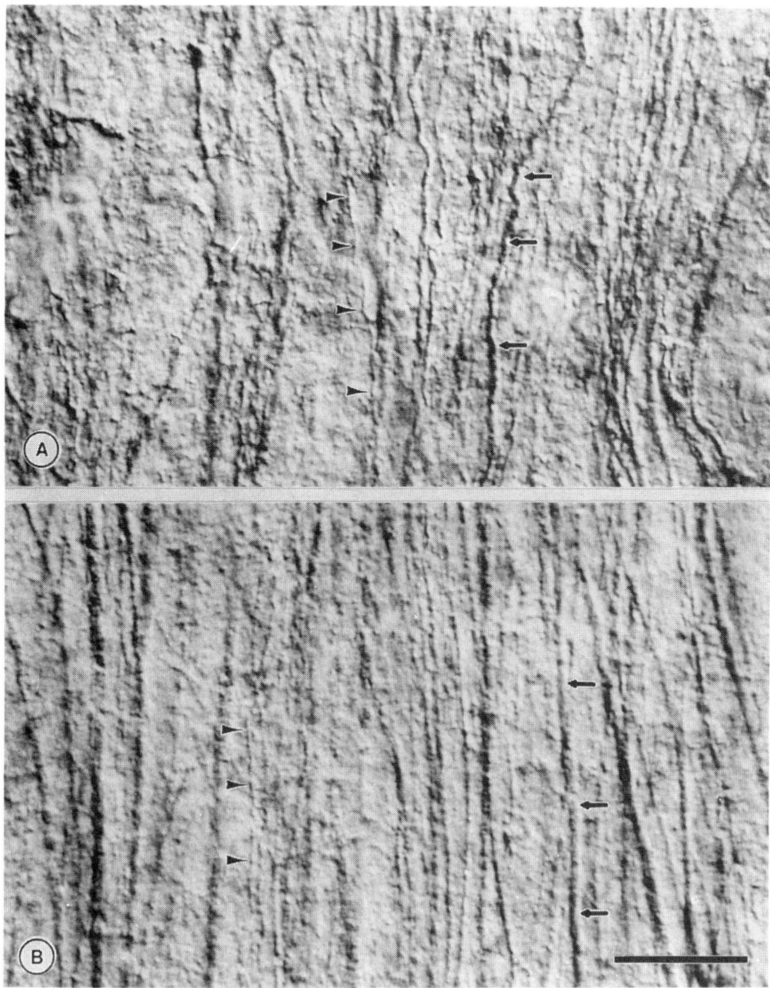

Figure 4–1. Light photomicrograph of glutamate-immunostained vertical fibers in layer II and upper portions of layer III in the anterior cingulate cortex of a control *(A)* and schizophrenic *(B)* subject. Both photomicrographs show abundant numbers of vertical processes with either a large *(arrows)* or small *(arrow heads)* caliber that probably represent apical dendrites of pyramidal neurons and incoming afferent axons, respectively. There appears to be an increased density of fibers, particularly those with a small caliber, in the anterior cingulate region of the schizophrenic subject.

Source. Reprinted from *Cerebral Cortex* (2:503–512, 1992) with permission of Oxford Press.

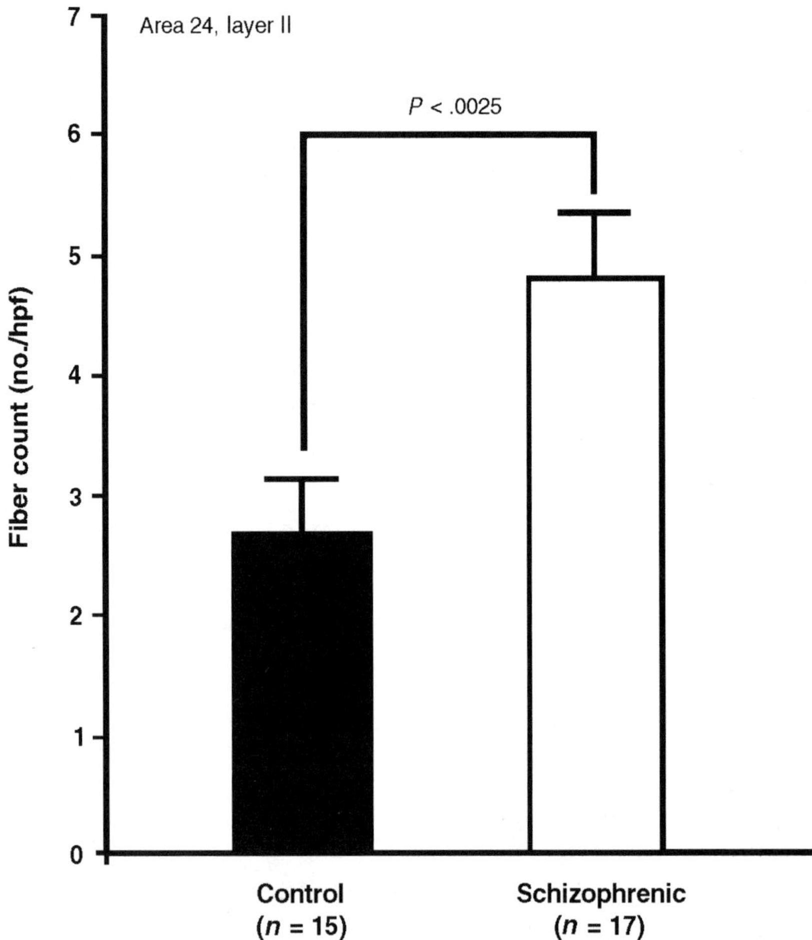

Figure 4–2. Average density (number per high-power field [hpf]) of glutamate-immunoreactive vertical fibers with a small caliber in anterior cingulate cortex (area 24) in control (n = 15) and schizophrenic (n = 17) subjects. The data are expressed as the "mean of means" for individual cases in the respective groups ± the standard error of the mean. There is a large increase (78%) in the density of glutamate-containing vertical axons in the schizophrenic subjects, which is quite significant when compared with similar data for the control group. Similar data for large-caliber vertical processes visualized in the same preparations showed only a slight increase in the schizophrenic subjects.
Source. Reprinted from *Cerebral Cortex* (2:503–512, 1992) with permission of Oxford Press.

fibers are thought to originate from pyramidal neurons in superficial layers of the cortex,[41] those that course in a rostral-to-caudal direction seem to arise from layer V,[42] making the prefrontal area a possible site of origin of the glutamate-containing vertical axons in superficial laminae of the cingulate region.[34]

It has also been suggested that the increased vertical fibers in the anterior cingulate region of schizophrenic subjects might have been derived from a process of anomalous reinnervation giving rise to abnormal connectivity in schizophrenic brain.[43] The decreased numbers of neurons observed in corticolimbic regions of schizophrenic subjects are not accompanied by volume loss and gliosis, making it probable that there is an increased amount of neuropil relative to neuronal cell bodies in patients with this disorder. Such an expansion of neuropil could theoretically arise from an exuberant sprouting of axon collaterals following an insult to the brain; however, such axonal processes would probably have the appearance of terminal arborizations, rather than straight vertical shafts.

Receptor Binding Studies

It is useful to consider whether there are neurochemical findings in support of the idea that a dysfunction of glutamatergic transmission may occur in individuals with schizophrenia. A reduction in the binding of [^{3}H]kainate and [^{3}H]glutamate has been observed in the hippocampal formation of schizophrenic subjects,[44] particularly in the area dentata, CA4, CA3, CA1, and the parahippocampal gyrus.[45] No change in non-*N*-methyl-D-aspartate (NMDA)-sensitive glutamate receptor binding was observed in the latter study. Consistent with these findings, a reduction in the amount of messenger RNA (mRNA) transcripts for an NMDA receptor gene has also been observed in the hippocampus of schizophrenic subjects, where sector CA3 showed the largest difference, but pronounced changes were also detected in the subiculum and CA1 subfield.[46] These latter findings are consistent with the idea that an increase of glutamatergic activity may be causing a compensatory downregulation of kainate-sensitive receptor binding in postsynaptic cells of the hippocampus.

It is noteworthy that an increase, rather than a decrease, of $[^3H]$kainate binding has been observed in the orbitofrontal cortex,[47] medial frontal cortex, and frontal eye field[48,49] of schizophrenic subjects. Although these findings might suggest that a compensatory increase of receptor binding has occurred in response to diminished glutamatergic activity, the concomitant finding of increased $[^3H]$aspartate receptor binding[47] has led to the suggestion that there may be an increase of glutamatergic innervation in the frontal cortex of individuals with schizophrenia.

An increase of phencyclidine (PCP) receptor binding activity has also been found in the frontal cortex,[50,51] entorhinal region, hippocampal formation, and putamen[50] of schizophrenic subjects. Because the PCP site noncompetitively blocks the activity of the NMDA receptor complex,[52] the increase of this binding activity could theoretically represent either an overall increase of NMDA-sensitive glutamate binding or a compensatory response of postsynaptic cells to limit the effect of glutamate on the NMDA receptor complex. Unfortunately, little is known about the regulation of PCP binding activity in relation to the NMDA receptor complex.

Taking together both the anatomical and receptor binding findings described here, the evidence concerning the glutamate system in individuals with schizophrenia cannot be interpreted straightforwardly. Several findings, including increased pyramidal neuron density in layer V of the prefrontal area, increased glutamate-containing afferent fibers in superficial laminae of the anterior cingulate region, and an increase of both kainate and aspartate binding in orbitofrontal cortex, suggest that excessive glutamatergic transmission may occur in the cortex. An apparent inconsistency emerges when similar reports for the hippocampal formation are taken into account. For example, the finding of decreased kainate receptor binding activity seems to be opposite that observed in the cortex, where it is increased. It is important to emphasize, however, that the interpretation of increased kainate binding in the cortex, although perhaps suggesting a decrease of glutamate release by presynaptic terminals, has been interpreted as representing an increase because of the associated increase of aspartate binding that is believed to be a marker for the presynaptic glutamate uptake site.[47] In contrast to the increased [^{3}H]kainate binding in the cortex, the decreased non-NMDA glutamate receptor binding in the hippocampus of schizophrenic subjects may also be consistent with an overall increase of glutamate release, resulting in a compensatory downregulation of receptor activity in the setting of an increased action of glutamate on postsynaptic receptors.

An alternative interpretation of decreased [^{3}H]kainate binding is that this has caused an excitotoxic dropout of pyramidal neurons on which the kainate receptors are found. Both of these mechanisms imply that there is a paradoxical increase of glutamatergic activity generated either directly within the hippocampus itself or indirectly by other regions that project to the hippocampal formation. Because both the frontal cortex[53] and anterior cingulate region[54,55] send abundant projections to the hippocampal formation, the latter possibility seems plausible, particularly because the evidence discussed here is consistent with an increase of outgoing glutamatergic activity from the cortex, giving rise to a reduced number of pyramidal neurons in the hippocampus.[8,12,14,20] The frontal cortex projects primarily to the subiculum and sector CA1,[53] whereas the afferents from the anterior cingulate region terminate primarily in the presubiculum,[54,55] and both inputs are probably mediated by NMDA-sensitive glutamate receptors.[40] Because changes in kainate-sensitive glutamate binding activity have been found to be most striking in the hilum and sector CA3, the most parsimonious explanation for their reduction in schizophrenic subjects would be a compensatory downregulation of activity occurring secondarily to an increase of glutamatergic activity projected to the presubiculum from the anterior cingulate region and to the subiculum and sector CA1 from the frontal cortex.

Thus, the evidence to date is consistent with a general model in which increased glutamatergic activity arises primarily in the cortex and is transmitted secondarily to the hippocampus. This perspective, however, does not necessarily provide an explanation for the increased PCP binding activity observed in both cortex and hippocampus. It is not clear how this receptor activity may reflect changes in glutamatergic activity processed through the NMDA receptor, although it is possible that dissociative anesthetic binding directly reflects NMDA-sensitive glutamate binding in such a fashion that if one is increased, then the other must be as well. An alternative possibility that must be considered is that the two binding sites are differentially regulated in such a way that postsynaptic neurons use PCP binding activity to offset increased excitatory activity mediated through the NMDA site. In other words, an increase of glutamatergic activity mediated by the NMDA receptor might stimulate a postsynaptic cell to alter the expression of genes related to the PCP receptor, so that the excitatory activity mediated through the NMDA receptor is diminished.

Evidence for GABAergic Dysfunction in Subjects With Schizophrenia

The idea that schizophrenia might involve a defect in GABA neurotransmission was first suggested by Roberts,[56] and it has been postulated that a reduction in inhibitory modulation could contribute to the loss of central filtering[57] and the so-called "over-inclusiveness" of cognitive processing seen in individuals with schizophrenia.[58,59] Consistent with this hypothesis, several studies have now reported alterations of the GABA system in postmortem brains of subjects with schizophrenia. For example, there is a lower concentration of GABA in the thalamus and nucleus accumbens of individuals with schizophrenia.[60] Moreover, a decrease in the specific activity of glutamate decarboxylase (GAD), the enzyme that synthesizes GABA, has been found in the frontal region,[61] whereas a reduction in the reuptake mechanism of GABA has been observed in both the frontal cortex[62] and the hippocampal formation[63] of patients with schizophrenia.

An increase of GABA receptor binding activity has been reported by two different groups. In one study, a classic "grind and bind" assay demonstrated an increase of [^{3}H]muscimol binding in the frontal cortex,[64] although the magnitude of the changes reported in this study was small. In a more recent microscopic study, the finding of a preferential reduction in the density of nonpyramidal neurons in the anterior cingulate and prefrontal cortices of schizophrenic subjects suggested that there might be an upregulation of $GABA_A$ receptors in these regions.[20] In a subsequent investigation, a high-resolution technique was employed to analyze receptor binding activity on individual neuronal cell bodies.[64] With this approach, it was possible to demonstrate a very marked (84% and 74%, respectively) increase of bicuculline-sensitive $[^3H]$muscimol binding to the $GABA_A$ receptor on pyramidal neuron cell bodies in layers II and III of the anterior cingulate region of schizophrenic subjects,[27] whereas neurons in deeper laminae of this region did not show such changes (Figure 4–3).

Even more recently, preliminary evidence has revealed a marked upregulation of $GABA_A$ receptor binding activity in the prefrontal cortex, and once again the changes were most marked on pyramidal neurons in layers II and III of schizophrenic subjects. Only one study to date has assessed binding to the benzodiazepine site where the activity was decreased;[66] however, it is not clear whether the benzodiazepine site may also show a differential regulation with respect to the $GABA_A$ receptor complex.[67]

Relationship of Ontogeny to Excitotoxicity

Significance of Layer II Findings for Schizophrenia

The marked increase in $GABA_A$ receptor binding detected on pyramidal neurons in layers II and III of the anterior cingulate and prefrontal cortices of schizophrenic subjects were quite striking,[27] particularly because other noteworthy changes have also been reported in superficial laminae of schizophrenic subjects.[32] For example, altered neuronal clusters have been found in layer II of the anterior cingulate region[18] and in the pre-alpha layer of the entorhinal area,[17] along with a decreased density of interneurons[20] and an increased density of vertical axons,[31,34] have all suggested that a disturbance in cortical ontogenesis may be related to the alterations in layer II of schizophrenic subjects.[17,20,27,28]

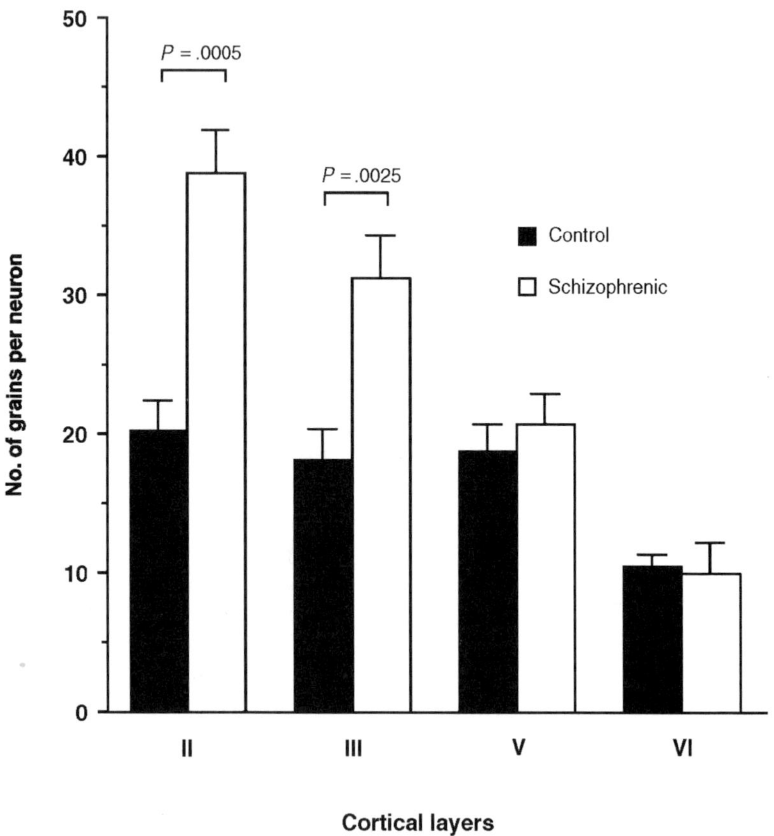

Figure 4–3. Specific γ-aminobutyric acid-A ($GABA_A$) receptor binding activity on individual neuronal cell bodies of anterior cingulate cortex from control (n = 8) and schizophrenic (n = 6) subjects. The data for neurons in layers II, III, V, and VI are indicated separately. Specific $GABA_A$ receptor binding activity was obtained by subtracting the number of grains present in cells incubated with [^{3}H]muscimol plus bicuculline from the number of grains present in cells incubated with [^{3}H]muscimol alone. A mean and standard error of the mean for total and inhibited binding were obtained separately for individual cases within the respective control and schizophrenic groups, and the specific binding activity for each case was determined by subtracting the inhibited grain count from the total grain count. The group means were then obtained by averaging the means for the individual cases. The numbers above the horizontal brackets indicate the level of significance for the differences between the two groups.
Source. From Benes et al., *Journal of Neuroscience* (12:924–929, 1992), with the permission of the Society for Neuroscience.

During cortical development, neurons are generated near the ventricular surface and migrate in an "inside-out" fashion so that those destined for deeper laminae arrive earlier and those destined for superficial laminae arrive later.[68,69] Layer II is the last cell-rich lamina to receive its full contingent of neurons.[69,70] The maturation of cortical neurons also follows a similar deep-to-superficial progression. At the time of birth in humans, pyramidal neurons in deeper laminae are quite mature, those in layer II are still actively developing, and inhibitory basket cells have only begun to differentiate.[71] It has been suggested that the relative immaturity of basket cells during the perinatal period of humans might render them more vulnerable to the effects of obstetrical complications,[32] which seem to occur with a particularly high frequency in subjects with schizophrenia.[72,73] Interestingly, exposure of young animals to high levels of adrenal steroid is associated with a reduction in brain weight.[74] Although the adrenal-pituitary axis is immature during the perinatal period,[75] circulating glucocorticoid hormone of maternal origin could impart a direct neurotoxic effect on the fetal brain. It has been reported that glucocorticoids can potentiate the excitotoxic effect of kainate,[76] although excitotoxicity in immature rats appears to be mediated through NMDA-sensitive glutamate receptors.[77,78] If a stress-induced mechanism does play a role in causing an injury in the neonatal brain, different subpopulations of neurons might theoretically show characteristic periods of peak vulnerability to excitotoxicity.[79] GABAergic neurons of the striatum[80] and hippocampus[81] are quite sensitive to excitotoxic injury during adulthood, and it is conceivable that, when inhibitory neurons of the cortex are immature, they may be particularly sensitive to excitotoxicity and/or neurotoxic levels of maternal glucocorticoid.

Pre- and Postnatal Development of Glutamatergic Transmission

There is a broad period of time during which associative glutamatergic systems of the human brain undergo developmental changes, although the particular intervals during which different pathways mature are often quite different. For example, corticocortical projections of the visual system in rat brain contain mature levels of glutamate at an earlier point than the corticostriatal projections from visual cortex.[82] At approximately 2 days before birth, the glutamate reuptake mechanism is 70% lower than what it will be by the end of the first 2 postnatal weeks; however, in the visual system,[83] glutamate uptake attains adult levels in the cortex earlier (day 15) than in the lateral geniculate nucleus (day 20).

High-affinity glutamate binding activity also shows important postnatal changes. Between postnatal days 10–15, glutamate receptor binding activity increases by 30%, to a level that is 10-fold higher than that encountered in adult animals.[84] After the second postnatal week, the amount of binding activity undergoes a gradual decline through day 25,[84] which marks the beginning of the weanling period. When rats are monocularly deprived of visual input, glutamate receptor binding is reduced in the lateral geniculate nucleus, where it remains low through adulthood;[84] however, in the visual cortex, activity-dependent changes of this type have not been observed.[84]

In the hippocampal formation, glutamate receptor binding activity also shows marked postnatal changes. Unlike the visual system, where there is normal binding activity between days 15 and 25 (see preceding discussion), the hippocampus shows a progressive increase of binding through postnatal day 23.[85] It has been postulated that this increase of glutamate receptor activity may be related to the occurrence of long-term potentiation during learning and memory in the hippocampus.[85]

It has long been suspected that myelination of associative cortical regions of human brain may continue well into adulthood,[86] and some investigators have speculated that changes of this type may continue even as late as the third or fourth decades of life.[87] Although empirical evidence for this concept had been lacking, two studies[88,89] have demonstrated that active myelination occurs in the superior medullary lamina, which lies along the surface of the parahippocampal gyrus during the second decade of life, when symptoms of schizophrenia typically begin to appear.[1] The superior medullary lamina includes fibers of the perforant pathway in more medial locations along the surface of the subiculum, whereas distal portions of the cingulum bundle are probably located in a more lateral position along the surface of the presubiculum. Because the changes in myelination that occur during adolescence are found primarily along the surface of the presubiculum,[89] the fibers showing these changes may have their origin in the cingulate gyrus[54,55] and, as such, are likely to be associative afferents that exert excitatory effects on the hippocampal formation.

Ontogenesis of Glutamatergic Transmission and Its Role in Excitotoxicity

It is intriguing to consider whether changes in myelination that would increase the conduction velocity along cingulum bundle fibers projecting to the presubiculum might influence the activity glutamatergic elements within the hippocampal formation and, if so, whether such changes might conceivably play a role in triggering the onset of schizophrenia during adolescence and early adulthood. Because such associative projections are believed to employ glutamate as a neurotransmitter,[33] increased activity flowing along such projections could potentially give rise to an excitotoxic injury. As noted above, data from rodent studies suggest that glutamate receptor binding activity may continue to increase in the hippocampal formation until the weanling period, which is equivalent to adolescence in humans. It seems plausible that a change in the myelination of associative inputs to the hippocampal formation during adolescence might increase glutamatergic effects on postsynaptic receptor binding activity. In individuals "at risk" for schizophrenia, glutamatergic transmission during adolescence could induce either a compensatory downregulation of glutamate receptor binding activity or a glutamate-mediated excitotoxic injury within the hippocampal formation of subjects with schizophrenia (see preceding discussion). Such an effect could help to explain the loss of volume[8,90,91] and neuronal loss[11,12,14] noted in the hippocampal formation of schizophrenic subjects.

It is important to consider whether such a pathophysiologic effect involving cortical projections to the subiculum, presubiculum, and sector CA1 would be confined only to neurons in those sectors directly receiving cortical inputs, or whether perhaps such changes could also be transmitted secondarily to neurons in other portions of the hippocampus, such as sector CA3, that lie downstream from them. It seems reasonable to assume that heightened glutamatergic activity in these relay areas of the hippocampal complex might also promote a downregulation of kainate-sensitive glutamate receptor binding in sector CA3 of subjects with schizophrenia.[44,45,46]

A Systems Level Approach to Modeling for Schizophrenia

On the basis of recent postmortem studies of schizophrenia, it is becoming increasingly apparent that this disorder may involve not only one brain region but rather several key components of the corticolimbic system. These regions include (but are probably not restricted to) the anterior cingulate cortex, the prefrontal region, the entorhinal area, and the hippocampal formation. Together, these regions are part of an extensively interconnected associational network involved in complex motivational, affective, and attentional behaviors that are disturbed in individuals with schizophrenia.[32] It seems appropriate to consider whether the various changes detected in individual regions could potentially influence the integration of activity within the corticolimbic system.

As indicated in Figure 4–4, a loss of GABAergic interneurons in the anterior cingulate cortex of schizophrenic subjects has been suggested by two separate findings: a decreased density of interneurons[20] and an increase of $GABA_A$ receptor binding activity.[27] Because both of these findings were most consistently and strikingly observed in layer II of schizophrenic subjects, the putative loss of GABAergic neurons has been postulated to occur during early brain development.[20,27,28,32] This proposed reduction of GABAergic activity in superficial laminae of the anterior cingulate, prefrontal, and possibly other cortical regions of schizophrenic subjects might contribute to the occurrence of abnormal amounts of excitatory activity in individuals with schizophrenia. Because there are extensive interconnections between neurons of layers II and V via collateral branches of pyramidal cell axons,[38] a decrease of inhibitory activity in layer II would probably result in an overall increase of excitatory downflow to layer V. Because pyramidal neurons of layer V in the anterior cingulate and those from layer V of the prefrontal area project to the hippocampal formation, an increase of excitatory outflow to presubiculum, subiculum, and subfield CA1 would be enhanced by the diminished inhibitory activity that is thought to occur in superficial cortical laminae of subjects with schizophrenia.

As noted previously, the density of pyramidal neurons is increased in layer V of the prefrontal area and decreased in the anterior cingulate in individuals with schizophrenia.[20] These findings suggest that the prefrontal area might play a more potent role in the occurrence of excitotoxicity in the hippocampal formation of subjects with schizophrenia. Unlike those in the prefrontal cortex, pyramidal neurons in layer V of the cingulate region seem to be decreased in density. Nevertheless, this region appears to receive a substantial increase in the number of glutamatergic projections to layer I, where important excitatory effects can be exerted directly on apical dendrites of pyramidal neurons—not only those in layers II and III, but also those in layer V. Thus, an increased excitatory inflow, together with reduced intrinsic inhibition in superficial layers, would promote increased excitatory activity in layers II and III, as well as in layer V. An increased excitatory outflow to the hippocampal formation of schizophrenic subjects could originate from both the anterior cingulate and the prefrontal cortices and result in either a compensatory downregulation of glutamate receptor binding activity or an outright loss of such receptors due to excitotoxic neuronal cell death.

In this setting, the proposed increase of glutamatergic activity into the hippocampal formation could be indirectly reflected back to the anterior cingulate and prefrontal cortices from the subiculum and subfield CA1. Could such a reverberation of excitatory activity be a proximate cause of injury to GABAergic interneurons in superficial layers of these two cortical regions? If this were the case, GABAergic activity in the cortex of schizophrenic subjects could be

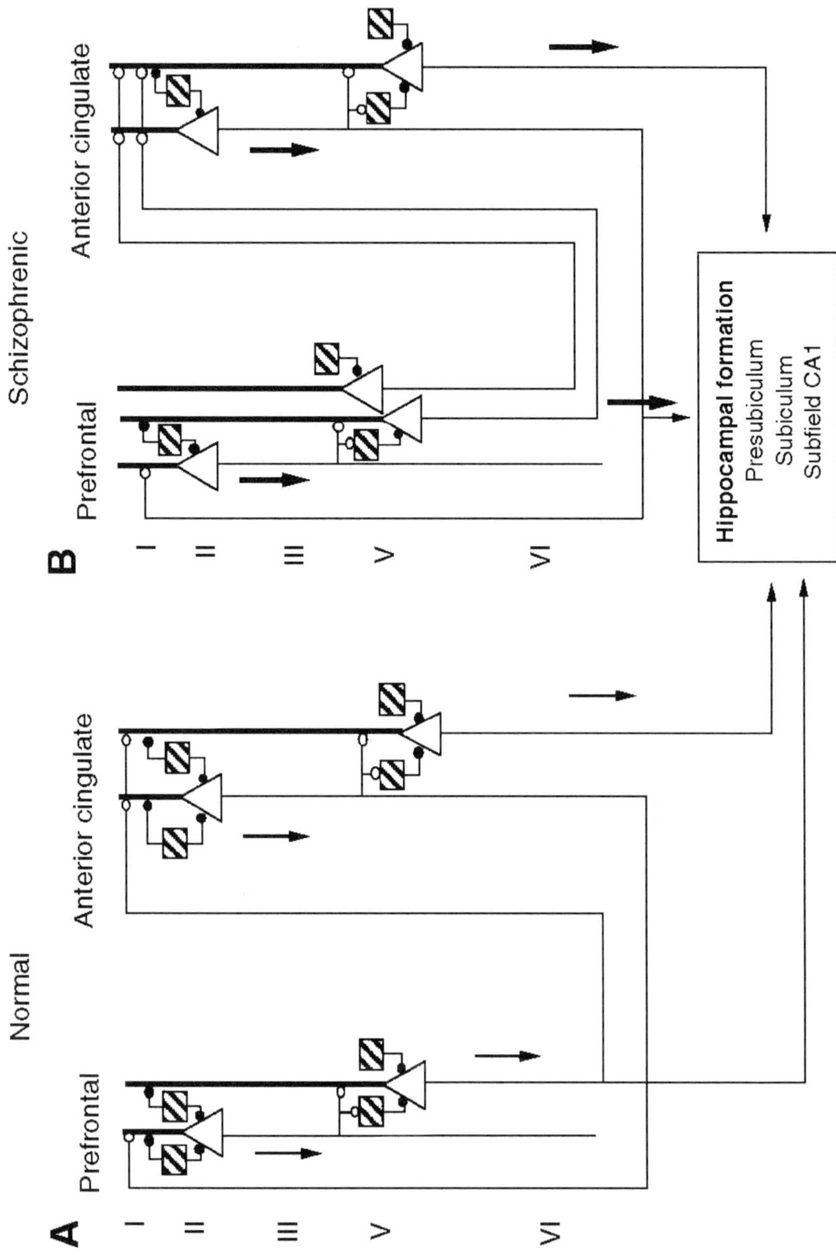
A
Normal
Prefrontal
Anterior cingulate
I
II
III
V
VI
B
Schizophrenic
Prefrontal
Anterior cingulate
I
II
III
V
VI
Hippocampal formation
Presubiculum
Subiculum
Subfield CA1

Figure 4–4 *(at left)*. Altered intrinsic circuitry within the prefrontal and anterior cingulate cortices of control *(A)* and schizophrenic *(B)* subjects and how these changes might effect the downflow of glutamatergic activity from these regions to the hippocampal formation. *Arrows* indicate control subjects; *bold arrows* indicate schizophrenic subjects.

***A:* Normal control circuit:**

1. GABAergic interneurons located in layers II and V provide an inhibitory input to pyramidal neurons.
2. Pyramidal neurons in layer V of the prefrontal area send an excitatory downflow of activity *(arrow)* toward layer I of the anterior cingulate region.
3. Pyramidal neurons in layer V of both the prefrontal and anterior cingulate cortices send descending glutamatergic activity *(arrows)* toward the hippocampal formation, where they terminate in the subiculum and presubiculum, respectively.

***B:* Schizophrenic circuit:**

1. There is a reduction in the number of GABAergic interneurons in layer II of both the prefrontal and anterior cingulate cortices that would exert a diminished inhibitory effect on the pyramidal neurons of this layer.
2. In layer V of the prefrontal cortex, there is no reduction in the number of interneurons but an increase in the number of pyramidal neurons that would give rise to a relative decrease in the amount of inhibitory activity exerted on the pyramidal neurons of this layer.
3. Pyramidal neurons in layer V of the prefrontal area would show an increase of excitatory outflow *(bold arrow)* directed toward layer I of the anterior cingulate region, where distal portions of apical dendrites of pyramidal neurons in deeper laminae are found. This effect in superficial layers would probably influence the firing of pyramidal neurons in layer V of this region.
4. Pyramidal neurons in layer V of both the prefrontal and anterior cingulate cortices would send an increased excitatory downflow of activity *(bold arrows)* toward the subiculum and presubiculum of the hippocampal formation via *N*-methyl-D-aspartate (NMDA)–sensitive glutamate receptors. Secondarily, this excitatory activity could influence kainate-sensitive glutamate receptor activity within other portions of the hippocampal formation, including subfields CA3 and CA4. A reduction of kainate receptor binding could be induced through either a compensatory downregulation of kainate receptor binding or a loss of kainate receptors as pyramidal neurons in these sectors are destroyed by excitotoxicity.

relatively normal until the onset of schizophrenia during adolescence, when an increase of myelination of associational fibers in the presubiculum[88,89] could result in an increased conduction of excitatory activity among the key components of the corticolimbic system.

This interpretation of the model would not explain, however, why pyramidal neurons in superficial laminae are spared a lethal excitotoxic injury. One possible explanation for such a differential effect might be that GABA neurons are rendered vulnerable to an excitotoxic injury during adolescence and adulthood by their smaller size, rather than by perinatal stress (see preceding discussion). If small neurons are more apt than pyramidal neurons to die in response to excitotoxicity, a pre- or perinatal injury may not be necessary to model for a loss of interneurons, although this would make it difficult to explain why changes are found preferentially in layer II of subjects with schizophrenia.

It was previously hypothesized[34] that glutamatergic afferents to superficial laminae of the anterior cingulate region might be a necessary component for the death of interneurons. The fact that the prefrontal area shows both a reduction in the density of interneurons[20] and increased $GABA_A$ receptor binding activity on pyramidal neurons[64] but does not show increased vertical axons[27] in layer II of schizophrenic subjects would argue against this idea. Thus, it does not seem likely that the proposed decrease of GABAergic activity is due to a direct excitotoxic effect arising from an increased number of associative axons. Could such an injury be triggered by an increase of activity conducted along excitatory axons, even when there are normal numbers of such fibers?

Conclusions

It is becoming increasingly clear that schizophrenia may involve both generalized changes in the brain as well as regionally specific alterations in key components of the corticolimbic system. Although the evidence published to date may be interpreted in different ways, when receptor binding studies are viewed together with other microscopic findings, paradoxically, both increases and decreases of glutamatergic activity may occur in individuals with schizophrenia. The direction of change in excitatory activity, however, may vary not only on a region-to-region basis but also according to the stage of the illness. Thus, there could initially be increased amounts of glutamatergic activity, followed by decreases, as compensatory postsynaptic changes in receptor binding activity and/or postsynaptic cell death occur. This may be particularly likely to occur in the hippocampal formation, where evidence in favor of both patterns can be found in the existing literature.

An important corollary question is whether postmortem brain changes in subjects with schizophrenia may be related to a perturbation of normal brain development. It is important to ask, however, whether such an ontogenetic perturbation occurs before, during, or perhaps even after the onset of illness in affected individuals. Important developmental changes in glutamatergic activity normally occur both pre- and postnatally, perhaps even during adulthood, and could contribute to the pathophysiology of this disorder. In this regard, the clinical observation that most schizophrenic individuals are relatively "normal" until adolescence or early adulthood underscores the importance of learning more about the postnatal development of the human brain and how normal maturational changes may interact with genetic and environmental risk factors for schizophrenia. To accomplish this, it will be necessary to define carefully the alterations of intrinsic neural circuits within the corticolimbic system of schizophrenic subjects and relate these changes to the normal ontogeny of these regions. In this way, it may eventually be possible to define the pathophysiology of schizophrenia in precise neural terms and to develop novel therapeutic strategies that may be applied early in the course of the illness to offset the deterioration in functioning that typically leads to a permanent "defect" state.

References

1. Kraeplin E: Dementia Praecox and Paraphrenia. Edinburg, Livingston, 1919

2. Dunlap CB: Dementia praecox: some preliminary observations on brains from carefully selected cases and a consideration of certain sources of error. Am J Psychiatry 80:403–420, 1924
3. Spielmeyer W: The problem of the anatomy of schizophrenia. J Nerv Ment Dis 72:241–244, 1930
4. Vogt O: Proposition de fonder une organision international e payor l'etude d'anatomie pathologique de la schizphrenie et d'autres psychoses dites fonctionelles, in Proceedings of the First International Congress of Neuropathology. Edited by Rosenberg. Rome, Italy, September 1952, pp 674–677
5. Corsellis JAN: Psychoses of obscure pathology, in Greenfield's Neuropathology. Edited by Blackwood W, Corsellis JAN. Chicago, Edward Arnold Publishers, 1976, pp 903–915
6. Weinberger DR, Torrey EF, Neophytides AN, et al: Structural abnormalities in the cerebral cortex of chronic schizophrenic patients. Arch Gen Psychiatry 36:935–939, 1979
7. Benes FM: The relationship between structural brain imaging and histopathologic findings in schizophrenia research. Harvard Review of Psychiatry 1:100–109, 1993
8. Bogerts B, Meertz E, Schonfeldt-Bausch R: Basal ganglia and limbic system pathology in schizophrenia: a morphometric study of brain volume and shrinkage. Arch Gen Psychiatry 42:784–791, 1985
9. Brown R, Colter N, Corsellis JAN, et al: Post-mortem evidence for structural brain changes in schizophrenia: differences in brain weight, temporal horn area and parahippocampal gyrus width as compared with affective disorder. Arch Gen Psychiatry 43:36–42, 1986
10. Benes FM, Davidson J, Bird ED: Quantitative cytoarchitectural studies of cerebral cortex of schizophrenics. Arch Gen Psychiatry 43:31–35, 1986
11. Bogerts B, Falkai P, Tutsch J: Cell numbers in the pallidum and hippocampus of schizophrenics, in Biological Psychiatry, Vol 27. Edited by Shagass C, et al. Amsterdam, Elsevier North-Holland, 1986, pp 1178–1180
12. Falkai P, Bogerts B: Cell loss in the hippocampus of schizophrenics. European Archives of Psychiatry and Neurological Sciences

236:154–161, 1986

13. Falkai P, Bogerts B, Rozumek M: Cell loss and volume reduction in the entorhinal cortex of schizophrenics. Biol Psychiatry 24:515–521, 1988
14. Jeste D, Lohr JB: Hippocampal pathologic findings in schizophrenia. Arch Gen Psychiatry 46:1019–1024, 1989
15. Pakkenberg B: Pronounced reduction of total neuron number in mediodorsal thalamic nucleus and nucleus accumbens in schizophrenics. Arch Gen Psychiatry 47:1023–1028, 1990
16. Kovelman JA, Scheibel AB: A neurohistological correlate of schizophrenia. Biol Psychiatry 19:1601–1621, 1984
17. Jakob H, Beckmann H: Pre-natal developmental disturbances in the limbic allocortex in schizophrenics. Journal of Neural Transmission 65:303–326, 1986
18. Benes FM, Bird ED: An analysis of the arrangement of neurons in the cingulate cortex of schizophrenic patients. Arch Gen Psychiatry 44:608–616, 1987
19. Roberts GW, Colter N, Lofthouse R, et al: Gliosis in schizophrenia: a survey. Biol Psychiatry 39:1043–1050, 1986
20. Benes FM, McSparren J, Bird ED, et al: Deficits in small interneurons in prefrontal and anterior cingulate cortex of schizophrenic and schizoaffective patients. Arch Gen Psychiatry 48:996–1001, 1991
21. Altschuler LL, Conrad A, Kovelman J, et al: Hippocampal pyramidal cell orientation in schizophrenia: a controlled neurohistology study of the Yakovlev collection. Arch Gen Psychiatry 44:1689–1701, 1987
22. Heckers S, Heinsen H, Heinsen Y, et al: Limbic structures and lateral ventricle in schizophrenia. Arch Gen Psychiatry 47:1016–1022, 1990
23. Benes FM, Sorensen I, Bird ED: Morphometric analyses of the hippocampal formation in schizophrenic brain. Schizophr Bull 17:597–608, 1991
24. Benes FM: Post-mortem structural analyses of schizophrenic brain: study designs and the interpretation of data. Psychiatr Dev 6:213–226, 1988
25. Weinberger DR: Implications of normal brain development for

the pathogenesis of schizophrenia. Arch Gen Psychiatry 44:660–669, 1987

26. Akbarian S, Bunney WE, Potkin SG, et al: Altered distribution of nicotinamide-adenine dinucleotide phosphate-diaphorase cells in frontal lobe of schizophrenics implies disturbances of cortical development. Arch Gen Psychiatry 50:227–230, 1993
27. Benes FM, Vincent SL, Alsterberg G, et al: Increased GABA-A receptor binding in superficial layers of cingulate cortex in schizophrenics. J Neurosci 12:924–929, 1992
28. Benes FM: Neurobiological investigations in cingulate cortex of schizophrenic brain. Schizophr Bull 19:537–549, 1993
29. Eccles JC: The cerebral neocortex: a theory of its operation, in Cerebral Cortex: Functional Properties of Cortical Cells, Vol 2. Edited by Jones EG, Peter A. New York, Plenum, 1984, pp 1–48
30. Majocha R, Marotta C, Benes F: Immunostaining of neurofilament protein in human post-mortem cortex: a sensitive and specific approach to the pattern analysis of human cortical cytoarchitecture. Can J Biochem 63:577–584, 1985
31. Benes FM, Majocha R, Bird ED, et al: Increased vertical axon numbers in cingulate cortex of schizophrenics. Arch Gen Psychiatry 44:1017–1021, 1987
32. Benes FM: Relationship of cingulate cortex to schizophrenia, in Neurobiology of Cingulate Cortex and Limbic Thalamus. Edited by Vogt BA, Gabriel M. Boston, Birkhauser, 1993, pp 581–605
33. Conti F, Fabri M, Manzoni T: Glutamate-positive cortico-cortical neurons in the somatic sensory areas I and II of cats. J Neurosci 8:2948–2960, 1988
34. Benes FM, Sorensen I, Vincent SL, et al: Increased density of glutamate-immunoreactive vertical processes in superficial laminae in cingulate cortex of schizophrenic brain. Cereb Cortex 2:502–512, 1992
35. Vogt BA, Pandya DA: Cingulate cortex of the rhesus monkey, II: cortical afferents. J Comp Neurol 262:271–289, 1987
36. Vogt BA, Pandya DN, Rosene DL: Cingulate cortex of the rhesus monkey, I: cytoarchitecture and thalamic afferents. J Comp Neurol 262:256–270, 1987
37. Dom R: Neostriatal and thalamic interneurons: their role in the

pathophysiology of Huntington's chorea, Parkinson's disease and catatonic schizophrenia. Acta Psychiatr Scand Suppl 265:103–123, 1976

38. Martin KAC: Neuronal circuits in cat striate cortex, in Cerebral Cortex: Functional Properties of Cortical Cells, Vol 2. Edited by Jones EG, Peters A. New York, Plenum, 1984, pp 241–284
39. Fairen A, DeFelipe J, Regidor J: Nonpyramidal neurons. Cereb Cortex 1:201–253, 1984
40. Monaghan DT, Cotman CW: Distribution of *N*-methyl-D-aspartate-sensitive L-[^{3}H]glutamate-binding sites in rat brain. J Neurosci 5:2905–2919, 1985
41. Jones EG: Laminar distribution of cortical efferent cells, in Cerebral Cortex, Vol 1. Edited by Peters A, Jones EG. New York, Plenum, 1984, pp 521–548
42. Galaburda AM, Pandya DN: The intrinsic architectonic and connectional organization of the superior temporal region of the rhesus monkey. J Comp Neurol 221:169–184, 1983
43. Stevens JR: Abnormal reinnervation as a basis for schizophrenia: an hypothesis. Arch Gen Psychiatry 49:238–243, 1992
44. Kerwin RW, Patel S, Meldrum BS, et al: Asymmetrical loss of glutamate receptor subtype in left hippocampus in schizophrenia. Lancet 1:583–584, 1988
45. Kerwin R, Patel S, Meldrum B: Quantitative autoradiographic analysis of glutamate binding sites in the hippocampal formation in normal and schizophrenic brain post-mortem. Neuroscience 39:25–32, 1990
46. Harrison PJ, McLaughlin D, Kerwin RW: Decreased hippocampal expression of a glutamate receptor gene in schizophrenia. Lancet 337:450–452, 1991
47. Deakin JF, Slater P, Simpson MD, et al: Frontal cortical and left temporal glutamatergic dysfunction in schizophrenia. J Neurochem 52:1781–1786, 1989
48. Nishikawa T, Takashima M, Toru M: Increased [^{3}H]kainic acid binding in the prefrontal cortex in schizophrenia. Neurosci Lett 40:245–250, 1983
49. Toru M, Watanabe S, Shibuya H, et al: Neurotransmitters receptors and neuropeptides in post-mortem brains of chronic schizo-

phrenic patients. Acta Psychiatr Scand 78:121–137, 1988

50. Kornhuber J, Mack-Burkhardt F, Riederer P, et al: [^{3}H]MK-801 binding sites in post-mortem brain regions of schizophrenic patients. Journal of Neural Transmission 77:231–236, 1989
51. Simpson MD, Slater P, Royston MC, et al: Alterations in phencyclidine and sigma binding sites in schizophrenic brains. Schiz Res 6:41–48, 1992
52. Harrison NL, Simmonds MA: Quantitative studies on some antagonists of *N*-methyl-D-aspartate in slices of rat cerebral cortex. Br J Pharmacol 84:381–391, 1985
53. Goldman-Rakic PS, Selemon LDM, Schwartz ML: Dual pathways connecting the dorsolateral prefrontal cortex with the hippocampal formation and parahippocampal cortex in the rhesus monkey. Neuroscience 12:719–743, 1984
54. Domesick VB: Projections from the cingulate cortex in the rat. Brain Res 12:296–230, 1969
55. Beckstead RM: An autoradiographic examination of corticocortical and subcortical projections of the mediodorsal projection (prefrontal) cortex in the rat. J Comp Neurol 184:43–62, 1979
56. Roberts E: An hypothesis suggesting that there is a defect in the GABA system in schizophrenia. Neurosciences Research Program Bulletin 10:469–482, 1972
57. Baleydier C, Maugiere F: The duality of the cingulate gyrus in monkey: neuroanatomical study and functional hypothesis. Brain 103:525–554, 1980
58. Cameron N: Reasoning, regression and communication in schizophrenics. Psychological Review Monographs 50:1–33, 1938
59. Detre P, Jarecki HG: Modern Psychiatric Treatment. Philadelphia, PA, JB Lippincott, 1971, pp 108–116
60. Perry TL, Buchanan J, Kish SJ, et al: Gamma-aminobutyric acid deficiency in brains of schizophrenic patients. Lancet 1:237, 1979
61. Bird ED, Spokes EGS, Iversen LL: Increased dopamine concentration in limbic areas of brain from patients dying with schizophrenia. Brain 102:347–360, 1979

62. Simpson MD, Slater P, Deakin JF, et al: Reduced GABA uptake sites in the temporal lobe in schizophrenia. Neurosci Lett 107:211–215, 1989
63. Reynolds GP, Czudek C, Andrews H: Deficit and hemispheric asymmetry of GABA uptake sites in the hippocampus in schizophrenia. Biol Psychiatry 27:1038–1044, 1990
64. Hanada S, Mita T, Nishinok N, et al: ^{3}H-Muscimol binding sites increased in autopsied brains of chronic schizophrenics. Life Sci 40:259–266, 1987
65. Benes FM, Vincent SL, SanGiovanni JP: High resolution imaging of receptor binding in analyzing neuropsychiatric diseases. Biotechniques 7:970–979, 1989
66. Squires RF, Lajtha A, Saederup E, et al: Reduced [^{3}H]fluntrazepam bindings in cingulate cortex and hippocampus of postmortem schizophrenic brains. Neurochem Res 18:219–223, 1993
67. Olsen RW: Drug interactions at the GABA receptor-inophore complex. Annu Rev Pharmacol Toxicol 22:245–277, 1982
68. Sidman R, Rakic P: Neuronal migration with special reference to developing human brain. Brain Res 62:1–35, 1973
69. Rakic P: Timing of major ontogenetic events in the visual cortex of the rhesus monkey, in Brain Mechanisms of Mental Retardation. Edited by Buchwald NA, Brazier M. New York, Academic Press, 1975, pp 3–40
70. Marin-Padilla M: Pre-natal and early post-natal ontogenesis of the human motor cortex: a Golgi study, I: the sequential development of the cortical layers. Brain Res 23:167–183, 1970
71. Marin-Padilla M: Pre-natal and early post-natal ontogenesis of the human motor cortex: a Golgi study, II: the basket-pyramidal system. Brain Res 23:185–191, 1970
72. Jacobsen B, Kinney DK: Peri-natal complications in adopted and non-adopted schizophrenics and their controls: preliminary results. Acta Psychiatr Scand 238:103–123, 1980
73. Parnas J, Schulsinger F, Teasdale W, et al: Peri-natal complications and clinical outcome. Br J Psychiatry 140:416–420, 1982
74. Cotterrell M, Balazs R, Johnson AL: Effects of corticosteroids on the biochemical maturation of rat brain: post-natal cell forma-

tion. J Neurochem 19:2151–2167, 1972

75. Sapolsky R, Meaney M: Maturation of the adrenocortical stress response: neuroendocrine control mechanisms and the stress hyporesponsive period. Brain Research Reviews 11:65–76, 1986
76. Stein-Behrens B, Elliott E, Miller C, et al: Glucocorticoids exacerbate kainic acid-induced extracellular accumulation of excitatory amino acids in the rat hippocampus. J Neurochem 1730–1734, 1992
77. Steiner HX, McBean GJ, Kohler C, et al: Ibotenate-induced neuronal degeneration in immature rat brain. Brain Res 307:117–124, 1984
78. Ikonomidou C, Mosinger LL, Shahid Sallett K, et al: Sensitivity of the developing rat brain to hyperbaric/ischemic damage parallels sensitivity to *N*-methyl-D-aspartate neurotoxicity. J Neurosci 9:2809–2818, 1989
79. Olney JW, Sesma MA, Wozniak DF: Glutamatergic, cholinergic and GABAergic systems in posterior cingulate cortex: interactions and possible mechanisms of limbic system disease, in The Neurobiology of Cingulate Cortex and Limbic Thalamus. Edited by Vogt BA, Gabriel M. Boston, MA, Birkhauser Publishing, 1993, pp 557–580
80. Schwarcz R, Coyle JT: Neurochemical sequelae of kainate injections in corpus striatum and substantia nigra of the rat. Life Sci 20:431–436, 1977
81. Zhang WQ, Rogers BC, Tandon P, et al: Systemic administration of kainic acid increases GABA levels in perfusate from the hippocampus of rats in vivo. Neurotoxicology 11:593–600, 1990
82. Johnston MV: Biochemistry of neurotransmitters in cortical development, in Cerebral Cortex. Edited by Jones PA. New York, Plenum, 1988, pp 211–236
83. Kvale I, Fosse VM, Fonnum F: Development of neurotransmitter parameters in lateral geniculate body, superior colliculus and visual cortex of the albino rat. Developmental Brain Research 7:137–145, 1983
84. Schliebs R, Kullman E, Bigl V: Development of glutamate binding sites in the visual structures of the rat brain: effect of visual pattern deprivation. Biomed Biophys Acta 45:4495–4506, 1986

85. Baudry M, Arst D, Oliver M, et al: Development of glutamate binding sites and their regulation by calcium in rat hippocampus. Developments in Brain Research 1:37–38, 1981
86. Flechsig P: Anatomie des menschlichen Gehirms und Ruckenmarks auf myelogenetischer Gundlange. Leipzig, G. Thieme, 1920
87. Yakovlev P, Lecours A: The myelinogenetic cycles of regional maturation of the brain, in Regional Development of the Brain Early in Life. Edited by Minkowski A. Oxford, Blackwell Scientific, 1967, pp 3–70
88. Benes FM: Myelination of cortical-hippocampal relays during late adolescence: anatomical correlates to the onset of schizophrenia. Schizophr Bull 15:585–594, 1989
89. Benes FM, Turtle M, Khan Y, et al: Myelination of a key relay zone in the hippocampal formation occurs in human brain during childhood, adolescence and adulthood. Arch Gen Psychol 51: 477–484, 1994
90. Suddath R, Christison G, Torrey EF, et al: Abnormalities in the brains of monozygotic twins discordant for schizophrenia. N Engl J Med 322:789–794, 1990
91. Shenton ME, Kikinis R, Jolesz FA, et al: Abnormalities of the left temporal lobe and thought disorder in schizophrenia: a quantitative magnetic resonance imaging study. N Engl J Med 327: 604–612, 1992

CHAPTER

5

Dissolution of Cerebral Cortical Mechanisms in Subjects With Schizophrenia

Patricia Goldman-Rakic, Ph.D.

Neuropsychological evidence and clinical observations have repeatedly implicated, directly or indirectly, the prefrontal cortex as a site of dysfunction in subjects with schizophrenia, on the basis of the similarity of impairments observed in demented patients and those with frontal lobe damage.[1–5] Although such findings have significantly advanced the empirical support for the "frontal lobe" hypothesis, countless other results in the literature leave considerable room for doubt about any singular explanation of this heterogeneous disorder.

Whatever the status of prefrontal involvement in individuals with schizophrenia, basic studies of its structure and function have provided support for three major conclusions. First, prefrontal cortex is specialized to direct or guide behavior by internalized representations of facts, events, and other memoranda.[4] Second, prefrontal cortex carries out its functions through interactions within a complex distributed network of reciprocating informational pathways.[6–8] Third, these informational networks are modulated by monoaminergic afferents originating in the brain stem.[9–11] Each of these points is covered in this chapter.

Prefrontal Cortex and Internal Representation

It has been argued elsewhere that guiding behavior by representations—that is, by ideas and concepts—normally requires working memory and that schizophrenic thought disorder could involve a breakdown in this basic capacity for "on-line" processing.[4,5] In my view, the fragmented, disjointed thought process that is thought disorder is reducible to an impairment of the operational mechanism(s) by which symbolic representations are both accessed from long-term memory and held "in mind" to guide behavior in the absence of instructive stimuli in the outside world. Working memory is the basic process for accomplishing this cognitive feat, and its dependence on the prefrontal cortex is a driving force for investigating the neurobiological mechanisms that could mediate this process in prefrontal cortex.

Working memory is a concept developed by cognitive psychologists to refer to a distinct process or ability to update and/or bring information to mind from long-term memory and/or to integrate incoming information for the purpose of making an informed decision, judgment, or response.[12] As explained by Baddeley,[12] the transient and active memory system referred to here as "working memory" evolved from the older concept, "short-term" memory.[4] Based on my own analysis,[4] working memory can be distinguished operationally from canonical or associative memory by several formal criteria, namely, its short duration, its limited capacity, and its neural substrate. The classical delayed-response tasks used extensively in animal research are prime examples of tasks that tax a subject's—both a monkey's and a human's—ability to hold information "in mind" for a short period of time and to update its memory buffer on a moment-to-moment basis. The relevant memorandum in spatial delayed-response tasks is the location or direction of an object. The relevant memorandum in the Wisconsin Card Sorting Test[13] is a categorical representation of the attributes of an object (e.g., its color or shape).

Studies in rhesus monkeys show that they are capable of remembering briefly presented visuospatial information over short delays—in the classical manual spatial delayed-response tasks,[4,14] as well as in the more demanding eight-item oculomotor version of that task.[15] The ability of monkeys to retain in working memory an item of spatial information is not unlike the capacity of a human to remember a seven-digit phone number or the name of someone to whom he or she has just been introduced. As is well established, lesions of the dorsolateral prefrontal cortex produce marked impairments on spatial delayed-response and spatial delayed alternation tasks,[16,17] and the cortical focus for these deficits is the principal sulcus (or Walker's area 46). A modification of this task has been employed in a number of studies of human cognition in schizophrenic patients[18] and in nonschizophrenic individuals studied by noninvasive imaging.[19,20]

That the dorsolateral prefrontal cortex plays a role in working memory is strongly supported by consistent results from numerous experimental approaches. In normal monkeys performing delayed-response tasks, portions of the principal sulcus are metabolically activated nearly 20% over the level of their involvement in associative memory tasks.[21] Single-unit analysis of neurons in the area of the principal sulcus has revealed three principal types of neurons that constitute the main elements of a prefrontal working memory circuit: those that register the stimulus to be recalled,[22] those that retain the information on line,[15] and those that use the information to guide the timing and/or direction of an appropriate response.[23] In addition, performance on delayed-response tasks[16,17,23,24] is selectively impaired by surgical removal of the principal sulcus, as well as by experimental depletion of catecholamines[9,11] and by pharmacological blockade of dopamine, subtype 1 (D_1) receptors[25] or reversible cooling of this area[26] (M. V. Chaffee and P. S. Goldman-Rakic, unpublished data, May 1995).

Importantly, none of these treatments applied to the principal sulcal area of prefrontal cortex alter associative memory (i.e., on tasks such as visual discrimination, in which stimulus-response associations are fixed and unchanging) or impair sensory-guided performance, when stimuli remain in view during delay periods of delayed-response tasks and the monkey has only to defer its response to a visible cue until the end of the delay. Thus, studies employing electrophysiological measurements and pharmacological, surgical, or reversible lesions of prefrontal circuits establish a strong dependence of spatial delayed-response performance, whether in a manual or oculomotor format, on the integrity of prefrontal circuits.

Recent studies have documented spatial working memory deficits in schizophrenic patients,[18] results that resemble findings obtained in rhesus monkeys with dorsolateral prefrontal lesions. These and similar findings in patients[27] provide important evidence for the selective involvement of the dorsolateral prefrontal cortex in the processing deficits of schizophrenic individuals. This parallelism is further strengthened by the recent findings in rhesus monkeys of involvement of the frontal eye field region of prefrontal cortex in smooth pursuit tracking.[28] Monkeys in which this region was surgically removed not only have reduced steady-state gain for pursuit directed ipsilateral to the effective lesions but also lack anticipatory pursuit prior to target movement. Like schizophrenic patients, monkeys with eye field lesions use large catch-up saccades to keep their eyes on track. Also similar to the tracking of schizophrenic subjects, the monkey's optokinetic following was normal, showing that the deficit could not be accounted for as a motor problem.

Imaging studies have begun to address the involvement of the prefrontal cortex in human working memory performance. In a recent positron emission tomography study, Jonides et al.[19] employed a task of spatial working memory modeled on the oculomotor paradigm described previously. The results showed activation of prefrontal cortex in working memory and extended previous evidence for a network organization of areas that support this function.[4,7] In another positron emission tomography study, Petrides et al.[29] imaged nonschizophrenic subjects as they were recalling the order of objects previously selected. Area 46 and adjacent area 9 were activated in this task, which requires memory of location and object features.

Andreasen et al.[30] used single-photon emission computed tomography to study blood flow in normal subjects and schizophrenic patients. According to these authors, blood flow was selectively increased in area 9. The localization of specific cytoarchitectonic regions in these studies must be interpreted cautiously, but together with other results, they emphasize how common is the activation of dorsolateral prefrontal areas in tasks tapping working memory. Moreover, an exact correspondence in the localization of spatial working memory function across human and nonhuman primates has been achieved by a recent experiment at Yale University, in which functional magnetic resonance imaging was used.[20] Functional magnetic resonance imaging offers high spatial resolution in individual subjects. In our study, subjects were shown a sequence of presentations on a television monitor every 1.7 seconds and had to judge whether a current stimulus (irregular shape) was in the same or a different location as a previous stimulus presented two trials back. Significant activation above control conditions was found in an area that corresponds to cytoarchitectonically defined area 46.[31] The same area 46 is where, in the nonhuman primate, memory cells are located and where lesions cause disruption in spatial working memory tasks. It seems clear from these new studies in human subjects both with and without the diagnosis of schizophrenia that there is an emerging consensus on the role of prefrontal cortex in the function of spatial working memory and that neurobiological studies of the dorsolateral prefrontal areas in nonhuman primates can provide a solid animal model for examination of the neural mechanisms that may be compromised in individuals with dementia.

Finally, working memory has been demonstrated in more than one knowledge domain and in more than one area of the prefrontal cortex. The multiplicity of special-purpose working-memory domains is supported by both functional and anatomical findings in nonhuman primates. The mechanisms for working memory are thus essentially replicated in different areas within the prefrontal cortex, each area processing different types of information. To state this as a principle of functional organization, informational domain, not process, is mapped across prefrontal cortex.

Direct evidence for this view has recently been obtained in my laboratory from studies of nonspatial memory, that is, memory for the features or attributes rather than the location of objects.[32] Recordings were obtained from neurons in areas 12 and 45 of Walker on the inferior convexity region in monkeys trained to perform delayed-response tasks in which spatial or feature memoranda had to be recalled on independent, randomly interwoven trials. Both spatial and feature trials required exactly the same eye movements at the end of the delay but differed in the nature of the mnemonic representation that guided those responses. The major finding was that most of the inferior convexity neurons encoded the features rather than the location of the stimulus.[32]

These results provide strong evidence that information about objects may be processed separately from those dedicated to the analysis of spatial location and vice versa. The finding that the prefrontal cortex contains a second area with working-memory functions supports the prediction that prefrontal areas are specialized for working-memory function and that the subdivisions of the prefrontal cortex represent different informational domains rather than different processes.[4] Furthermore, I have postulated that a working-memory component is present in the Wisconsin Card Sorting Test commonly used with human subjects.[4] Although the relevant features of the stimuli (color, size, shape) are all present in the environment at the time of response, they contain no information about the correct response. Rather, it must be provided from representational memory—in this case, the instructions or concepts of color, shape, and number guide the response choice. The deficits in schizophrenic subjects in the Wisconsin Card Sorting Test have been attributed specifically to dysfunction in the dorsolateral prefrontal cortex.[3,33–35] On the basis of the studies in nonhuman primates discussed here,[32] it can be surmised that dysfunction of dorsolateral areas 12 and 45 may be the relevant component of dorsolateral prefrontal cortex that is the focus of the impairment in patients with larger frontal lobe lesions.

The literature on cognitive deficits in individuals with schizophrenia supports the conclusion that schizophrenic patients are consistently impaired on tests that invoke working memory and further supports clinical observations on the similarity between patients with prefrontal damage and those with schizophrenia. Furthermore, the specific deficits can be produced by selective lesions in distinctly different subareas of the dorsolateral prefrontal cortex. Considerable evidence suggests that spatial processing in rhesus monkeys may be carried out in a dorsolateral subdivision of the prefrontal cortex, principally Walker's area 46; nonspatial processing in areas 12/45 on the inferior convexity; and eye tracking associated principally with area 8 (Figure 5–1). It follows that dysfunction in one of these areas could be the pathophysiological basis of the corresponding deficit in schizophrenic subjects and that the heterogeneity of dysfunction in individual patients may be related to the extent and number of prefrontal areas that are compromised.

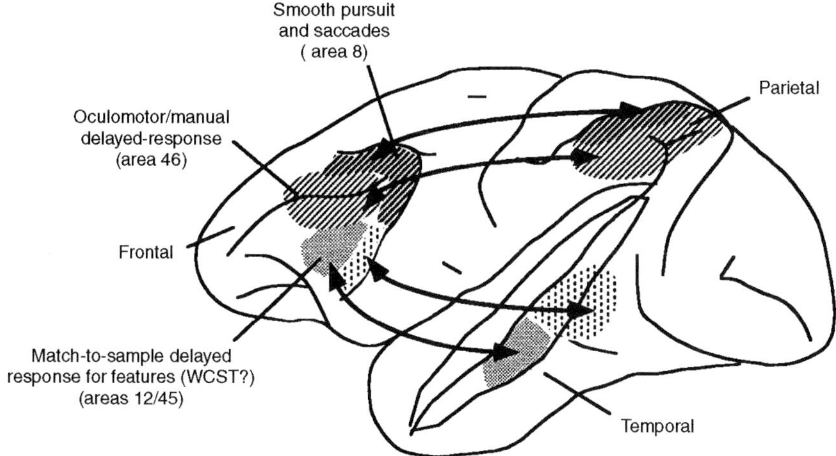

Figure 5–1. Diagram summarizing the functional divisions of the dorsolateral prefrontal cortex that can be linked to deficits observed in schizophrenic patients. Also shown diagrammatically are the connections of these prefrontal areas with the subdivisions of posterior parietal and temporal lobe sensory association regions with which they are anatomically interconnected. Large regions of prefrontal cortex remain as yet uncharted with respect to specific deficits that can be related to symptoms of dementia. The findings summarized here provide evidence for the nonhuman primate as a model system for analysis of thought and affective disorders in humans. WCST = Wisconsin Card Sorting Test.

Dopamine Systems, Neuroleptics, and Neuropathology

The therapeutic potencies of typical neuroleptic drugs usually correlate with their ability to bind dopaminergic D_2 receptors.[36,37] It was this fact that led me to explore the dopamine system in relation to prefrontal function as far back as the mid 1970s. Biochemical assays[38] and behavioral analysis of 6-hydroxydopamine intracerebral injections directly into the prefrontal areas[9] have established a role for dopamine in prefrontal function. More recent studies from my laboratory have been dedicated to characterizing the distribution of dopamine terminals in the cortex, with particular emphasis on the prefrontal areas.[39,40]

In our studies, we have identified the synaptic targets of the cortical dopamine innervation in both monkeys and humans and have uncovered a specialized synaptic architecture in which dopamine synapses are opposed to the same spine heads as are excitatory synapses, presumptively from cortico-cortical-bearing axons (Figure 5–2). I believe that this mechanism may explain how dopamine can effect a change in a cell's capacity or efficiency in integrating its myriad inputs. Disruption of this mechanism could help to explain how dopamine dysfunction could affect cortical processes in general and internally generated representations in particular.[41]

I next explored the dopamine receptors in prefrontal cortex, using quantitative receptor autoradiography and layer-by-layer analysis of receptor distributions as well as immunocytochemistry. The results revealed a high concentration of the D_1 family of receptors in the prefrontal cortex relative to D_2 receptors[42,43] that may be of particular functional importance in regulating prefrontal working memory processes. In addition, I have localized the main intracellular distribution of D_1 receptors in prefrontal cortex to the spines of pyramidal cells, which, as described previously, are the target of dopamine afferents.[44] Injections of the D_1 antagonists SCH23390 or SCH39166 intracerebrally[10,25] or systemically[45] in monkeys result in deficits in working-memory tasks. Similar impairments have also

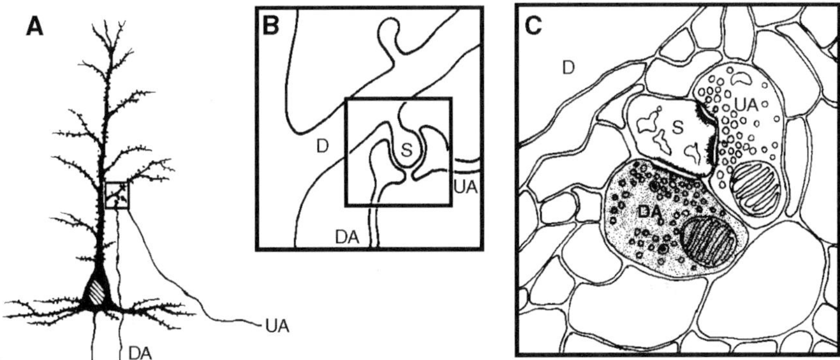

Figure 5–2. Diagram of synaptic arrangements involving the dopamine input to the cortex. *A:* Afferents labeled with a dopamine (DA)–specific antibody terminate on the spine of a pyramidal cell in the prefrontal cortex, together with an unidentified axon (UA). *B:* Enlargement of axospinous synapses illustrated in panel A showing apposition of the DA input and a presumed excitatory input that makes an asymmetrical synapse on the same dendritic (D) spine. *C:* Diagram of ultrastructural features of the axospinous synapses illustrated in panel B; the dopamine terminal (darkened profile representing DA immunoreactivity) forms a symmetrical synapse; the unidentified profile forms an asymmetrical synapse with the postsynaptic membrane. S = spine.
Source. Adapted from Reference 41.

now been reported for humans with dopamine insufficiency.[46–49]

I expected that neuroleptic drugs might act in the cortex in a different way than in the neostriatum, where D_2 and D_1 receptors are more nearly in balance. To examine this question, I treated monkeys chronically with clozapine, haloperidol, or remoxipride.[50] The chronic studies revealed that each of the distinctly different drugs decreased the density of D_1 receptors (by 30%–34%) and modestly increased the density of D_2 receptors (by 11%–18%) in the prefrontal and temporal cortex, where dopamine is most concentrated. These changes were not observed in the visual, motor, or somatosensory cortex. The remarkably similar and regionally specific effects of these three drugs on cortical dopaminergic receptors in the prefrontal cortex suggests common therapeutic targets for typical and atypical neuroleptics in the treatment of schizophrenia. Such data are particularly important in view of mounting evidence of the cerebral cortical involvement in schizophrenia.

Finally, given the functional evidence for prefrontal dysfunction in schizophrenic subjects, it is important to assess the integrity of its cells and circuits in humans with schizophrenia. I have examined the dorsolateral prefrontal cortex in postmortem studies, using a three-dimensional counting method.[51] I found widespread changes in several parameters of cortical architecture. Neuronal density was about 17% higher in schizophrenic subjects than in control subjects; the cortex was 9% thinner; and cell somata were significantly smaller, particularly in layer V in prefrontal cortex and in visual cortex, the two areas examined so far. In prefrontal cortex, nonpyramidal as well as pyramidal neurons were affected, but the density of glial cells was normal.

I cannot yet say whether involvement of the prefrontal cortical in the pathophysiology of schizophrenia is associated with the working-memory impairments or thought disorder expressed in the disease. However, prefrontal circuitry and its ultrastructure, neurotransmitter complementation, and mechanisms of development cannot help but shed light on the dissolution of both structures and functions in this major mental disorder.

References

1. Levin S: Frontal lobe dysfunctions in schizophrenia, I: eye movement impairments. J Psychiatr Res 18:27–55, 1984
2. Levin S: Frontal lobe dysfunctions in schizophrenia, II: impairments of psychological and brain functions. J Psychiatr Res 18:57–72, 1984
3. Weinberger DR, Berman KF, Zec RF: Physiological dysfunction of dorsolateral prefrontal cortex in schizophrenia, I: regional cerebral blood flow (rCBF) evidence. Arch Gen Psychiatry 43:114–125, 1986
4. Goldman-Rakic PS: Circuitry of the prefrontal cortex and the regulation of behavior by representational knowledge, in Hand-

book of Physiology, Vol 5. Edited by Plum F, Mountcastle V. Bethesda, MD, American Physiological Society, 1987, pp 373

5. Goldman-Rakic PS: Prefrontal cortical dysfunction in schizophrenia: the relevance of working memory, in Psychopathology and the Brain. Edited by Carroll BJ, Barrett JE. New York, Raven Press, 1991, pp 1–23
6. Selemon LD, Goldman-Rakic PS: Topographic intermingling of striatonigral and striatopallidal neurons in the rhesus monkey. J Comp Neurol 297:359–376, 1990
7. Goldman-Rakic PS: Topography of cognition: parallel distributed networks in primate association cortex. Annu Rev Neurosci 11:137–156, 1988
8. Goldman-Rakic PS, Chafee M, Friedman H: Allocation of function in distributed circuits, in Brain Mechanisms of Perception and Memory: From Neuron to Behavior, Part IV. Edited by Ono T, Squire LR, Raichle ME, et al. New York, Oxford University Press, 1993, pp 445–456
9. Brozoski T, Brown RM, Rosvold HE, et al: Cognitive deficit caused by regional depletion of dopamine in prefrontal cortex of rhesus monkey. Science 205:929–932, 1979
10. Sawaguchi T, Goldman-Rakic PS: The role of D1-dopamine receptor in working memory: local injections of dopamine antagonists into the prefrontal cortex of rhesus monkeys performing an oculomotor delayed-response task. J Neurophysiol 71:515–528, 1993
11. Arnsten AFT, Goldman-Rakic PS: Alpha2-adrenergic mechanisms in prefrontal cortex associated with cognitive decline in aged nonhuman primates. Science 230:1273–1276, 1985
12. Baddeley A: Working Memory. London, Oxford University Press, 1986
13. Heaton R: Wisconsin Card Sorting Test. Odessa, TX, Psychological Assessment Resources, 1985
14. Fuster JM: The Prefrontal Cortex, 2nd Edition. New York, Raven Press, 1989, p 255
15. Funahashi S, Bruce CJ, Goldman-Rakic PS: Mnemonic coding of visual space in the monkey's dorsolateral prefrontal cortex. J Neurophysiol 61:331–349, 1989

16. Goldman PS, Rosvold HE: Localization of function within the dorsolateral prefrontal cortex of the rhesus monkey. Exp Neurol 27:291–304, 1970
17. Goldman PS, Rosvold HE, Vest B, et al: Analysis of the delayed alternation deficit produced by dorsolateral prefrontal lesions in the rhesus monkey. J Comp Physiol Psychol 77:212–220, 1971
18. Park S, Holzman PS: Schizophrenics show spatial working memory deficits. Arch Gen Psychiatry 49:975–982, 1992
19. Jonides J, Smith EE, Koeppe RA, et al: Spatial working memory in humans as revealed by PET. Nature 363:623–625, 1993
20. McCarthy G, Blamire AM, Puce A, et al: Functional magnetic resonance imaging of human prefrontal cortex activation during a spatial working memory task. Proc Natl Acad Sci U S A 91:8690–8694, 1994
21. Friedman HR, Goldman-Rakic PS: Coactivation of prefrontal cortex and inferior parietal cortex in working memory tasks revealed by 2DG functional mapping in the rhesus monkey. J Neurosci 14:2775–2788, 1994
22. Funahashi S, Bruce CJ, Goldman-Rakic PS: Visuospatial coding in primate prefrontal neurons revealed by oculomotor paradigms. J Neurophysiol 63:814–831, 1990
23. Funahashi S, Bruce CJ, Goldman-Rakic PS: Neuronal activity related to saccadic eye movements in the monkey's dorsolateral prefrontal cortex. J Neurophysiol 65:1464–1483, 1991
24. Passingham RE: Delayed matching after selective prefrontal lesions in monkeys (*Macac mulatta*). Brain Res 92:89–102, 1975
25. Sawaguchi T, Goldman-Rakic PS: D1 dopamine receptors in prefrontal cortex: involvement in working memory. Science 251:947–950, 1991
26. Alexander GE, Goldman PS: Functional development of the dorsolateral prefrontal cortex: an analysis utilizing reversible cryogenic depression. Brain Res 143:233–249, 1978
27. Fukushima J, Fukushima K, Chiba T, et al: Disturbances of voluntary control of saccadic eye movements in schizophrenic patients. Biol Psychiatry 23:670–677, 1988
28. MacAvoy MG, Bruce CJ, Gottlieb JP: Smooth pursuit eye movement representation in the primate frontal eyefield. Cereb Cor-

tex 1:95–102, 1991
29. Petrides M, Alivisatos B, Evans AC, et al: Dissociation of human mid-dorsolateral from posterior dorsolateral frontal cortex in memory processing. Proc Natl Acad Sci U S A 90:873–877, 1993
30. Andreasen NC, Rezai K, Alliger R, et al: Hypofrontality in neuroleptic-naive patients and in patients with chronic schizophrenia: assessment with xenon 133 single-photon emission computed tomography and the Tower of London. Arch Gen Psychiatry 49:943–958, 1992
31. Rajkowska G, Goldman-Rakic PS: Cytoarchitectonic definition of prefrontal areas in the normal human cortex, II: variability in locations of areas 9 and 46 and relationship to the Talairach coordinate system. Cereb Cortex, in press
32. Wilson FAW, O'Scalaidhe SP, Goldman-Rakic PS: Dissociation of object and spatial processing domains in primate prefrontal cortex. Science 260:1955–1958, 1993
33. Milner B: Effects of different brain lesions on card sorting. Arch Neurol 9:100–110, 1963
34. Milner B: Some effects of frontal lobectomy in man, in The Frontal Granular Cortex and Behavior. Edited by Warren JM, Akert K. New York, McGraw-Hill, 1964, pp 313
35. Milner B, Petrides M, Smith ML: Frontal lobes and the temporal organization of memory. Human Neurobiology 4:137–142, 1985
36. Creese I, Burt DR, Snyder S: Dopamine receptor binding predicts clinical and pharmacological potencies of antipsychotic drugs. Science 192:481–483, 1976
37. Hess EJ, Creese I: Biochemical characterization of dopamine receptors, in Dopamine Receptors, Vol 8. Edited by Creese I, Fraser CM. New York, Alan R. Liss, 1987, pp 1–27
38. Brown RM, Goldman PS: Catecholamines in neocortex of rhesus monkeys: regional distribution and ontogenetic development. Brain Res 124:576–580, 1977
39. Williams SM, Goldman-Rakic PS: Characterization of the dopaminergic innervation of the primate frontal cortex using a dopamine-specific antibody. Cereb Cortex 3:199–222, 1993
40. Smiley JF, Goldman-Rakic PS: Heterogeneous targets of dopamine synapses in monkey prefrontal cortex demonstrated by se-

rial section electron microscopy: a laminar analysis using the silver-enhanced diaminobenzidine sulfide (SEDS) immunolabeling technique. Cereb Cortex 3:223–238, 1993

41. Goldman-Rakic PS, Leranth C, Williams SM, et al: Dopamine synaptic complex with pyramidal neurons in primate cerebral cortex. Proc Natl Acad Sci U S A 86:9015–9019, 1989
42. Goldman-Rakic PS, Lidow MS, Gallager DW: Overlap of dopaminergic, adrenergic, and serotonergic receptors and complementarity of their subtypes in primate prefrontal cortex. J Neurosci 10:2125–2138, 1990
43. Lidow MS, Goldman-Rakic PS, Gallager DW, et al: Distribution of dopaminergic receptors in the primate cerebral cortex: quantitative autoradiographic analysis using [^{3}H]raclopride, [^{3}H]spiperone, and [^{3}H]SCH23390. Neuroscience 40:657–671, 1991
44. Smiley JF, Levey AI, Ciliax BJ, et al: D1 dopamine receptor immunoreactivity in human and monkey cerebral cortex: predominant localization in dendritic spines. Proc Natl Acad Sci U S A 91:5720–5724, 1994
45. Arnsten AFT, Cai JX, Murphy BL, et al: Dopamine D1 receptor mechanisms in the cognitive performance of young adult and aged monkeys. Psychopharmacology 116:143–151, 1994
46. Gothan AM, Brown RG, Marsden CP: "Frontal" cognitive function in patients with Parkinson's disease "on" and "off" levodopa. Brain 111:299–321, 1988
47. Lees AJ, Smith E: Cognitive deficits in the early stages of Parkinson's disease. Brain 106:257–270, 1983
48. Levin BE, Llabre MM, Weiner WJ: Cognitive impairments associated with early Parkinson's disease. Neurology 39:557–561, 1989
49. Lange KW, Robbins TW, Marsden CD, et al: L-Dopa withdrawal in Parkinson's disease selectively impairs cognitive performance in tests sensitive to frontal lobe dysfunction. Psychopharmacology 107:394–404, 1992
50. Lidow MS, Goldman-Rakic PS: A common action of clozapine, haloperidol and remoxipride on D1- and D2-dopaminergic receptors in the primate cerebral cortex. Proc Natl Acad Sci U S A 91:4353–4356, 1994

51. Selemon LD, Rajkowska G, Goldman-Rakic PS: Abnormally high neuronal density in two widespread areas of the schizophrenic cortex: a morphometric analysis of prefrontal area 9 and occipital area 17. Arch Gen Psychiatry (in press)

CHAPTER

Linkage and Molecular Genetics of Infantile Autism

Roland D. Ciaranello, M.D.

Autism is a severe developmental disorder with onset usually within the first 3 years of life. It is characterized by marked social deficits, delay in language development, and a restricted range of stereotyped, repetitive behaviors. The prevalence of autism is about 1 in 2,000 births, and the ratio of affected boys to girls is about 3:1.[1] About 125,000 Americans are

---

This work was supported by a program project grant from the National Institute of Mental Health (MH 39437), a Research Scientist Award to the author (MH 00219), the Scottish Rite Foundation, the Solomon and Rebecca Baker Foundation, the Spunk Fund, the National Alliance for Research in Schizophrenia and Affective Disorders (NARSAD), and the endowment fund of the Nancy Pritzker Laboratory.

I gratefully acknowledge the role of the many collaborators who carried out the research described here, in particular Drs. Donna Spiker, Joachim Hallmayer, Linda Lotspeich, Dona Wong, Helena Kraemer, and Luigi Cavalli-Sforza at Stanford University; Drs. Brent Petersen, William McMahan, Peter Nicholas, and Carmen Pingree of the University of Utah; and Dr. Edward Ritvo of the University of California, Los Angeles.

afflicted with autism, and nearly 4,000 American families have two or more autistic children. The direct cost of services utilized by autistic individuals exceeds $3 billion annually. Because the disorder usually strikes in infancy and autistic children live a normal life span, the social burden of autism is substantial.

Causes of Autism

Several nongenetic agents, including prenatal rubella or cytomegalovirus infection, have been implicated in the etiology of autism.[2] In addition, several metabolic and other genetic disorders also occur in association with autism. Although the exact causes of autism are unknown in most cases, studies in families and twins strongly support a genetic etiology, particularly in families in whom multiple cases occur.[3, 3a] The recurrence rate among siblings of autistic individuals is 2.7%, which is about 50 times higher than the risk in the general population.[1] In families with multiple autistic members, the recurrence risk for subsequent siblings is 8.6%, and the relative risk is greater than 200.[4] The concordance rate pooled across several twin studies is 64% in monozygotic twins and 9% in dizygotic twins.[1,5]

The mode of transmission of inherited cases of autism is unknown, but it does not appear to follow classical mendelian models. Among the factors that hinder the establishment of a clear mode of inheritance are the difficulty in identifying parental carriers of an autism gene, stoppage rules, and the confounding presence of nongenetic phenocopies.[2] In various reports, autosomal dominant, autosomal recessive, and mixed major locus and multifactorial modes of transmission have all been postulated.[1,6]

Linkage analysis with polymorphic DNA markers is currently the best available and most commonly used strategy for finding disease genes.[7,8] The high relative risk figures cited above for autism are quite favorable, making a linkage strategy feasible.[9] Several problems, however, must be considered in planning a linkage analysis. These include the presence of phenocopies, which are diagnostically indistinguishable from genetic cases and lead to misclassification errors; genetic heterogeneity (two or more genes may independently cause a disorder, but only one is responsible in any individual case); and polygenic inheritance (the additive action of two or more genes is required to cause the disorder in each individual). In linkage analysis, diagnostic accuracy and a correct assignment of both the affected and the unaffected phenotypes are essential. There has been considerable debate in the literature over what constitutes the autistic phenotype for genetic purposes and whether it should be strictly defined, that is, limited solely to autistic disorder or broadened to include related syndromes such as pervasive developmental disorder, Asperger's syndrome, and even cognitive and communication disturbances.[10–14] In contrast, there has been almost no consideration in the literature of how the unaffected phenotype should be defined.

Genetic heterogeneity in autism has not been studied and, in the absence of any identified gene or linkage marker, is a problem of unknown magnitude. Genetic heterogeneity can arise by mutation at different sites within a single gene locus (allelic heterogeneity) or by mutation in individual genes whose protein products subserve related functions (nonallelic or locus heterogeneity). Allelic heterogeneity is illustrated by Duchenne's muscular dystrophy, which arises from mutations toward the 5′ end of the dystrophin gene and is clinically severe. Mutations nearer the 3′ end of the dystrophin gene result in a clinically milder disease and were once thought to constitute a distinct syndrome called Becker's muscular dystrophy.

Cystic fibrosis, Lesch-Nyhan syndrome, and phenylketonuria are all examples of diseases that exhibit allelic heterogeneity. Phenylketonuria exhibits locus heterogeneity as well; the disease can be caused by mutation in the phenylalanine hydroxylase gene or in the gene for the enzyme tetrahydropteridine reductase, which is involved in the formation of the pterin cofactor essential to the phenylalanine hydroxylase reaction.[15,16] As the biochemical bases for more genetic diseases are uncovered, both types of genetic heterogeneity are increasingly likely to be observed. Unless otherwise specified, the term *genetic heterogeneity* usually refers to locus heterogeneity. Locus heterogeneity can be detected by linkage analysis, whereas allelic heterogeneity cannot.

X-Linked Inheritance and Autism

That autism predominantly affects males has long fueled speculation about sex-linked inheritance. This has been reinforced by the occurrence of autism in two X-linked disorders, Norrie's disease and fragile X syndrome. Among the genetic disorders associated with autism, fragile X mental retardation is the most common. The proportion of fragile X-positive cases among autistic individuals varies widely from study to study. Rates as high as 50% and as low as 0% have been reported.[12,17] These large discrepancies appear to be due to differences in ascertainment strategy, diagnostic criteria for autism, varying thresholds for the cytogenetic diagnosis of fragile X syndrome, and possibly variability in the diagnosis of autism among centers. To date, only one study has used a standardized instrument, the Autism Diagnostic Interview (ADI), to assess the occurrence of fragile X syndrome in an autistic sample.[18] In that study, a prevalence of fragile X syndrome of 2.7% was reported in a sample of 75 autistic individuals, whereas the prevalence was 0.1% in the general population.[19]

Autosomal Inheritance and Autism

A number of autosomal disorders, primarily single-gene metabolic diseases, have been associated with autism. Among these are phenylketonuria, tuberous sclerosis, adenylosuccinate lyase deficiency, histidinemia, and type II mucopolysaccharidosis. These associations are rare, however, and it is not possible to determine the percentage of cases of autism they comprise. Although autism occurs predominantly in males, most investigators have assumed that autosomal transmission predominates. There have been only a few linkage studies in autism, with no positive findings and no published studies using DNA markers. A recent report of an association of autism with the *h(ras)* locus on chromosome 11 has appeared, but linkage was not examined.[20]

The importance of finding genes responsible for autism lies in their value as diagnostic markers and in providing essential information about the regulation of brain development. In most cases, signs and symptoms of autism may be detected in infancy, but often the disorder cannot be diagnosed with confidence before 4–5 years of age. Brain development in children, however, is not complete until mid-childhood. Thus there is a substantial period during which therapeutic interventions could be made that might take advantage of the plasticity of the developing brain. A reliable and accurate biologic marker could be used to identify children at risk for autism prenatally or at birth if it were used in screening high-risk families. The same marker would be invaluable in helping determine the boundaries of the autistic phenotype. There is much debate, for example, about whether autistic children's siblings who exhibit communication or cognitive disabilities have a mild form of autism and whether these disabilities are part of an autistic spectrum. Similarly, there are important questions about whether the parents of autistic children have a subclinical form of the disorder that does not preclude their marrying and having children.[3,13,14] It is extremely difficult with currently available tools to prove that these are phenotypic variants of autism. Screening members of high-risk families for mutations in a gene responsible for autism would answer these questions.

Finally, there is much to be learned about normal and abnormal brain development, and a knowledge about the molecular structure and biologic function of a gene causing autism would be an invaluable tool in this effort. Some years ago, my co-workers and I put forth the hypothesis that autism reflects a disturbance in the terminal (neuritic differentiation) stages of brain development and that the genetic defect is in a protein involved in control of synaptic connectivity.[2,21,22] Identifying a gene responsible for autism would permit direct studies of its function in brain development in both humans and experimental animals.

Studies in the Genetics of Infantile Autism

Overview and Discussion of Major Issues

For the past 4 years, my colleagues and I have been recruiting families for our study of the genetics of infantile autism. In the process of designing and conducting this study, we have made a number of strategic decisions, many of which evolved as the study progressed. In many cases, these were informed by events in psychiatric genetics, some of which suggested that changes or even reversals in strategy were necessary. These strategies pertain to the following issues, which are briefly highlighted in the following sections and are expanded upon in the description of the results.

Multiplex families. The proportion of phenocopies to genetic cases of autism is unknown. Phenocopies could be an important confounding factor in a linkage analysis; we expected that these would more likely occur in families with a single autistic offspring than in multiplex families. For this reason, we have collected only multiplex families for our linkage study. Our target for this study is 200 multiplex families; we have already evaluated 48, and 92 families are enrolled who are awaiting assessment.

Selection of diagnostic instruments. In recent years, experience in psychiatric genetics indicates the importance of uniform, reliable, well-documented diagnoses collected "blinded" to related individuals. For our study, we chose two standardized instruments: the ADI[23] and the Autism Diagnostic Observation Schedule (ADOS).[24] The ADI is an investigator-based structured interview containing items designed to capture symptoms of autism in four areas: social interaction and behavior, language and communication, interests and daily routines, and age at onset. The interview is administered to the parent of the autistic individual and takes 2–3 hours to complete. The ADOS is a structured behavior observation instrument administered to the autistic child and takes 20–45 minutes to complete. After completing tasks designed to elicit social, language, and communication behaviors, the examiner rates the child on a number of rating scales.

The ADI is currently the best available instrument for use in a genetic linkage study for the following reasons:

- It is a structured interview with consistent questions about all the behaviors used to diagnose autism. This ensures consistency across interviewers who gather the diagnostic data. Furthermore, we can document the nature and reliability of data on individual types of clinical signs.
- It requires the interviewer to elicit specific examples from the parent or caregiver, which are then used to evaluate specific signs. Such an interviewing technique yields the most valid data because the interviewer rather than the parent makes the interpretation about the quality of the behavior.[25]
- It allows us to gather information systematically on both present and past signs and symptoms. The data from the 4- to 5-year-old period is used in the application of the diagnostic criteria. In this way, children who are evaluated at very different ages can still be compared on a common metric.
- It includes all the information on individual signs needed to apply the DSM-III-R[26] and ICD-10[27] criteria, as well as those proposed for inclusion in DSM-IV.[28]
- Both the ADI and the ADOS are easily videotaped. Thus, we can have a second or third diagnostician independently and blindly verify each assessment. This permits ongoing quality control of diagnoses and assessment of reliability on individual symptoms and on various diagnostic criteria.

The ADI scoring algorithm allows quantification of the data on the interview items for each of the 16 diagnostic criteria of autism in the ICD-10 system. Multiple interview items are summed to yield a score for each criterion, and the criteria scores within each of the four areas are then summed to yield a score for each. The diagnosis of autism is made if the child meets the prespecified cutpoint in all four areas.

Definition of affected status. There has been considerable discussion in the literature about the limits of the autistic phenotype, whether mild or subclinical forms exist, whether parents can be subclinically affected, and whether cognitive and communication disorders fall within the autistic spectrum.[12–14] On the basis of the data described here, we decided to use a strict definition of autism. An autistic individual is defined as one meeting ADI cutoffs in all four areas, and only autistic subjects are included in the linkage analysis. A multiplex family is defined as one having two or more members who meet full ADI definitions of autism. Subjects falling into an ambiguous or uncertain diagnostic category are excluded from the linkage analysis, even though they meet clinical definitions of syndromes related to autism (e.g., pervasive developmental disorder). This is a conservative strategy; it almost certainly excludes subjects and families with an autism genotype who express only a partial phenotype. However, we feel this approach minimizes misclassification errors, which have proven to be a major obstacle in psychiatric genetic studies.[29]

Definition of unaffected status. For linkage purposes, it is also important to correctly identify unaffected individuals. The term *unaffected* refers to an individual who does not possess an autism gene. Because this cannot be known, it is approximated by a lack of positive signs on assessment. We attempted to minimize inclusion of false-negatives by defining unaffected subjects as those below the ADI thresholds in all four areas of the instrument and by excluding ambiguous ("uncertain") cases from the linkage analysis. Although this reduced misclassification errors, it did not entirely eliminate them. The inability to specify unaffected status with certainty is a problem that can be avoided only by using an "affecteds-only" analysis, so this is also an important element in our strategy.

Linkage analysis. Linkage of polymorphic DNA markers to disease states has been an extremely powerful and successful tool for finding disease genes. Linkage analysis works best for single-gene disorders and requires the specification of genetic models. In the absence of heterogeneity, linkage can be detected with relatively small samples. Affecteds-only analysis is a nonparametric form of linkage analysis that does not rely on prespecified models of inheritance. This method is sensitive to heterogeneity and requires quite large sample sizes.[9] Affecteds-only analyses are becoming the method of choice for complex disorders, but their major limitation remains the need for a large sample size. We have chosen to employ both methods in our design. We are collecting multiplex autism families and carrying out a conventional linkage analysis, but we will also utilize an affecteds-only analysis when our sample reaches an appropriate size (about 100 families).

Recruitment and Evaluation of Multiplex Families

To determine an optimal sample size for this study, we carried out several simulations testing different models of major locus transmission ranging from autosomal dominant with varying estimates of penetrance to autosomal recessive (see Table 6–10). The power calculations suggested that, in the absence of genetic heterogeneity, 40 families would be sufficient to detect linkage to a major autism locus. We set a target sample size of 200 families because 1) 200 families will allow us to detect linkage if heterogeneity due to as many as four independent genes is present, 2) our simulations suggest that 200 families is an adequate number for affecteds-only analyses with moderate genetic heterogeneity, and 3) we have modeled autism as a monogenic disorder. However, there are compelling arguments to consider oligogenic models. The likelihood of detecting a contributing gene by linkage analysis in oligogenic inheritance depends on the number of genes involved and the overall contribution each makes. Larger sample sizes are more likely to lead to the identification of such genes, although if more than three additive genes are required for autism, 200 families may still be an insufficient number.

Recruitment methods. We recruited families through newsletter advertising, referral from other autism researchers or clinicians, and national lectures and meetings. We also sought subjects by screening 5,000 families in the national registry of over 14,000 families compiled by Dr. Bernard Rimland at the Autism Research Institute in San Diego. To date, we have identified 140 presumptively multiplex families who have consented to participate in the study and have completely evaluated and confirmed the multiplex status of 48. Based on the results described here, we expect that about 15% of families recruited for the study will not meet our criterion of having two ADI autistic members. Therefore, we expect to evaluate 230 families to obtain a multiplex sample of 200.

Initial screening procedures. For a family to be eligible for the study, a qualified clinician must have determined that at least two children in the family are autistic, and those diagnostic records must be available for our review. Our preliminary eligibility screening consists of a telephone interview with a parent to explain the nature of the study, to obtain background information on the family members, to verify the presence of records that confirm a clinical diagnosis of autism in at least two children, and to determine availability for the diagnostic assessments. Diagnostic and medical records as well as written consents to participate are obtained before diagnostic appointments are scheduled. Families are excluded from the linkage study if any member has a disorder known to be associated with autism, such as fragile X syndrome, Norrie's syndrome, neurofibromatosis, phenylketonuria, or tuberous sclerosis. (Families whose autistic children have these disorders are retained in the data base for later evaluation and inclusion in other studies.) Families with monozygotic autistic twins are identified during recruitment and enrolled for inclusion in other studies.

Diagnostic instruments. All referred families who give informed consent and who meet the eligibility criteria are seen for evaluations. Almost all the data collection takes place in hospitals, clinics, or schools; a few assessments were conducted in subjects' homes. Parents, usually the mothers, are interviewed with the ADI about each child in the family. Children under age 17 years also receive the ADOS.[24] The diagnosis of autism (affected) is made if the child meets the prespecified cutpoint in all four areas of the ADI. We classify children who meet some but not all four cutpoints as uncertain, whereas children meeting none of the cutpoints are classed as not autistic (unaffected). All diagnostic evaluations are videotaped for review by additional, blinded evaluators.

Blindness in diagnoses. The mathematical basis of linkage analysis assumes conditional independence of phenotypes within a family. It is also conditional on independence of errors in diagnosis and genotyping. Blindness is therefore important in the design of linkage studies.[30] To achieve the greatest possible blinding of evaluators, different interviewers are used whenever possible for each child in a family. We have achieved this in 73% of families with two affected children, whereas in larger families independent interviews for all children were achieved 21% of the time. The ADOS was administered, by either the ADI interviewer or another trained person, after the ADI was completed. The ADI interviewers do not have access to other clinical records or other family members' ADI data when administering or scoring a given ADI.

Intelligence test scores are obtained from existing school or clinical records. Nonverbal or performance IQ scores are used when available; otherwise, full-scale IQ scores are used to classify children as mentally retarded (IQ < 70) or nonretarded (IQ > 70).

Fragile X syndrome and cytogenetic testing. All autistic children are tested for the fragile X mutation, as described in the following section. The presence of cytogenetic abnormalities has been described in autism, although no consistent abnormalities have been noted. We conduct chromosome analyses on one affected proband from each of our multiplex families. So far, 37 autistic children have been investigated. In one child we found a centromeric translocation on chromosome 3. The parents, as well as an affected cousin, showed no cytogenetic abnormalities, however. This subject, then, represents a de novo translocation, and the association may be coincidence. No other defects have been found. Because a chromosomal defect could be invaluable in locating a gene involved in autism, we will continue to screen one affected member from each family.

Initial Results

We have conducted several studies to answer specific questions about designing a genetic study and to test particular hypotheses. The results of our diagnostic assessments on the first 44 families are described in the following section and by Spiker et al.[31] These families reside in California, Utah, Florida, Michigan, Illinois, Indiana, Maryland, and New Hampshire. Fifteen of these families participated in the UCLA-University of Utah Epidemiologic Survey.[4,32]

Comparison of Referral and ADI Diagnoses

There has been much discussion in the literature about the use of chart or referral diagnoses in psychiatric genetic studies. In genetic studies, it may be difficult and costly for the research team to examine every subject. To what extent can the evaluations done by professionals outside the study be used in linkage analyses? To assess this question, we compared our ADI diagnoses with the clinical diagnoses carried out by our referring sources (Table 6–1, A and B). The referral diagnosis of autism matched the ADI diagnosis in 90 of 97 cases (sensitivity = 0.93) and in 32 of 44 nonautistic cases (specificity = 0.73). We excluded seven presumptively multiplex families (15%) because one child in the subject pair met all ADI cutpoints but the other did not. In each case, this latter sibling was classified as uncertain. In most cases he or she would have been given a clinical diagnosis of pervasive developmental disorder not otherwise specified, a category many autism researchers believe is a part of the autistic syndrome. Although these families are excluded from the linkage analysis, data from them is retained in the data base for future studies. They are not included in the figures cited in Table 6–1.

These data are of interest in several respects. They suggest that there is good agreement in classifying children as autistic but poor agreement in identifying nonautistic, or unaffected, subjects. There was a tendency by our referring sources to overestimate the number of autistic subjects. Similarly, 12 children referred as unaffected ex-

Table 6–1A. Relationship between presumptive (referral) diagnosis and ADI diagnosis for children in presumed autism multiplex families (N = 44 families)

			Presumptive diagnoses	
Stanford ADI diagnoses	***N***	**Autistic**	**Nonautistic**	**Uncertain**
Autistic	90	90	0	0
Nonautistic	32	0	32	0
Uncertain	20	7	12	1
Total	142	97	44	1

Table 6–1B. Relationship between referral diagnosis and ADI diagnosis for children in strictly defined multiplex families (N = 37 families)

			Presumptive diagnoses	
Stanford ADI diagnoses	***N***	**Autistic**	**Nonautistic**	**Uncertain**
Autistic	83	83	0	0
Nonautistic	26	0	26	0
Uncertain	8	0	7	1
Total	117	83	33	1

Table 6–1A shows the relation between the referral diagnosis and ADI diagnosis for all 44 families. Table 6–1B provides the same information after seven families who had one but not two autistic children were excluded. Numbers in parentheses are the referral diagnoses for subjects in each diagnostic category.

ceeded one or more ADI cutpoints and were classed by us as uncertain. It is particularly clear that a presumptive assessment of unaffected cannot be accepted without confirmation. We concluded from these data that it is necessary for our research team to carry out its own diagnostic assessments.

The distribution of children among these three groups is also of interest. At the outset of this work, we hypothesized that ADI analysis of all children in multiplex families would yield a broad distribution of phenotypes, spanning more or less a continuum from unaffected to affected, without clear breakpoints. We expected to find a large group of children falling into an ambiguous, or uncertain, phenotype. This was of great concern to us, because such a phenotypic distribution would present a severe challenge to a linkage analysis. The data, however, demonstrated that children were either autistic (71%) or nonautistic (22%), with only a small uncertain group. These proportions were not greatly affected by excluding the 7 families who were not strictly multiplex; taking all 44 families, the autistic group was 63%, the nonautistic group was 22%, and the uncertain group was 14% of all children.

Clinical Characteristics of Autism Multiplex Families

Table 6–2 shows the ages, sexes, and family sizes of the 37 autism multiplex families. Thirty-three (89%) of the families had two autistic children, two had four, and two had five. Fifteen families (40.5%) had no nonautistic children. Thirty-four of the families were white, and three were black.

Table 6–2. Ages, sex, and family size in 37 autism multiplex families

Diagnosis	Age (years) Mean ± SD	Age (years) Median	Sex Male *n*	Sex Female *n*	Male-to-female ratio
Autistic (*N* = 83)	13.6 ± 9.2	11	59	24	2.45
Nonautistic (*N* = 26)	16.2 ± 9.9	14	14	12	1.16
Uncertain (*N* = 8)	13.8 ± 6.9	13	3	5	0.60

No. of autistic children per family (total no. of families)	No. of nonautistic children per family: 0	1	2	3	4	5	6
2 (33)	14	10	5	3	0	0	1
4 (2[a])	1	1	0	0	0	0	0
5 (2)	0	1	1[b]	0	0	0	0

[a]Includes one family with four autistic children, two of whom are monozygotic twins.
[b]One child in this family died at age 18 months.

Clinical Characteristics of Autistic, Unaffected, and Uncertain Groups

The next set of studies was aimed at further defining the affected and unaffected phenotypes. There is general consensus that an autistic spectrum exists, with variation both in severity and clinical expression.[33,34] If this is true, then who in a linkage study should be included as affected? Authors of numerous studies have attempted to define the boundaries of the autism phenotype. Classically autistic subjects, those meeting criteria for pervasive developmental disorder, as well as those with developmental language disorders, have all been included in the definition of affected in various studies.[3,11,12,14,18]

Table 6–3 shows the ADI area scores by diagnostic status and indicates that autistic children can be readily distinguished from the other two groups. Children in the nonautistic group showed some overlap with the uncertain group when their median and range scores were examined. However, nonautistic children were below the ADI cutoffs in all areas, whereas children in the uncertain group met one or more ADI cutoffs.

From the data in Table 6–3, we concluded that a conservative or strict definition of autism is best used to define affected status, because autistic subjects can be clearly delineated from the other two groups. Because the uncertain group is very small, it is best treated as "unknown" and excluded from linkage analysis. The loss of power resulting from this is modest, and the risk of false-positive classification is minimized. Accordingly, we consider only those children who meet all ADI criteria as affected, and we conduct the linkage analysis only on the autistic and nonautistic groups.

Characteristics of Unaffected Siblings in Autism Multiplex Families

We next sought to examine further the unaffected phenotype by studying the clinical characteristics of the 26 nonautistic siblings. The ADI area scores for this group are shown in Table 6–4. Although

Table 6–3. ADI area scores for children in autism multiplex sibling families

ADI area	Autistic (n = 83 in 37 families)	Nonautistic (n = 26 in 22 families)	Uncertain (n = 8 in 6 families)
Social total			
Range	17–44	0–9	0–14
Median	36	1	1.5
Language total[a]			
Verbal			
No. of children	58	26	8
Range	11–29	0–8	0–7
Median	21	0.5	0
Nonverbal			
No. of children	25	0	0
Range	9–16	—	—
Median	15	—	—
Ritual total			
Range	3–12	0–2	0–4
Median	8	0	1.5
No. (%) onset present[b]	83 (100)	0 (0)	6 (75)

Note. N = 37 families, 117 children. Social cutpoint = 12, range = 0–44. Language cutpoint for verbal subjects = 10, range = 0–30; cutpoint for nonverbal subjects = 8, range = 0–16. Rituals cutpoint = 3, range = 0–12.
[a]Verbal = having phrase speech by age 5 years; nonverbal = not having phrase speech by age 5 years.
[b]Meets onset criteria; developmental delays or deviance before age 3 years.

we judged this group both clinically and by the ADI area scores as being nonautistic, there were a few slightly elevated but still subthreshold scores.

These observations indicate that there is no empirical reason to consider the nonautistic children as anything other than unaffected. However, some caution may be warranted. Rutter and Schopler,[33] Folstein and Piven,[3] and others have observed the occurrence of cognitive and communication disorders in the siblings of

Table 6–4. Distributions of ADI area scores for nonautistic children in autism multiplex sibling families

Area score	Total ADI score [N (%)]		
	Social	**Language**	**Rituals**
0	6 (23.1)	13 (50.0)	21 (80.8)
1	9 (34.6)	5 (19.2)	4 (15.4)
2	4 (15.4)	3 (11.5)	1 (3.8)
3	2 (7.7)	0 (0)	
4	1 (3.8)	2 (7.7)	
5	2 (7.7)	2 (7.7)	
6	1 (3.8)	0 (0)	
7	0 (0)	0 (0)	
8	0 (0)	1 (3.8)	
9	1 (3.8)	0 (0)	
Total	26	26	26

Note. N = 22 families, 26 children. Social cutpoint = 12, range = 0–44. Language cutpoint for verbal subjects = 10, range = 0–30; cutpoint for nonverbal subjects = 8, range = 0–16. Rituals cutpoint = 3, range = 0–12.

autistic individuals.[3,12,13,14] Because these individuals often exhibit deficits in reciprocal social interactions in later life, it has been proposed that cognitive and communication disorders in families with one or more autistic members reflect a mild form of autism and that all share a common genotype.

We did not evaluate the siblings or other family members of our autistic probands for cognitive or communication disorders, so although we can say that they are not autistic, we cannot say they are unaffected, that is, that they lack an autism gene. Thus, there remains the possibility that "nonautistic" and "unaffected" are not synonymous. By defining autistic and nonautistic as we have and excluding the uncertain group from the linkage analysis, we can minimize false-negative errors, but the problem can be avoided only by an affecteds-only analysis. Therefore, our plan is to collect a sufficient number of families to allow such an analysis. We will begin this analysis when the sample size reaches 100; in the interim, we are carrying out a conventional linkage strategy as well.

Characteristics of Uncertain Siblings in Autism Multiplex Families

The data in Table 6–3 suggest that children in the uncertain group were more like their nonautistic than their autistic siblings. To examine this further, we studied the individual ADI area scores. Table 6–5 shows the ADI area scores for the eight children in six families who were classified as uncertain because they met one or more, but not all, of the ADI cutpoints. One of these (identification no. 258-3) was referred to the study with an uncertain diagnosis; the remainder were considered unaffected by their referring source. Five met only the ADI cutpoint for age at onset, indicating that parents or professionals identified some developmental problem, usually language delays or behavioral irritability, before the subject was 3 years of age. Two subjects met only the ADI cutpoint for ritualistic behaviors. One (no. 258-3) met the social, rituals, and age-at-onset cutpoints and also had language deficits but with a subthreshold score. This child would be given the clinical diagnosis of pervasive developmental disorder not otherwise specified. It is clear from this analysis that the uncertain category is itself heterogeneous. There is no justification

Table 6–5. ADI scores for uncertain cases

Subject ID	Age (years)	Sex	Verbal type	Total ADI area scores: Social	Language	Rituals	Onset[a]
258-3	3	Male	V	12	7	4	Yes
337-2	20	Female	V	2	1	3	No
337-7	10	Female	V	0	0	3	No
381-2	26	Female	V	5	0	1	Yes
346-3	14	Female	V	3	1	0	Yes
346-4	12	Male	V	1	0	2	Yes
328-4	15	Female	V	0	0	0	Yes
265-3	10	Male	V	0	0	0	Yes

Note. Siblings of autistic subjects who were classed as "uncertain" shown here. Social cutpoint = 12, range = 0–44. Language cutpoint = 10 for verbal subjects, range = 0–30; cutpoint = 8 for nonverbal subjects, range = 0–16. Rituals cutpoint = 3, range = 0–12. V = verbal, NV = nonverbal status on ADI: presence versus absence of phrase speech by age 5 years.
[a]Meets onset criteria: developmental delays or deviance <3 years.

for including it as part of the affected group, and there may be some danger in including it as part of the unaffected group. We have concluded that the best strategy for dealing with this small group is to exclude it from the linkage analysis.

Linkage Studies

Immortalizing Lymphocytic Cell Lines

Blood samples are obtained from all available family members at the time of evaluation, shipped to Stanford by Federal Express, and transformed immediately upon arrival. Lymphoblast cell lines for restriction fragment length polymorphism (RFLP) and polymerase chain reaction (PCR) analysis are established using a slightly modified protocol by Anderson and Gusella.[35] To date, blood has been drawn from 371 individuals.

X Linkage and Autism

The preponderance of males among autistic individuals supports the possibility of X-linked inheritance. We are examining two hypotheses concerning X-linkage in autism: linkage to the fragile X locus and linkage to a locus elsewhere on the X chromosome.

Fragile X Syndrome and Autism

Approximately 2.7% of autistic children exhibit the cytogenetic defect fragile X syndrome.[18] The molecular biology of the fragile X site has now been well established, and a candidate gene (*FMR-1*) responsible for the phenotype has been isolated.[36,37] The vast majority of fragile X subjects have an amplification of a $(CGG)_n$ trinucleotide repeat that occurs in the 5′-untranslated region of the *FMR-1* transcript, as detected by either Southern blotting or PCR analysis.[38] Males in whom the $(CGG)_n$ repeat is greater than 600 base pairs (bp) almost invariably show clinical and cytogenetic expression of the disease.

In individuals with fragile X syndrome, extreme cytogenetic and phenotypic variability are the rule. Males have been found who have both an expanded CGG repeat and who show the fragile X phenotype clinically, yet are cytogenetically normal.[39] Amplification of the CGG repeat has been detected in individuals who did not show any signs of the fragile X phenotype either cytogenetically or clinically.[40] Finally, subjects have been described who had neither an amplification of the CGG repeat nor a fragile site by cytogenetic methods, but who had clinical manifestation of the fragile X phenotype. In these individuals, molecular analysis of the *FMR-1* gene showed a deletion within the *FMR-1* gene in one case[41] and a point mutation in another.[42]

A tenable hypothesis to emerge from the preceding observations is that autism is a variant of fragile X syndrome in which the usual phenotypic and cytogenetic manifestations may be absent. This could arise in one of the following ways:

- An increase in the CGG repeat in the *FMR-1* gene, which for unknown reasons is not expressed in the usual cytogenetic or phenotypic fashion, but which instead exhibits the clinical features of autism
- A mutation elsewhere in the fragile X site that does not involve the CGG repeat
- A deletion of segments of both the FMR-1 gene and an unknown neighboring gene that is involved in autism

A deletion spanning both genes would lead to both autism and fragile X syndrome. The null hypothesis is that autism and fragile X syndrome are unrelated and their co-occurrence is simply coincidental; it may be related to the mental retardation that characterizes both syndromes.[43]

These hypotheses are amenable to testing with existing methodologies, and we have examined two of them in our studies to date. Testing them requires exclusion of families with cytogenetic or phenotypic evidence of fragile X syndrome. We studied 35 of the 37 multiplex families described previously (blood from two other families was not available at the time this study was conducted). To test the hypothesis that a mutation in the CGG region in the *FMR-1* gene is involved in the etiology of familial autism, we examined the size of the CGG repeat in 79 autistic children from these families. To examine the possibility of a mutation elsewhere in the *FMR-1* gene, we carried out a linkage analysis for autism, using microsatellite markers that are tightly linked to the *FMR-1* gene.[44]

Southern Blot Typing of the CGG Repeat in *FMR-1*

Blood was drawn from 208 children, their parents, and, if available, their grandparents. Lymphoblastoid cell lines were established as described by Anderson and Gusella,[35] with minor modifications. DNA was extracted according to the protocol of Steffen and Weinberg.[45] Samples containing 5 μg of genomic DNA were digested overnight with the restriction enzymes *Eag*I and *Eco*RI, as described by Rousseau et al.[46] Restriction fragments were separated by electrophoresis on 1% agarose gels for 16 hours at 1–1.5 V/cm. Lambda phage-derived size markers were included in one lane to permit sizing of the fragments. After the DNA was denatured with sodium hydroxide and neutralized for 1 hour, the DNA was transferred to nylon filters by the method of Southern.[47] The probe StB12.3 was radiolabeled with [^{32}P]adenosine triphosphate (specific activity = 3,000 Ci/mMol; Amersham Corp.) by the oligolabeling method[48] for 5 hours. The filters were prehybridized in 50% formamide, 5× SSPE (150 mM sodium chloride, 10 mM sodium phosphate, 1 mM EDTA [ethylenediaminetetraacetic acid], disodium salt), 1× Denhardt's solution overnight at 42°C and hybridized for 24 hours with 0.6–2.0 $\times 10^7$ cpm of labeled probe. After being washed, filters were exposed to film (Kodak XAR-5) with intensifying screens (DuPont Lightning Plus) at −70°C for 3 and 14 days.

Using the *Eco*RI/*Eag*I double digest allows us to analyze both amplification of the CGG repeat and methylation of DNA.[46] When DNA from unaffected individuals is digested with *Eco*RI/*Eag*I and probed with StB12.3, one or two bands are typically seen. Females show characteristic 5.2- and 2.8-kb bands, the 5.2 band arising from the failure of *Eag*I to cut DNA from the methylated (inactive) X chromosome, and the 2.8 kb band from the nonmethylated (active) X chromosome. Males show a single 2.8-kb band. The analysis of methylation is useful to distinguish between large premutations without clinical expression and small full mutations. Premutations in males are detected by an increase in size of the unmethylated fragment by 70 to about 500 bp. In females, premutations give a very distinctive four-band pattern that is easily detected. Full mutations are generally in the range of 1–3 kb and are rarely missed.

In none of the subjects examined did we detect any increase in the size of the 2.8- or 5.2-kb fragment. All females showed the expected 5.2- and 2.8-kb band pattern, whereas males showed only the 2.8-kb band. Fragile X-positive control subjects (received from the Cytogenetics Laboratory at Stanford University Medical Center) could easily be detected by an increase in the size of the fragment. Thus, we found no molecular evidence for the occurrence of fragile X syndrome in this sample of autistic children.

Linkage to *FMR-1*

To study the linkage of autism to *FMR-1*, we used two highly polymorphic markers. DXS548 is known from physical mapping to be 150 kb away from *FMR-1*; no recombination of this marker and the *FMR-1* locus has been described. FRAXA1 is located within the *FMR-1* complementary DNA (cDNA), about 5 kb from the 5′ end of the gene. Three families were excluded from linkage analysis; these consisted of affected cousin pairs in which father-to-son transmission was evident on inspection of the pedigrees. We carried out genotyping on 177 individuals, including 74 autistic children and 22 unaffected children. For the statistical analysis, autism was treated as an X-linked dominant trait. Because the penetrance of the disease gene is unknown, calculations were carried out with four different penetrance values (Table 6–6). The affected status of the parents was considered unknown in all models. Individuals with the diagnosis "uncertain" were omitted from the calculations. Linkage analysis was carried out with the software package LINKAGE.[49] Two-point analysis was performed with the program MLINK.

Two-point lod scores between the DXS548 probe or the FRAXA1 probe and autism for the 32 families are shown in Tables 6–7 and 6–8. In all four genetic models, linkage between the fragile X locus and autism could be excluded with high confidence for at least Θ = 0% and Θ = 5% recombination. The multipoint analysis for both markers for each family is shown in Table 6–9.

Conclusions

We found no evidence to support the hypothesis of a $(CGG)_n$ amplification in individuals with autism. It is thus unlikely that an unusual variant of fragile X syndrome accounts for even a minor fraction of the genetic cases of autism. We also did not find evidence for premutations in the *FMR-1* gene in any subject. The techniques we

Table 6–6. Genetic models used to calculate lod scores

Model	Penetrance: Male	Penetrance: Female	Gene frequency
1	0.80	0.13	0.000375
2	0.50	0.083	0.0006
3	0.30	0.05	0.001
4	0.10	0.016	0.003

Note. Autism was treated as an X-linked dominant disease. The male penetrance values were fixed, and the female penetrances were calculated based on a male-to-female ratio of 3:1. Gene frequencies were calculated assuming a prevalence of autism of 4/10,000.

Table 6–7. Two-point lod scores between autism and DXS548

	Recombination fraction					
Male	0.00	0.05	0.10	0.20	0.30	0.40
Model 1	–30.520	–5.899	–3.251	–1.069	–0.258	–0.022
Model 2	–26.936	–5.472	–2.925	–0.887	–0.171	–0.008
Model 3	–24.393	–5.349	–2.870	–0.857	–0.154	–0.011
Model 4	–19.877	–5.532	–2.983	–0.912	–0.176	–0.006

Table 6–8. Two-point lod scores between autism and FRAXA1

	Recombination fraction					
Male	**0.00**	**0.05**	**0.10**	**0.20**	**0.30**	**0.40**
Model 1	−22.733	−4.790	−2.879	−1.205	−0.453	−0.103
Model 2	−20.839	−4.716	−2.834	−1.190	−0.450	−0.103
Model 3	−19.163	−4.722	−2.844	−1.199	−0.454	−0.104
Model 4	−15.760	−4.707	−2.850	−1.207	−0.459	−0.106

Note. The following primers were chosen to amplify the region containing the CA repeat DXS548:[54] RS46-CA1 24 (5′–3′) AGA GCT TCA CTA TGC AAT GGA ATC; RS46-CA2 24 (5′–3′) GTA CAT TAG AGT CAC CTG TGG TGC. The primer sequences for the locus FRAXA1[55] were as follows: FRAXA.PCR1.1 28 (5′–3′) GAT CTA ATC AAC ATC TAT AGA CTT TAT T and FRAXA.PCR1.2 25 (5′–3′) AGA TTG CCC ACT GCA CTC CAA GCC. T polymerase chain reactions[3a] were carried out in a 25-μl volume containing 75 ng of human genomic DNA as template, 200 μM each dGTP and dTTP, 5 μM each dATP and dCTP, 2 μCi each α[^{35}S]dCTP (Amersham Corp.) and α[^{35}S]dATP (Amersham Corp.), 50 mM KCl, 10 mM Tris, 1.5 mM $MgCl_2$, and 1 U of *Taq* polymerase (Boehringer Mannheim Corp.). For specific amplification of the FRAXA1 CA repeat, a higher $MgCl_2$ concentration of 5.5 mmol was required. After an initial denaturation step of 5 minutes at 94°C, samples were overlaid with mineral oil and amplified in 25 temperature cycles consisting of 1 minute at 94°C, 1 minute at 60°C (62°C for FRAXA1), and 1 minute at 72°C. Four microliters of the amplified product was mixed with formamide sample buffer and analyzed on a 6% denaturing polyacrylamide sequencing gel. Samples were electrophoresed at 80 W for 2 and 3 hours, dried without fixation, and exposed to XAR film (Kodak) overnight at room temperature with no intensifying screen. Genotype assignments were done by investigators who were blinded to the affected status of the subjects.

applied should detect most premutations, although we cannot entirely exclude small premutations in females. The results of our genotyping analysis are in agreement with those of cytogenetic studies in autistic children from simplex families.[50]

We also used linkage analysis to examine the hypothesis that a mutation lies elsewhere within the *FMR-1* region. From the multipoint analysis for both these markers, we could unequivocally rule out linkage in 12 families, whereas 14 families were uninformative for both markers. Five had slightly positive lod scores, and one was slightly negative. Tests for heterogeneity with the program HOMOG[8] were negative. Because the overall lod scores for the two probes

Table 6–9. Multipoint lod scores for DXSA548 and FRAXA1 in individual multiplex families

Family no.	DXS548	FRAXA1	DXS548/FRAXA1
1	–3.125	–3.125	–3.125
2	–3.125	0.000	–3.125
3	–3.125	–3.125	–3.125
4	–3.250	0.000	–3.250
5	0.000	0.000	0.000
6	0.000	0.000	0.000
7	0.000	0.000	0.000
8	–0.176	0.000	–0.176
9	0.725	0.000	0.725
10	0.000	0.000	0.000
11	–3.125	–3.125	–3.125
12	0.000	0.000	0.000
13	0.000	0.000	0.000
14	0.000	–3.125	–3.125
15	0.176	0.000	0.176
16	0.000	0.000	0.000
17	–3.301	0.222	–3.301
18	0.000	0.000	0.000
19	–0.033	0.301	0.229
20	0.523	0.000	0.523
21	0.000	0.000	0.000
22	0.119	0.000	0.119
23	0.000	0.000	0.000
24	–2.223	0.000	–2.223
25	0.000	–3.426	–3.426
26	0.000	0.000	0.000
27	0.000	0.000	0.000
28	0.000	0.000	0.000
29	0.000	0.000	0.000
30	–4.204	–4.204	–4.204
31	–3.125	–3.125	–3.125
32	–3.250	0.000	–3.250

Note. Lod scores for linkage analysis between DXS548/FRAXA1 and autism in 32 multiplex families are shown. Calculations were carried out for model 1 at a recombination fraction of 0%.

were highly negative, it is likely that linkage to *FMR-1* can be ruled out in multiplex families, although the possibility remains that a small (about 10%) number of families might show linkage, so additional families and probes will be tested.

Autism and X Linkage

To test the hypothesis that autism is associated with other genes located on the X chromosome, we have been carrying out a linkage analysis examining other X markers. We have just begun this study and are planning to type 20 markers in the 32 families. We expect to have completed this study by the end of this year.

Testing for Linkage to Autosomal Markers: Genotyping

The molecular basis for RFLPs is usually a difference of a single nucleotide between individuals, leading to the creation or deletion of a restriction enzyme site. Another type of polymorphism results from differences in the number of repeats of short oligonucleotide sequences. The human genome contains many sequences of the type $(CA)_n$, where n is usually between 10 and 60.[51] Variability in the length of the dinucleotide repeat makes these sequences much more polymorphic than RFLPs. Polymorphic trimeric and tetrameric repeats are also found in the human genome. Such differences in the number of short sequences (often called microsatellites) can be detected by polyacrylamide gel electrophoresis after amplification by PCR. It is estimated that there are up to 500,000 microsatellite repeats distributed throughout the human genome, with an estimated average spacing of about 7,000 bp. In the last 2 years, microsatellite maps covering nearly the whole human genome have been established.[52] Because of their high heterozygosity, microsatellite markers have become the preferred type of polymorphism for carrying out linkage analysis.

Recently the CA repeat technique has been automated with single dye-labeled primers and a fluorescent-based detection system. This has the advantage of eliminating the costs and biohazards of radioactivity and radioactive waste disposal, which have become considerable in the past few years. By using this technique, we can analyze up to 12 different loci in a single lane with discrimination based on either size or color. We are currently testing combinations of loci to increase even further the number of loci combined in one lane. An internal size standard ladder is included in each lane and allows automatic sizing of alleles. This also eliminates lane-to-lane and gel-to-gel comparison differences.

So far, we have analyzed 30 loci in the members of 34 families by using the automated technology. We have typed another 60 RFLP or CA markers in subsets of these families. In CA typing, one primer of each set is fluorescein labeled at the 5′ terminus. The labeled oligonucleotide is purified in our laboratory by reverse-phase chromatography. The purified product is quantified by ultraviolet spectrometry. PCR reactions[38] are carried out in a 12.5-μl volume containing 100 ng of human genomic DNA as template, 200 nM oligonucleotide primer each, 200 μM each deoxyguanosine triphosphate (dGTP) and deoxythymidine triphosphate (dTTP); deoxyadenosine triphosphate (dATP) and deoxycytidine triphosphate (dCTP), 50 mM KCl, 10 mM Tris [tris(hydroxymethyl)aminomethane], 1.5 mM $MgCl_2$, and 0.5 U of *Taq* polymerase. Samples are amplified in a Perkin Elmer Cetus System 9600 thermocyler for 25 temperature cycles consisting of 10 seconds at 95°C, 60 seconds at 55°C, and 75 seconds at 72°C. For certain primer pairs, the cycling conditions have to be adapted. Between 0.1 and 1 ml per reaction is loaded onto a 6% polyacrylamide-bisacrylamide, 7 M urea, and 0.04% TEMED (*N*, *N*, *N*′, *N*′-tetramethylethylenediamine) DNA sequencing gel. To keep the loading volume per lane small, aliquots of several reaction products are mixed and ethanol precipitated before loading. Fluorescent products are automatically detected and quantified with the ABI 373A-DNA sequencer. The readings are analyzed with the GENESCAN 672 microsatellite software package.

Testing of Models and Calculating Lod Scores

In the absence of a defined mode of inheritance for a complex disorder, Risch et al.[53] proposed carrying out an exploratory linkage analysis testing several different models. We have tested five linkage models: two dominant, one recessive, and two intermediate models (Table 6–10). For the purely recessive model, the penetrance for homozygous males was set at 80%, and for the two dominant models, we assumed 80% and 20% penetrance for the male heterozygotes. Two intermediate dominant models were defined with penetrance values for the male heterozygotes of 5% and 1.25% and for the male homozygotes of 80% and 80%. The male penetrances were fixed according to the specified model. Calculations of gene frequencies were based on an assumed prevalence of autism of 4/10,000. Penetrances for females were calculated according to a male-to-female ratio of autism of 3:1.

Table 6–10. Genetic models defined for the calculations of lod scores

Model	Genotype	Penetrances		Gene frequency
		Male	Female	
Recessive	aa	0.00	0.00	A: 0.0224
	Aa	0.00	0.00	a: 0.9776
	AA	0.80	0.26	
Intermediate				
I	aa	0.00	0.00	A: 0.0117
	Aa	0.0125	0.004	a: 0.9883
	AA	0.80	0.26	
II	aa	0.00	0.00	A: 0.0039
	Aa	0.05	0.02	a: 0.9610
	AA	0.80	0.26	
Dominant				
I	aa	0.00	0.00	A: 0.0010
	Aa	0.20	0.07	a: 0.9990
	AA	0.80	0.80	
II	aa	0.00	0.00	A: 0.0005
	Aa	0.80	0.27	a: 0.9995
	AA	0.80	0.80	

Note. Male penetrances were fixed, and female penetrances were calculated assuming a male-to-female ratio of autism of 3:1, based on data from 28 multiplex families. Gene frequencies were calculated based on a frequency of autism of 4/10,000.

Results

We began the project by systematically typing entire chromosomes. To date, we have generated exclusion maps for chromosomes 9, 14, and 7. We have also carried out extensive RFLP typings on chromosomes 13, 9, and 15. The lod scores so far are negative for all models calculated and for all markers. We have thus excluded approximately 15% of the genome from linkage to autism. The most highly negative lod scores are calculated under the recessive model. Concurrent testing for heterogeneity has not disclosed any to date.

References

1. Smalley SL, Asarnow RF, Spence A: Autism and genetics: a decade of research. Arch Gen Psychiatry 45:953–961, 1988
2. Lotspeich LJ, Ciaranello RD: The neurobiology and genetics of infantile autism. Int Rev Neurobiol 35:87–129, 1993
3. Folstein SE, Piven J: Etiology of autism: genetic influences. Pediatrics 87:767–773, 1991
3a. Smalley SL: Genetic influences in autism. Psychiatr Clin North Am 14:125–139, 1991
4. Ritvo ER, Freeman BJ, Pingree C, et al: The UCLA-University of Utah epidemiologic survey of autism: prevalence. Am J Psychiatry 146:194–199, 1989
5. Steffenburg S, Gillberg C, Hellgren L, et al: A twin study of infantile autism in Denmark, Finland, Iceland, Norway, and Sweden. J Child Psychol Psychiatry 30:405–416, 1989
6. Jorde LB, Hasstedt SJ, Ritvo ER, et al: Complex segregation analysis of autism. Am J Hum Genet 49:932–938, 1991
7. Cavalli-Sforza LL, King MC: Detecting linkage for genetically heterogeneous diseases and detecting heterogeneity with linkage data. Am J Hum Genet 38:599–616, 1986
8. Ott J: Analysis of Human Genetic Linkage, Revised Edition. Baltimore, MD, Johns Hopkins University Press, 1991, pp 203–215
9. Risch N: Linkage strategies for genetically complex traits, III:

the effects of marker polymorphism on analysis of affected relative pairs. Am J Hum Genet 46:242–253, 1990

10. Wing L: Language, social and cognitive impairments in autism and severe mental retardation. J Autism Dev Disord 11:31–44, 1981
11. Wing L: The continuum of autistic characteristics, in Diagnosis and Assessment in Autism. Edited by Schopler E, Mesibov GB. New York, Plenum, 1988, pp 91–110
12. Bolton P, Rutter M: Genetic influences in autism. International Review of Psychiatry 2:67–80, 1990
13. Piven J, Gayle J, Chase GA, et al: A family history study of neuropsychiatric disorders in the adult siblings of autistic individuals. J Am Acad Child Adolesc Psychiatry 29:177–183, 1990
14. Piven J, Chase GA, Landa R, et al: Psychiatric disorders in the parents of autistic individuals. J Am Acad Child Adolesc Psychiatry 30:471–478, 1991
15. Sugita R, Takahashi S, Ishii K, et al: Brain CT and MR bindings in hyperphenylalaninemia due to dihydropteridine reductase deficiency (variant of phenylketonuria). J Comput Assist Tomogr 14:699–703, 1990
16. Takashima S, Chan F, Becker LE: Cortical dysgenesis in a variant of phenylketonuria (dihydropteridine reductase deficiency). Pediatr Pathol 11:771–779, 1991
17. Payton JB, Steele MW, Wenger SL, et al: The fragile X marker and autism in perspective. J Am Acad Child Adolesc Psychiatry 28:417–421, 1989
18. Piven J, Gayle J, Landa R, et al: The prevalence of fragile X in a sample of autistic individuals diagnosed using a standardized interview. J Am Acad Child Adolesc Psychiatry 30:825–830, 1991
19. Webb TP, Bundey SE, Thake A, et al: The frequency of fragile X among schoolchildren in Coventry. J Med Genet 23:396–399, 1986
20. Herault J, Perrot A, Barthelemy C, et al: Possible association of c-Harvey-Ras-1 (HRAS-1) marker with autism. Psychiatry Res 46:261–267, 1993
21. Ciaranello RD, VandenBerg SR, Anders TF: Intrinsic and extrin-

sic determinants of neuronal development: relations to infantile autism. J Autism Dev Disord 12:115–146, 1982
22. Rubenstein JLR, Lotspeich L, Ciaranello RD: The neurobiology of developmental disorders, in Advances in Clinical Child Psychology. Edited by Lahey BJ, Kazdin AE. New York, Plenum, 1990, pp 1–52
23. Le Couteur A, Rutter MCL, Rios P, et al: Autism diagnostic interview: a standardized investigator-based instrument. J Autism Dev Disord 19:363–387, 1989
24. Lord C, Rutter M, Good S, et al: Autism Diagnostic Observation Scale: a standardized observation of communicative and social behavior. J Autism Dev Disord 19:185–212, 1989
25. Payne SL: The Art of Asking Questions. Princeton, NJ, Princeton University Press, 1951
26. American Psychiatric Association: Diagnostic and Statistical Manual of Mental Disorders, 3rd Edition, Revised. Washington, DC, American Psychiatric Association, 1987
27. World Health Organization: International Classification of Diseases, 10th Edition. Geneva, Switzerland, World Health Organization, 1992
28. American Psychiatric Association: Diagnostic and Statistical Manual of Mental Disorders, 4th Edition. Washington, DC, American Psychiatric Association, 1994
29. Ciaranello RD, Ciaranello AL: Genetics of major psychiatric disorders, in Annual Review of Medicine. Edited by Creger WP, Coggins CH, Hancock EW. Palo Alto, CA, Annual Review, 1991, pp 151–158
30. Kraemer HC: Evaluating Medical Tests: Objective and Quantitative Guidelines. Newbury Park, CA, Sage Publications, 1992
31. Spiker D, et al: The genetics of autism: characteristics of affected and unaffected children from 37 multiplex families. Submitted for publication
32. Ritvo ER, Jorde LB, Mason-Brothers A, et al: The UCLA–University of Utah epidemiologic survey of autism: recurrence risk estimates and genetic counseling. Am J Psychiatry 146:1032–1036, 1989
33. Rutter M, Schopler E: Classification of pervasive developmental

disorders: some concepts and practical considerations. J Autism Dev Disord 22:459–482, 1992

34. Szatmari P: The validity of autistic spectrum disorders: a literature review. J Autism Dev Disord 22:583–600, 1992
35. Anderson MA, Gusella JF: The use of cyclosporin A in establishing EBV-transformed lymphoblastoid cell lines. In Vitro 11:856–858, 1984
36. Oberlé I, Rousseau F, Heitz D, et al: Instability of a 550-base pair DNA segment and abnormal methylation in fragile X syndrome. Science 252:1097–1102, 1991
37. Verkerk AJMH, Nelson DL, Sutcliff JS, et al: Identification of a gene (FMR-1) containing a CGG repeat coincident with a breakpoint cluster region exhibiting length variation in fragile X syndrome. Cell 65:905–914, 1991
38. Saiki RK, Bugaswan TL, Horn GT, et al: Analysis of enzymatically amplified β-globin and HLA-DQalpha DNA with allele-specific oligonucleotide probes. Nature 324:163–166, 1986
39. Tarleton J, Wong S, Schwartz C: Direct analysis of the FMR-1 gene provides an explanation for an exceptional case of a fragile X negative, mentally retarded male in a fragile X family. J Med Genet 29:919–920, 1992
40. Macpherson JN, Nelson DL, Jacobs PA: Frequent small amplifications in the FMR-1 gene in fra(X) families: limits to the diagnosis of premutations. J Med Genet 29:802–806, 1992
41. Gedeon AK, Baker E, Robinson H, et al: Fragile X syndrome without CCG amplification has an FMR1 deletion. Nat Genet 1:341–344, 1992
42. De Boule K, Verkerk AJMH, Reyniers E, et al: A point mutation in the FMR-1 gene associated with fragile X mental retardation. Nat Genet 3:31–35, 1993
43. Fisch GS: Is autism associated with the fragile X syndrome? Am J Hum Genet 43:47–55, 1992
44. Hallmayer J, Pintado E, Lotspeich L, et al: Exclusion of linkage between the fragile X gene and familial autism. Submitted for publication.
45. Steffen D, Weinberg RA: The integrated genome of murine leukemia virus. Cell 15:1003–1010, 1978

46. Rousseau F, Heitz D, Biancalna V, et al: On some technical aspects of direct DNA diagnosis of the fragile X syndrome. Am J Med Genet 43:197–207, 1992
47. Southern EM: Detection of specific sequences among DNA fragments separated by gel electrophoresis. J Mol Biol 98:503–517, 1975
48. Feinberg AP, Vogelstein B: A technique for radiolabeling DNA restriction endonuclease fragments to high specific activity. Anal Biochem 132:6–13, 1983
49. Lathrop GM, Lalouel JM: Easy calculations of lod scores and genetic risk on small computers. Am J Hum Genet 36:460–465, 1984
50. Einfeld S, Hall W: Behavior phenotype and the fragile X syndrome (editorial). Am J Med Genet 43:56–60, 1992
51. Weber DE, May PE: Abundant class of human DNA polymorphisms which can be typed using the polymerase chain reaction. Am J Hum Genet 44:388–396, 1989
52. Weissenbach J, Gyapay G, Dib C, et al: A second-generation linkage map of the human genome. Nature 359:794–801, 1992
53. Risch N, Claus E, Giuffra L: Linkage and mode of inheritance in complex traits, Genetic Analysis Workshop 6: Proceedings of a Workshop held at Gulf Park. Edited by Elston RC. Long Beach, MS, October 10–12, 1988

CHAPTER

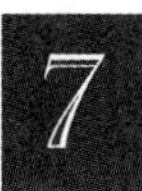

Epidemiology and Behavioral Genetics of Schizophrenia

Ming T. Tsuang, M.D., Ph.D., D.Sc., F.R.C.Psych.
Stephen V. Faraone, Ph.D.

To the clinician and researcher alike, schizophrenia is a paradoxical disorder. Although a clinically heterogeneous illness, it defies subclassification. Patients with schizophrenia exhibit extreme dysfunctions in perception, thinking, behavior, and emotions; nevertheless, the cerebral source of these anomalies has remained elusive. It has been known for some time that genes play a role in the etiology of schizophrenia, but the search for specific mutations has been frustrated by diagnostic dilemmas. Despite these problems, the past two decades have witnessed great strides in the diagnosis and treatment of this disorder. In this chapter, we describe the epidemiological and ge-

Preparation of this chapter was supported in part by Grants 1 R01MH41879-01, 5 UO1 MH46318-02, and 1 R37MH43518-01 from the National Institute of Mental Health to Ming T. Tsuang and by the Veterans Administration's Medical Research, Health Services Research and Development, and Cooperative Studies Programs.

netic work that has facilitated scientific and clinical progress and that promises someday to yield the secrets of the etiology of this disorder.

Epidemiology

Psychiatric epidemiology is the study of the distribution of disorders in well-defined populations. Its goal is to identify risk factors that explain why some populations are at higher risk for psychiatric illness than others. To attain this goal, three fundamental questions are asked:

1. How many people from a well-defined population will be diagnosed with an illness at a specified point or period in time (i.e., what is the prevalence)?
2. How many people from the population will experience onset of the illness during a specified period of time (i.e., what is the incidence)?
3. What proportion of the population will develop the disorder at some time during their entire lifetime (i.e., what is the lifetime prevalence)?

Prevalence Rate

The *prevalence rate* of a disorder is the number of people diagnosed with the disorder divided by the total number of persons examined in the population under study. The computed rate depends on several factors: the definition of the disorder, the total number examined in the population, and the method used to choose who to examine. Ideally, the sample used to compute prevalence should be representative of the population as a whole.

Epidemiologists usually report the prevalence rate as the number of cases per 1,000 people surveyed within a year. This is called the *one-year prevalence per 1,000*. Many studies of schizophrenia from around the world have found these rates to range from a low of 0.6 per 1,000 to a high of 17 per 1,000. Most studies find rates between 3 and 10 per 1,000.[1–4]

The prevalence rates for schizophrenia do not depend on any obvious demographic differences among countries. Whether we consider east or west, developed countries or less developed countries, or other classifications, the 1-year prevalence of schizophrenia is approximately 0.5%. In other words, schizophrenia is found in approximately one-half of 1% of the population at any point in time. The highest prevalence (17 per 1,000) was reported from a Swedish sample in 1978.[5] The population studied lived in northern Sweden; it is isolated from the rest of the country and located in a bleak, austere environment. The high prevalence there might indicate that such environments are suitable, and even attractive, for the socially withdrawn and isolated life-style of many schizophrenic patients.

Incidence Rate

Another way of reporting the rate of schizophrenia in a population is to estimate the number of new cases to appear in the population during a specified period of time; this is called the *incidence rate*. Prevalence rates (as discussed previously) include both new and old cases because once schizophrenia has emerged, it usually runs a chronic, unremitting course. Thus, once patients are classified as schizophrenic, they usually remain schizophrenic.

One problem faced in studies of the incidence of schizophrenia is how to define the onset of the illness. In many cases, its onset is slow, starting with subtle signs of social withdrawal and unusual thinking or behavior. Because the time of onset is difficult to determine, reported incidence rates are usually based on a patient's first visit to psychiatric services for schizophrenic symptoms.

The incidence rate is usually expressed as the number of new cases in a given period per 100,000 population. For schizophrenia, incidence rates range from a low of 0.10 to a high of 0.70.[6,7] As is the case for prevalence figures, the incidence of schizophrenia is not highly variable over time or across geographical areas.

Lifetime Risk

Most schizophrenic individuals first become ill between ages 20 and 39 years. We call this the "high-risk period" for schizophrenia. Men tend to be younger than women at the time of onset.[8] Due to the variability of age at onset, prevalence and incidence rates vary according to the age and sex composition of the population studied. The age distribution is particularly important when estimating the probability or risk of a person becoming schizophrenic throughout his or her lifetime. We call this the *lifetime risk*. To estimate lifetime risk, the age distribution of the population surveyed should be taken into account. A variety of statistical methods are available for this purpose.[9]

The lifetime risk for schizophrenia ranges from 0.3% to 3.7%, depending on the definition of schizophrenia and the method of survey used.[6,7] Taken together, studies of the lifetime risk for schizophrenia in the general population suggest that it is around 1%. In other words, approximately 1 in every 100 people will develop a schizophrenic disorder at some time in their life.

Risk Factors

Schizophrenia has been found in all cultures throughout the world. When differences among countries have been observed, these are usually due to diagnostic differences, not differences in true rates of illness. For example, in the 1960s, a team of U.S. and British researchers set out to determine why the incidence of schizophrenia in hospitals the United States (28.0 per 100,000 population) significantly exceeded that of Great Britain (17.9 per 100,000 population). In British hospitals, mood disorders were diagnosed much more often than in U.S. hospitals (36 versus 7 per 100,000). The U.S.-U.K. project was begun to determine the source of these differences.[10] This project showed that when identical methods of diagnosis and assessment were used, the incidence of schizophrenia did not differ significantly between U.S. and British hospitals.

Authors of epidemiological studies have found that schizophrenic patients usually belong to lower socioeconomic groups.[11]

Because low social class is associated with many disadvantages, such as poor nutrition and limited access to health care, researchers set out to determine whether economic deprivation increased the risk for schizophrenia. This work suggests that the excess of schizophrenic individuals in the lowest socioeconomic group is a result, not a cause, of schizophrenia.[12,13] Because the disease hampers educational and occupational attainment, schizophrenic patients born to families in a high social class tend to fall in social status, and those born into economic hardship seldom escape it. For example, Goldberg and Morrison[14] found that the social class distribution of the fathers of schizophrenic individuals did not differ from that of the general population. Male schizophrenic patients tended to have lower job achievement than did fathers, brothers, and other male relatives. Whereas fathers tended to rise in job status, schizophrenic sons tended to fall into jobs of lower and lower status or to become disabled. Thus, it appears that, although low socioeconomic status is known to have deleterious effects, it is primarily an effect of schizophrenia rather than its cause.

Gender differences in schizophrenia have received a good deal of attention.[15] Among schizophrenic individuals, men have an earlier age at onset and poorer premorbid history. Women are more likely to display affective symptoms, paranoia, and auditory hallucinations. They are less likely to have the negative symptoms of schizophrenia.

The gender differences in schizophrenic symptomatology make it difficult to determine whether rates of the disorder vary by gender. Goldstein[15] concluded that recent studies indicate a higher incidence for males than females. There also appears to be a higher prevalence among males, but both assertions are tentative because many epidemiological studies have not rigorously addressed the issue of gender in schizophrenia.

Family Studies

It is convenient to divide family studies of schizophrenia into those completed before and after the advent of structured diagnostic criteria. Many of the earlier studies were completed by European investigators in the first half of the 20th century. A review of these early studies[16] showed that the risks for schizophrenia in relatives of schizophrenic probands were 5.6% for parents, 10.1% for siblings, and 12.8% for offspring. Notably, the risk for parents is less than that for siblings, but under any genetic model these risks should be the same. The difference occurs because, by definition, parents have reproduced, and the presence of schizophrenia has an adverse affect on the probability of doing so. In the early studies, the risks to second-degree relatives ranged from 4.2% for half-siblings to 2.4% for uncles and aunts. First cousins, a type of third-degree relative, had an average risk of 2.4%.

Kendler[17] pointed out that the early family studies of schizophrenia usually did not include a control group that would allow the comparison of rates within a single study. In these studies, the rates observed in the family study were compared with data from other studies on rates of schizophrenia in the general population. Differences in diagnostic practices across studies, however, make it difficult to interpret such findings. In addition, many of the early studies provided no description of how diagnoses were assigned. We do not know whether diagnoses were based on interview, records, or informants. Another methodological problem was the potential lack of blindness on the part of diagnosticians. If the diagnoses of relatives were made by individuals who were aware of the probands' diagnosis, diagnostic decisions may have been biased.

Recent studies in which more rigorous research methods and narrower, criterion-based definitions of schizophrenia have been used are also consistent with the genetic hypothesis. However, they report risk figures that are somewhat lower than those seen in earlier studies. Tsuang et al.[18] reported the risk of schizophrenia to first-degree relatives of schizophrenic individuals to be 3.2%, whereas the risk for relatives of nonpsychiatric control subjects was 0.6%. Guze et al.[19] reported comparable figures of 3.6% and 0.56%, respectively. In both studies, the increased risk for schizophrenia among relatives of schizophrenic individuals remained statistically significant despite the lower prevalence figures.

In modern family studies of schizophrenia, the reported rates of schizophrenia in relatives are approximately one-third of those found in the earlier European studies. This difference is probably due to differences in diagnostic procedures. For example, the figure of 3.2% obtained by Tsuang et al.[18] when using stringent Washington University criteria increases to 3.7% when DSM-III[20] criteria are applied. It increases to 7.8% when the category of schizophrenia is broadened to include individuals with atypical schizophrenia (e.g., schizoaffective disorder or psychosis not otherwise specified). Thus, as Faraone and Tsuang[21] noted, the risk figures for schizophrenia based on modern criteria are similar to those obtained by the earlier European studies when atypical cases are included.

The exclusion of cases of atypical schizophrenia from family studies may also explain why two modern family studies failed to find familial transmission in schizophrenia. Pope et al.[22] found no cases of schizophrenia among first-degree relatives of their schizophrenic probands. Abrams and Taylor[23] found the risk for schizophrenia to be only 1.6% among 128 first-degree relatives of schizophrenic individuals. Although certain methodological problems may explain these results,[24] it is also possible that they are due to diagnostic practices.

Despite the caveats noted, contemporary figures as well as those reported in earlier studies suggest that the risk for schizophrenia in first-degree relatives of schizophrenic patients exceeds the observed rate in the general population by 5 to 10 times. Thus, it is reasonable to conclude that schizophrenia is a familial disorder. Because environmental factors can cause familial transmission, however, twin and adoption studies must be examined to verify a genetic hypothesis of familial transmission for schizophrenia.

Twin Studies

There are two types of twins: monozygotic (MZ) and dizygotic (DZ). MZ twins have identical genes. DZ twins are as genetically alike as ordinary brothers and sisters; they share only half of each other's genes. In a twin pair, if both have schizophrenia, they are said to be "concordant" for schizophrenia; if one is schizophrenic and the other is not, they are said to be "discordant." The concordance rate is usually expressed as the percentage of concordant pairs out of a total number of pairs of twins in which one is reported to be schizophrenic. The concordance rate assesses the probability that a twin has schizophrenia, given that his or her co-twin is known to have schizophrenia.

If genes were entirely responsible for causing schizophrenia, the concordance rates for MZ and DZ twins would be 100% and 50%, respectively. A significantly higher concordance rate for schizophrenia in MZ than in DZ twin pairs would be strong evidence that a genetic component of schizophrenia exists. On the other hand, if schizophrenia were entirely due to environmental factors, there would be no difference between the concordance rates of monozygotic and dizygotic twin pairs.

Kendler[25] pooled the results of twin studies from different parts of the world and found concordance rates of about 53% for MZ twin pairs and 15% for DZ twin pairs. This is solid evidence that schizophrenia has a hereditary component. However, the fact that the concordance rate for MZ twin pairs is not 100% indicates that environmental factors also play a crucial role in the etiology of schizophrenia. When concordance rates are translated into "heritabilities" (the proportion of the liability to schizophrenia due to genetic factors), 70% of the variance is attributed to genetic factors. Thus, there is a substantial role for environmental factors in the expression of schizophrenia.

Several possibilities exist. Some forms of schizophrenia may be caused completely by environmental factors, such as birth complications or viral infection. Alternatively, it may be that all cases of schizophrenia require a genetic susceptibility that is expressed in only some environmental circumstances.

A nongenetic explanation for the higher concordance in MZ than in DZ twin pairs is that the former are exposed to more similar environmental factors than are the latter. This hypothesis can be tested by looking at twins at birth who are raised in different environments. A high concordance rate for MZ twin pairs reared apart would refute the theory that sharing the same predisposing environment leads to the higher concordance rate in MZ twin pairs. Seventeen such MZ twin pairs have been observed;[16] 11 (65%) were concordant for schizophrenia. Although not conclusive, this strengthens the hypothesis that both genes and environment play a causal role in the development of schizophrenia.

Adoption Studies

Like twin studies, adoption studies can also disentangle genetic and environmental sources of etiology. Essentially, adoption studies are carried out to determine whether biological or adoptive relationships explain the familial transmission of disease. Heston[26] examined 47 children who had been separated from their biological, schizophrenic mothers within 3 days of birth. These children were raised by adoptive parents with whom they had no biological relationship. This author also examined a control group of 50 persons who had been separated from nonschizophrenic mothers. Both groups studied were adults at the time of examination. If genes caused schizophrenia, then the biological children of schizophrenic mothers should have a higher risk for schizophrenia, regardless of who raised them as children. In contrast, if the parenting relationship caused schizophrenia, then separating children from a schizophrenic parent should prevent them from having schizophrenia. Heston's results supported a genetic etiology of schizophrenia: five children of schizophrenic mothers became schizophrenic, whereas none of the children of nonschizophrenic mothers became schizophrenic.

Kety et al.[27] carried out adoption studies of schizophrenia in Denmark. In the Greater Copenhagen area, 5,500 children had been separated from their biological families by adoption between 1923 and 1947. Of these children, 33 who later became schizophrenic were studied, along with 33 nonschizophrenic adoptees. The investigators examined the biological relatives of these schizophrenic and nonschizophrenic adoptees. They diagnosed 21% of the biological relatives of schizophrenic adoptees with schizophrenia or a related disorder. In contrast, only 11% of the biological relatives of nonschizophrenic individuals had schizophrenia. There were no differences between the rates of schizophrenia in the adoptive relatives of the schizophrenic and nonschizophrenic adoptees. One component of this study was similar to the study by Heston.[26] Children born to schizophrenic families but raised by nonschizophrenic families were compared with children born to and raised by nonschizophrenic parents. Schizophrenia and related disorders were found in 32% of the former group but in only 18% of the latter group.

The sample used by Kety et al. also included some persons who had been born to nonschizophrenic parents but raised by a schizophrenic parent. If being reared by a schizophrenic parent caused schizophrenia, then these persons should be likely to develop schizophrenia. This was not the case, however; being raised by a schizophrenic parent did not predict schizophrenia in children who were not genetically predisposed to the disorder (i.e., who did not have a schizophrenic biological parent).

These adoption studies show that genetic factors mediate the transmission of schizophrenia. However, these studies also have some limitations. Most important, although the adopted children had been separated from their mothers soon after birth, they had spent 9 months in the mother's uterus. During that time, the mother could have transmitted to the fetus some nongenetic biological or psychosocial factor that might have resulted in the child's schizophrenia 15 years later.

Fortunately, the Danish researchers could examine whether or not in utero influences might have explained their results. Kety et al.[27] found that 13% of paternal half-siblings of schizophrenic adoptees had schizophrenia, whereas only 2% of paternal half-siblings of nonschizophrenic adoptees had the illness. Paternal half-siblings have different mothers, so these results cannot be explained by in utero effects. Indeed, the fact that a higher rate of schizophrenia was found among these half-siblings from the father's side than in the half-siblings of the control subjects is compelling evidence for the genetic basis of schizophrenia.

Mathematical Models of Genetic Transmission

Although family, twin, and adoption studies have conclusively shown that genes play a role in the etiology of schizophrenia, it has been difficult to clearly define the mechanism of genetic transmission. Several possibilities exist. At one extreme, it may be that a mutation in a single gene causes schizophrenia. At the other extreme, there is the possibility that many genes act in combination with one another and with the environment to cause the illness. The transmission of genes obeys known biological laws, and these laws have a clear mathematical description. It is therefore theoretically possible to use the results of family, twin, and adoption studies to determine whether one, several, or very many genes are the cause of schizophrenia.

It is clear that a classic mendelian model of inheritance will not adequately describe the genetic transmission of schizophrenia. For example, if schizophrenia were caused by a fully penetrant dominant gene (penetrance is defined as the probability that an individual with the genotype will actually express the trait of interest), one would expect that 50% of the offspring of one schizophrenic parent would become schizophrenic. The observed value, however, is much lower. If schizophrenia were caused by a fully penetrant recessive gene, one would expect that 100% of the children of two schizophrenic parents would become schizophrenic. The observed value, however, is 36.6%. Thus, more complex models are needed to describe the genetic transmission of schizophrenia. Quantitative or mathematical modeling studies provide a strategy for doing so. Such studies are discussed briefly in this section. (For details, see the review by Faraone and Tsuang.[28])

Single major locus (SML) models propose that the pair of genes present at a single locus is responsible for the transmission of schizophrenia. Results of SML analyses have not consistently supported single-gene transmission. SML models accurately predict the prevalence in the general population, the prevalence in offspring of schizophrenic parents, and the incidence in siblings of schizophrenic individuals. However, segregation analyses that provide statistical tests of model adequacy rule out single-gene transmission. Those that cannot rule out the model note that the risks to MZ twins and the offspring of two schizophrenic parents are under-predicted by the SML model. The negative statistical results are compelling, but the rejection of a genetic model may merely indicate that some of the nongenetic assumptions of the model are not correct.

An innovative approach to the modeling of single-gene disorders was suggested by Matthysse et al.[29] and Holzman et al.[30] Its foundation lies in a statistical technique known as *latent structure analysis*. The model assumes the existence of a latent trait that is not directly observable and, depending on its site of involvement in the brain, can cause schizophrenia or other phenotypic manifestations. It is hypothesized that the latent trait displays mendelian transmission, whereas the observable traits (e.g., schizophrenia and schizotypal personality disorder) do not necessarily conform to such a genetic pattern.

Matthysse et al.[29] have suggested that schizophrenia and smooth-pursuit eye movement dysfunctions may be transmitted as independent phenotypic manifestations of a single latent trait (i.e., a gene). Applying the latent structure model to two different samples (a Chicago-Boston sample of the parents of psychotic probands and a Norwegian sample of the offspring of discordant MZ and DZ twins), the authors concluded that smooth-pursuit eye movement dysfunctions and schizophrenia might be considered expressions of a single underlying trait that is transmitted by an autosomal dominant gene. Their results were not definitive, however, because even the latent-trait model cannot account for the risk to MZ twins and the risk to children of two schizophrenic parents.[31] Nevertheless, the work of Matthysse et al.[29] indicates that the addition of neurobiological assessments to psychiatric studies of schizophrenic families may be useful in finding genes that predispose certain individuals to developing schizophrenia.

The failure to find an SML model that unequivocally accounts for the familial transmission of schizophrenia has led to the testing of polygenic models. When these models are used, it is assumed that genes found at more than one locus are responsible for the familial pattern of the disorder. There are two types of polygenic models.

Oligogenic models postulate a relatively limited number of loci (e.g., fewer than 10), whereas multifactorial polygenic (MFP) models propose a large, unspecified number of loci (e.g., more than 100).

Studies in which SML and oligogenic models were compared have shown no dramatic differences between the abilities of the two models to account for the familial transmission of schizophrenia. Furthermore, the oligogenic models are similar to the SML model in predicting that most individuals with the schizophrenic genotype will not develop schizophrenia. Simulation studies by Risch[32] suggest that multilocus models that include gene interactions may be needed to account for the familial pattern of illness in schizophrenia.

Unlike oligogenic models, MFP models do not specify the number of loci involved in schizophrenia. Instead they assume that there are many interchangeable loci and that genes at these loci have small, additive effects on an individual's predisposition for developing schizophrenia. This model assumes that all individuals have some unobservable "liability" or predisposition to develop schizophrenia. Gottesman and Shields[16,33] noted five points in favor of MFP models:

1. Like other MFP disorders, schizophrenia is found with various degrees of severity.
2. The risk for schizophrenia is greater for persons with many schizophrenic relatives than for persons with few schizophrenic relatives.
3. A person's risk for schizophrenia increases as a function of the severity of a schizophrenic relative's illness.
4. Nonschizophrenic individuals from the schizophrenia spectrum can be conceptualized as having a liability close to, but not exceeding, the threshold for schizophrenia.
5. MFP disorders are expected to respond slowly to natural selection.

Furthermore, the MFP model is more adequate than the SML model if, as is the case for schizophrenia, concordance in MZ twins is substantially greater than that in DZ twins. Thus, the results of twin studies of schizophrenia are consistent with the MFP model.

Overall, the results from the MFP model are more promising than those from the SML model. In particular, results of path analytic MFP studies support the hypothesis that schizophrenia is, to a large extent, a disorder with a mostly genetic multifactorial etiology. Under this model, genetic factors account for 60%–70% of the familial pattern of schizophrenia. Environmental factors are important to a much lesser degree. Overall, the results suggest that the MFP model deserves serious consideration. These results cannot rule out, however, the possibility of a mixed model in which an SML component and an MFP component both exist. Attempts to fit such a mixed model, however, have not been able to determine the mode of transmission.[34,35]

Linkage Analysis

The frustration of scientists unable to describe the mechanism of transmission of schizophrenia was initially relieved during the 1980s by rapid developments in the laboratory science of molecular genetics. These developments made it possible for schizophrenia researchers to use a better methodology, known as linkage analysis, for finding genes. Although it had been theoretically possible to find genes with linkage analysis for several decades, these new developments made such progress feasible. In fact, with the molecular genetic technologies currently available, there is no question that it is possible to find the genes responsible for many disorders. The list of disorders for which there is already an identified genetic source grows every year. This list includes Huntington's disease, Alzheimer's disease, cystic fibrosis, Duchenne's muscular dystrophy, myotonic dystrophy, familial colon cancer, von Recklinghausen neurofibromatosis, and mental retardation due to fragile X syndrome.

The biological events that occur when gametes are created provide the foundation for linkage analysis. Most crucial in this regard is the crossing-over of chromosomes. Due to crossing-over, an individual's chromosomes are not identical to any of the original chromosomes of his or her parents. When gametes are formed, the original chromosomes in each parent's pair cross over each other and exchange segments of their DNA. After crossing-over, the resulting two chromosomes each consist of a combination of genes that differs from each of the original parental chromosomes. It is said that two genetic loci *recombine* when they are separated by an odd number of crossovers. Two loci are *linked* when, due to their physical proximity, they are not separated by crossing-over. If two loci are very far apart, the probability of an odd number of crossovers between them is equal to the probability of an even number. As a result, the probability of recombination is 50%. Therefore, genes on the same chromosome that are very far apart from one another are transmitted independently, as are genes on different chromosomes.[36]

With linkage analysis, it can be determined whether a putative disease gene is closely linked to a known genetic marker. A genetic marker is a measurable human trait controlled by a single gene with a known chromosomal location. The marker must be polymorphic (i.e., more than one version of the gene exists with high frequency), and its mode of inheritance must be known. In early linkage studies, genetically controlled traits were used as genetic markers. Examples include color blindness, blood groups, enzymes, proteins, and systems such as human leukocyte antigen that control immune response. Such markers, however, are relatively rare. Linkage analysis became a powerful tool when molecular geneticists developed methods to define DNA markers throughout the genome.

An early example of a DNA marker is the restriction fragment length polymorphism (RFLP).[37] Restriction endonucleases cut DNA into pieces. The locations of the cuts are determined by the sequence of the nucleotides in the DNA. There are four nucleotides: adenine (A), guanine (G), cytosine (C), and thymine (T). For example, the restriction endonuclease known as *Alu*I cuts DNA between the nucleotides guanine and cytosine wherever the nucleotide sequence AGCT occurs. The size of the resulting fragments is determined by the particular sequence of base pairs in the gene. Because these fragments can be measured in the laboratory, family members can be classified according to the length of the fragment that results from cutting their DNA with *Alu*I. Today, RFLPs are being replaced by new DNA markers that are easier to assess and, because they have greater variability, are more powerful for linkage analysis.

The statistical methods of linkage analysis capitalize on both the occurrence of crossing-over and the availability of polymorphic genetic markers. They seek to compute a statistic indicating the probability that the cosegregation of genetic markers and disease within pedigrees exceeds what would be expected from the play of chance alone.

In the 1980s, the potential for finding schizophrenia genes caused much excitement in scientific circles. Indeed, some preliminary findings implicated a gene on chromosome 5. Interest in chromosome 5 was initially motivated by the report of a single family in which two cases of schizophrenia each had a distinct abnormality of this chromosome.[38]

After that report appeared, Sherrington et al.[39] studied seven British and Icelandic families with schizophrenic members in at least three generations. Using the new molecular genetic technologies to track the inheritance pattern of schizophrenia in these families, these investigators demonstrated genetic linkage to the part of chromosome 5 that had been previously implicated in schizophrenia. Taken together, these two findings suggested that a schizophrenia gene would be found.

Unfortunately, other linkage studies could not replicate this linkage finding, and some clearly excluded the chromosome 5 locus as being involved in schizophrenia.[40–45] What can we make of these conflicting results? Some argued that, if more than one gene can cause schizophrenia, then both the positive and the negative findings could be correct. As increasing numbers of studies fail to find linkage to chromosome 5, however, it becomes more reasonable to conclude that the original positive finding may be a false result due to the play of chance. This now seems likely, given that the group that produced the original finding of linkage found that evidence for it diminished when they extended their original sample.[46]

Recent data implicated a pseudo-autosomal locus in the etiology of schizophrenia. The pseudo-autosomal region is a small portion of the Y chromosome that crosses over with the X chromosome during meiosis. Because this genetic region exhibits crossing-over as if it were an autosome rather than a sex chromosome it is called *pseudo-autosomal*. If a gene from the pseudo-autosomal region causes schizophrenia, we would expect the following pattern of sex-specific transmission: Pairs of siblings with schizophrenia should be more likely to have the same sex if the father is schizophrenic, but no such sex concordance would be expected if the mother is schizophrenic. Because this pattern was found among schizophrenic families, the pseudo-autosomal region was proposed to be the locus for a schizophrenia gene.[47] Support for the pseudo-autosomal hypothesis was found by Collinge et al.,[48] who used the linkage analysis method of affected sibling pairs. They reported a significant linkage between schizophrenia and a pseudo-autosomal telomeric locus among 83 sibships with two or more members with schizophrenia or schizoaffective disorder. Unfortunately, other investigators have excluded linkage to the pseudo-autosomal region.[49]

A similar situation is seen for studies of linkage to chromosome 22. Pulver et al.[50] reported a potential linkage to chromosome 22. The finding was not statistically significant but might have indicated a gene that accounted for only a small proportion of schizophrenia. Two other groups found evidence consistent with this finding,[51,52] yet a second sample reported by Pulver et al.[53] excluded linkage to chromosome 22 loci.

A number of issues remain unresolved. One important problem is whether schizophrenia is a single disorder or is genetically heterogeneous. If schizophrenia is genetically heterogeneous, it may prove very difficult to elucidate the relevant genetic mechanisms. One heterogeneity model that has received some support is the familial/sporadic approach, which suggests that some cases of schizophrenia are primarily or exclusively genetic and some are primarily or exclusively of environmental etiology.[54–56] Another unresolved issue is the boundary of phenotypic expressions of the schizophrenia genotype.[57–59] The existence of symptom-free MZ co-twins of schizophrenic probands suggests that one possible outcome of a schizophrenia genotype is an unaffected phenotype.

Finding genes responsible for genetically complex illnesses like schizophrenia is a new challenge for both geneticists and mental health researchers. The many problems that arise in such studies are receiving close attention by ongoing linkage studies of schizophrenia supported by the National Institute of Mental Health and the Department of Veterans Affairs (in the United States) and the European Science Foundation (in Europe). Moreover, many independent investigators are collecting samples of schizophrenic pedigrees suitable for linkage analysis.[41,43,50,60–67]

It may be that previous attempts to detect linkage to schizophrenia have failed due to the use of relatively small samples. It is difficult to determine exactly how many pedigrees of what size would be needed to detect linkage, but there is a consensus in the literature that the detection of schizophrenia genes will require very large samples. Computing an exact number requires us to know the mode of inheritance of the gene and the degree of genetic heterogeneity. Because both of these factors are unknown, attempts to assess statistical power can be only suggestive, not definitive. Goldin and Gershon[68] calculated the number of schizophrenic sib pairs needed to detect linkage. Their autosomal dominant model assumed a population prevalence of 1%, no genetic heterogeneity, and no phenocopies (subjects without the pathogenic gene who develop the disease). Under these conditions, 50 pairs achieved 80% power when the DNA marker was located at the pathogenic gene, whereas 120 pairs achieved 80% power for a value when it was more distant. These power calculations, however, were based on a significance level of .05; this is much less stringent than the traditional linkage significance cutoff of 3, which is approximately equal to .001.[36] If the .001 significance level is used, the number of affected sib pairs needed increases by about 1.7-fold.[68] Thus 200 sib pairs (400 individuals), rather than 120 pairs (240 individuals), would be needed to achieve 80% power when the DNA marker is not located exactly at the pathogenic gene. Risch[32] computed similar results.

Chen et al.[69] assessed the statistical power for linkage studies of schizophrenia by simulating schizophrenia pedigrees. In these simulations, the known demographic, epidemiologic, and familial features of the disorder were used to create pedigrees that one would expect to ascertain in a linkage study of schizophrenia. They then evaluated the power of the pedigrees using simulation methodology. They assumed that penetrance was incomplete (0.189) and age dependent, 16% of cases were phenocopies, and DNA markers were moderately informative. Their results indicated that, when 50% of pedigrees were linked, 1,600 individuals from 160 pedigrees achieved a power of .72, assuming the gene and marker were close but not next to one another. To achieve 85% power, 2,000 individuals from 200 pedigrees were required. At 25% heterogeneity, the detection of linkage was very difficult: 2,000 individuals from 200 pedigrees achieved a power of only 45% even when the marker was located at the pathogenic gene. Similar results were reported in a simulation study by Levinson.[70]

Suarez et al.[71] examined the power to detect linkage under oligogenic inheritance. Their simulations showed the need for large samples to detect linkage. Moreover, they showed that, under oligogenic inheritance, even larger samples would be needed to replicate a linkage finding. For example, if it is assumed that six loci cause a disorder, completely informative markers are available, and the true recombination fraction is 0, 200 families would be needed to replicate a linkage finding for a disorder that, like schizophrenia, has a 1% population prevalence. In these simulations, a fixed pedigree structure was used that included four siblings, two parents, and four grandparents. Thus, 2,000 individuals would be needed to replicate the linkage. In contrast, only 40 families (400 individuals) would be needed to detect linkage.

Because family, twin, and adoption studies point to a genetic etiology of schizophrenia, it seems likely that our current inability to find consistently replicable linkages is due to the complex inheritance of schizophrenia and/or high levels of genetic heterogeneity. Thus, more work with larger samples will be required before aberrant genes can be identified. As others have suggested,[53,70] finding genes for schizophrenia with linkage analysis may require an unprecedented level of cooperation and collaboration among schizophrenia researchers.

Schizophrenia Spectrum Disorders

Genetic studies suggest that there is a spectrum of disorders that are similar to schizophrenia and are caused by the same genes. These disorders are called *schizophrenia spectrum disorders*. A disorder is said to be in the schizophrenia spectrum if it occurs more frequently among the biological relatives of schizophrenic patients than among the relatives of people who do not have schizophrenia.

Psychotic Spectrum Disorders

Approximately 9% of the first-degree relatives of schizophrenic patients will have some psychotic disorder that does not meet the criteria for either schizophrenia or a mood disorder.[16,72] Two prominent examples are schizoaffective disorder and psychosis not otherwise specified. As the name suggests, schizoaffective disorder is diagnosed in patients who exhibit features of both schizophrenia and affective disorders (also known as mood disorders). The affective symptoms of these patients include depression, irritability, and mania. In schizoaffective patients, these symptoms are as prominent as the schizophrenic symptoms. In DSM-IV,[73] the diagnosis of schizoaffective disorder requires that an episode of mood disorder is present for a substantial portion of the psychotic episode. Patients are often classified in this category when the diagnostician finds equal support for diagnoses of schizophrenia and mood disorder.

Psychosis not otherwise specified is a residual diagnostic category. After diagnostic rules are carefully applied, many psychotic patients do not meet the criteria for schizophrenia, schizoaffective disorder, or other psychotic diagnoses. The main identifying characteristic of these patients is that they have psychotic symptoms but do not fit into any more rigorously defined category. In many cases, the diagnosis of psychosis not otherwise specified serves as a temporary category for patients whose disorder is of recent onset until the course of their symptoms reveals their diagnosis.

Both schizoaffective disorder and psychosis not otherwise specified are more common among the relatives of schizophrenic patients than among the relatives of nonschizophrenic people. Thus, these two disorders satisfy the requirements for schizophrenia spectrum disorders. Curiously, schizoaffective disorder is also found among the relatives of patients with bipolar disorder. This has led some investigators to conclude that schizophrenia and bipolar disorder may share genes in common. In this view, the two disorders are at opposite ends of a "continuum of psychosis," and the schizoaffective patients lie in the middle. This idea is controversial and is now the subject of much research.

Schizotypal Personality Disorder

The search for mild forms of schizophrenia started nearly a century ago, when psychiatrists observed that many of the relatives of schizophrenic patients had eccentric personalities. They also noticed poor social relations, anxiety in social situations, and limited emotional responses among the family members of schizophrenic patients. Less frequently, psychiatrists also observed mild forms of thought disorder, suspiciousness, magical thinking, illusions, and perceptual aberrations.

Psychiatric genetic researchers have focused on the familial prevalence of three personality disorders: schizotypal, schizoid, and paranoid personality disorders. Numerous studies have documented the increased prevalence of schizotypal personality disorder in the biological relatives of chronic schizophrenic probands. These results have demonstrated consistency across family studies,[74–76] adoption studies,[77,78] and twin studies.[79,80] Although two studies failed to find a higher rate of schizotypal personality disorder among relatives of schizophrenic probands,[81,82] most studies suggest that the biological relatives of schizophrenic patients demonstrate subthreshold pathology in the form of schizotypal personality disorder.[83,84] The incidence of such disorders in schizophrenic families has been estimated to be 4.2%–14.6%.[75,76,85] If "probable" schizotypal personality disorder is included, estimates may run as high as 26.8%.[75]

Results for schizoid and paranoid personality disorders have been somewhat more controversial and contradictory. Baron et al.[75] found higher rates of paranoid personality disorder in the relatives of schizophrenic probands (7.3%) than in control probands (2.7%). Their results have been criticized,[86] however, for artificially inflating estimates of paranoid personality disorder in relatives on the grounds that the sample of probands with schizophrenia as defined by Research Diagnostic Criteria may have also included probands with delusional disorders. It has been suggested, based on family studies, that schizophrenia and delusional disorder are not genetically related.[87–89] In addition, Winokur[89] found increased rates of paranoid traits in relatives of patients with delusional disorder, but not in the relatives of schizophrenic patients. Kendler et al.[90] showed that rates of paranoid personality disorder as defined by DSM-III criteria are not increased in the relatives of schizophrenic patients but are higher in the relatives of probands with delusional disorder than in the relatives of control probands. Thus, there is not strong evidence favoring paranoid personality disorder as a member of the schizophrenia spectrum; further work is needed to clarify conflicting findings.

Schizoid personality disorder has received relatively little interest and examination despite its apparent similarities to traits (e.g., social isolation and affective impoverishment) cited in the literature as relevant to family member pathology in schizophrenia. Kety et al.[27,91] and the Danish adoption studies are most frequently cited as providing the evidence that potentially refutes a schizoid-schizophrenia genetic link. A more recent replication in an adoption sample[78] indicated findings similar to the earlier report by Kety et al. The recent findings, however, of Baron et al.,[75] who used DSM-III criteria for schizoid personality disorder, failed to uncover statistically significant differences, although the relatives of schizophrenic patients did show a higher rate of schizoid personality disorder than control relatives (1.6% versus 0%). Baron et al., however, incorporated the category "probable schizotypal personality disorder," which required only two of the necessary four DSM-III criteria for inclusion. The family members of schizophrenic patients demonstrated a significantly higher rate of probable schizotypal personality disorder than did the family members of control subjects (12.1%

versus 6.5%). Because a symptom overlap exists between the DSM-III criteria for schizotypal and schizoid personality disorders (e.g., affective constriction and social isolation), it is possible that family members who would otherwise have met the criteria for schizoid personality disorder were instead diagnosed as "probable schizotypal" personality disorder. Finally, Kendler et al.[76,90] reported an increased prevalence of a combined "schizotypal-schizoid" personality disorder in biological relatives of schizophrenic patients, but their results do not allow for a distinction between "schizotypal" and "schizoid" traits. Thus, as with paranoid personality disorder, strong evidence has yet to be presented in establishing a link between schizophrenia and schizoid personality disorder. Clearly, among Axis II disorders, schizotypal personality disorder is the strongest candidate for a relatively mild illness that is genetically related to schizophrenia.

Clinical Implications

Unlike clinical research in other areas, genetic research has not produced new therapies for psychiatric patients. There is little doubt that, in the long run, the discovery of etiological genes will lead to treatments that are more effective. At the very least, the discovery of genetic markers will lead to the very early identification of children at risk for schizophrenia. This raises the possibility of designing primary prevention and other early intervention strategies.

Although the major clinical contributions of genetic research in schizophrenia may be decades away, this line of research has led to advances in diagnosis, treatment, and genetic counseling that should be useful to the practicing clinician.

Diagnosis

Because schizophrenia is familial, the art of diagnosis should be extended from diagnosing patients to diagnosing entire families. Indeed, we have found that a comprehensive psychiatric family history is one of the most illuminating sources of information in a diagnostic interview. By determining what psychiatric illnesses occur in the patient's family, the clinician may be more precise in the diagnosis of the patient.

The psychiatric family history is most helpful for atypical patients who are not clearly schizophrenic or mood disordered. It is also useful when few data about the patient are available. Nevertheless, such data should be routinely collected because, in all cases, it helps the clinician develop and test diagnostic hypotheses.

The use of family history data is straightforward and intuitive. For example, consider the case of a 30-year-old patient who is admitted to a hospital for the first time with both the psychotic symptoms of schizophrenia and the affective symptoms of bipolar disorder, but without clearly meeting the criteria for any disorder. If the patient has two bipolar siblings, a provisional diagnosis of bipolar disorder would certainly be in order. If these siblings were schizophrenic, the diagnosis of schizophrenia would prevail.

Treatment

In addition to the indirect effects of diagnosis on treatment, the genetics of a disorder should influence treatment in three ways. First, if a patient has relatives with the disorder, the patient's response to specific biological treatments should be considered in choosing a therapy. Although little is known about the pharmacogenetics of psychotropic drugs, in some cases biologically related schizophrenic individuals may respond best to the same medication. Controlled research is needed, however, before practice guidelines can be established in this area.

The second influence of genetic findings on treatment is in the area of medication compliance. Many schizophrenic patients actively resist taking psychotropic medication; others find it difficult to maintain their prescribed regimen. These problems can be mitigated by discussing the genetic etiology of a disorder when teaching a patient about his or her illness. Many patients hold naive beliefs about the etiology of their schizophrenia; they are quick to attribute it to life circumstances, past events, or their own psychological inadequacies. Such beliefs (sometimes delusional) may make it difficult for a patient to accept the biological roots of their problems. For many psychiatric disorders, genetic data provide the quickest and most convincing means of showing patients how biology plays a role in their condition. Although this is often easier when other relatives are known to be ill, it is also useful when the patient is the only family member affected.

A third therapeutic use of genetic data is as part of the educational component of family therapy, especially those therapies that do not assume that the illness was directly or indirectly caused by deviant family interaction. An educational component can be used in attempts to reduce the family's self-blame for the illness. Once families learn about the genetic and biological bases of the illness, they can discard guilty feelings and more productively cooperate in the treatment of their relative. Understanding biological bases also helps families accept the necessity of medication.

Genetic Counseling

Many patients, along with their relatives, are concerned about the potential recurrence of schizophrenia among other family members. Ideally, genetic counseling should be based on genetic markers from linkage analysis or risk figures from a known model of genetic transmission. These data can then be applied to an individual's pedigree to determine that individual's risk for a disorder. Unfortunately, such information is not available for schizophrenia.

In the absence of knowledge of the mode of transmission of schizophrenia, we can use the available family study data to make predictions. For example, it is reasonable to tell a schizophrenic patient that the risk to siblings for severe psychotic illness is approximately 10%. The risk to an identical twin would be approximately 55%. Unfortunately, little is known about complicated family structures (e.g., the risk to a child who has a schizophrenic father and a schizophrenic sibling). In such cases, it is reasonable to assume some increment in risk, but the size of the increment cannot be specified.

If linkage analyses are successful, they may lead to dramatic improvements in our ability to make specific predictions about the onset of psychiatric disorders. After a linkage has been confirmed, we can identify individuals within a pedigree who are marker positive and disease negative but who have not yet passed through the period of risk for the illness. We would then predict that these individuals would later manifest the disorder. Thus, linkage analysis carries with it the promise of substantially increasing our understanding of etiology, with hopes of providing leads toward primary prevention.

References

1. Babigian HM: Schizophrenia: epidemiology, in Comprehensive Textbook of Psychiatry, Vol II. Edited by Freedman AM, Kaplan HI, Sadock BJ. Baltimore, MD, Williams & Wilkins, 1980, pp 1113–1121
2. Beiser M, Iacono WG: An update on the epidemiology of schizophrenia. Can J Psychiatry 35:657–668, 1990
3. Eaton WW: Epidemiology of schizophrenia. Epidemiol Rev 7:105–126, 1985
4. Jablensky A: Epidemiology of schizophrenia: a European perspective. Schizophr Bull 12:52–73, 1986
5. Böök JA, Wetterberg L, Modrzewska K: Schizophrenia in a North Swedish geographical isolate, 1900–1977: epidemiology, genetics and biochemistry. Clin Genet 14:373–394, 1978
6. Tsuang MT, Faraone SV, Day M: The schizophrenic disorders, in The Harvard Guide to Modern Psychiatry. Edited by Nicholi AM. Cambridge, MA, Belknap Press, 1988, pp 259–295
7. Tsuang MT, Faraone SV: Schizophrenia, in Medical Basis of Psychiatry. Edited by Winokur G, Clayton P. Philadelphia, PA, Harcourt Brace Jovanovich, 1994, pp 81–114
8. Goldstein JM, Tsuang MT, Faraone SV: Gender and schizophrenia: implications for understanding the heterogeneity of the illness. Psychiatr Res 28:243–253, 1989

9. Faraone SV, Tsuang MT: Methods in psychiatric genetics, in Textbook in Psychiatric Epidemiology. Edited by Tohen M, Tsuang MT, Zahner GEP. New York, Wiley (in press)
10. Cooper JE, Kendell RE, Gurland BJ, et al: Psychiatric Diagnosis in New York and London: A Comparative Study of Mental Hospital Admissions. London, Oxford University Press (Institute of Psychiatry, Maudsley Monographs No 20), 1972
11. Cooper B: Epidemiology, in Schizophrenia: Towards a New Synthesis. Edited by Wing JK. New York, Grune & Stratton, 1978
12. Dohrenwend BP, Levav I, Shrout PE, et al: Socioeconomic status and psychiatric disorders: the causation-selection issue. Science 255:946–952, 1992
13. Dunham HW: Community and Schizophrenia: An Epidemiological Analysis. Detroit, MI, Wayne State University Press, 1965
14. Goldberg EM, Morrison SL: Schizophrenia and social class. Br J Psychiatry 109:785–802, 1963
15. Goldstein JM: The impact of gender on understanding the epidemiology of schizophrenia, in Gender and Psychopathology. Edited by Seeman MV. Washington, DC, American Psychiatric Association (in press)
16. Gottesman II, Shields J: Schizophrenia: The Epigenetic Puzzle. Cambridge, MA, Cambridge University Press, 1982
17. Kendler KS: The genetics of schizophrenia: an overview, in Handbook of Schizophrenia: Nosology, Epidemiology and Genetics of Schizophrenia. Edited by Tsuang MT, Simpson JC. New York, Elsevier, 1988, pp 437–462
18. Tsuang MT, Winokur G, Crowe RR: Morbidity risks of schizophrenia and affective disorders among first-degree relatives of patients with schizophrenia, mania, depression and surgical conditions. Br J Psychiatry 137:497–504, 1980
19. Guze SB, Cloninger RC, Martin RL, et al: A follow-up and family study of schizophrenia. Arch Gen Psychiatry 40:1273–1276, 1983
20. American Psychiatric Association: Diagnostic and Statistical Manual of Mental Disorders, 3rd Edition. Washington, DC, American Psychiatric Association, 1980
21. Faraone SV, Tsuang MT: Familial links between schizophrenia

and other disorders: application of the multifactorial polygenic model. Psychiatry: Interpersonal and Biological Processes 51:37–47, 1988
22. Pope HG, Jones JM, Cohen BM, et al: Failure to find evidence of schizophrenia in first degree relatives of schizophrenic probands. Am J Psychiatry 139:826–830, 1982
23. Abrams R, Taylor MA: The genetics of schizophrenia: a reassessment using modern criteria. Am J Psychiatry 140:171–175, 1983
24. Kendler KS: Familial aggregation of schizophrenia and schizophrenia spectrum disorders. Arch Gen Psychiatry 45:377–383, 1988
25. Kendler KS: Overview: a current perspective on twin studies of schizophrenia. Am J Psychiatry 140:1413–1425, 1983
26. Heston LL: Psychiatric disorders in foster home-reared children of schizophrenic mothers. Br J Psychiatry 112:819–825, 1966
27. Kety SS, Rosenthal D, Wender PH, et al: The types and prevalence of mental illness in the biological and adoptive families of adopted schizophrenics. J Psychiatr Res 1:345–362, 1968
28. Faraone SV, Tsuang MT: Quantitative models of the genetic transmission of schizophrenia. Psychol Bull 98:41–66, 1985
29. Matthysse S, Holzman PS, Lange K: The genetic transmission of schizophrenia: application of mendelian latent structure analysis to eye tracking dysfunctions in schizophrenia and affective disorder. J Psychiatr Res 20:57–76, 1986
30. Holzman PS, Kringlen E, Matthysse S, et al: A single dominant gene can account for eye tracking dysfunctions and schizophrenia in offspring of discordant twins. Arch Gen Psychiatry 45:641–647, 1988
31. McGue M, Gottesman II: A single dominant gene still cannot account for the transmission of schizophrenia. Arch Gen Psychiatry 46:478–479, 1989
32. Risch N: Linkage strategies for genetically complex traits, I: multilocus models. Am J Hum Genet 46:222–228, 1990
33. Gottesman II, Shields J: Schizophrenia and Genetics: A Twin Study Vantage Point. New York, Academic Press, 1972
34. Risch N, Baron M: Segregation analysis of schizophrenia and re-

lated disorders. Am J Hum Genet 36:1039–1059, 1984
35. Vogler GP, Gottesman II, McGue MK, et al: Mixed model segregation analysis of schizophrenia in the Lindelius Swedish pedigrees. Behav Genet 20:461–472, 1990
36. Ott J: Analysis of Human Genetic Linkage, 2nd Edition. Baltimore, MD, Johns Hopkins University Press, 1991
37. Botstein D, White RL, Skolnick M, et al: Construction of a genetic linkage map in man using restriction fragment length polymorphisms. Am J Hum Genet 32:314–331, 1980
38. Bassett AS, McGillivray BC, Jones BD, et al: Partial trisomy of chromosome 5 cosegregating with schizophrenia. Lancet 1:799–801, 1988
39. Sherrington R, Brynjolfsson J, Petursson H, et al: Localization of a susceptibility locus for schizophrenia on chromosome 5. Nature 336:164–167, 1988
40. Aschauer HN, Aschauer-Treiber G, Isenberg KE, et al: No evidence for linkage between chromosome 5 markers and schizophrenia. Hum Hered 40:109–115, 1990
41. Detera-Wadleigh SD, Goldin LR, Sherrington R, et al: Exclusion of linkage to 5q11-13 in families with schizophrenia and other psychiatric disorders. Nature 340:391–393, 1989
42. Diehl S, Su Y, Bray J, et al: Linkage studies of schizophrenia: exclusion of candidate regions on chromosomes 5q and 11q (abstract). Psychiatric Genetics 1991; 2:14–15
43. Kaufmann CA, DeLisi LE, Lehner T, et al: Physical mapping, linkage analysis of a putative schizophrenia locus on chromosome 5q. Schizophr Bull 15:441–452, 1989
44. Hallmayer J, Maier W, Ackenheil M, et al: Evidence against linkage of schizophrenia to chromosome 5q11-q13 markers in systematically ascertained families. Biol Psychiatry 31:83–94, 1992
45. McGuffin P, Sargeant M, Hetti G, et al: Exclusion of a schizophrenia susceptibility gene from the chromosome 5q11-q13 region: new data and a reanalysis of previous reports. Am J Hum Genet 47:524–535, 1990
46. Gurling HMD: New microsatellite polymorphisms fail to confirm chromosome 5 linkage in Icelandic and British schizophrenia families. Paper presented at the meeting of the American Psy-

chopathological Association, New York, March 1992
47. Crow TJ, DeLisi LE, Johnstone EC: Concordance by sex in sibling pairs with schizophrenia is paternally inherited: evidence for a pseudoautosomal locus. Br J Psychiatry 155:92–97, 1989
48. Collinge J, DeLisi LE, Boccio A, et al: Evidence for a pseudoautosomal locus for schizophrenia using the method of affected sibling pairs. Br J Psychiatry 158:624–629, 1991
49. Parfitt E, Asherson P, Sargeant M, et al: A linkage study of the pseudoautosomal region in schizophrenia (abstract). Psychiatric Genetics 1991; 2:92–93
50. Pulver AE, Karayiorgou M, Wolyneic P, et al: Sequential strategy to identify a susceptibility gene for schizophrenia on chromosome 22q12-q13.1: Part I. Am J Med Genet 54:36–43, 1994
51. Coon H, Holik J, Hoff M, et al: Analysis of chromosome 22 markers in 9 schizophrenia pedigrees. Am J Med Genet 54:72–79, 1994
52. Polymeropoulos MH, Coon H, Byerley W, et al: Search for a schizophrenia susceptibility locus on human chromosome 22. Am J Med Genet 54:93–99, 1994
53. Pulver AE, Karayiorgou M, Lasseter VK, et al: Follow-up of a report of a potential linkage for schizophrenia on chromosome 22q12-q13.1: Part II. Am J Med Genet 54:44–50, 1994
54. Lyons MJ, Kremen WS, Tsuang MT, et al: Investigating putative genetic and environmental forms of schizophrenia: methods and findings. International Review of Psychiatry 1:259–276, 1989
55. Lyons MJ, Faraone SV, Kremen WS, et al: Familial and sporadic schizophrenia: a simulation study of statistical power. Schizophr Res 2:345–353, 1989
56. Tsuang MT, Lyons MJ, Faraone SV: Heterogeneity of schizophrenia: conceptual models and analytic strategies. Br J Psychiatry 156:17–26, 1990
57. Tsuang MT, Lyons MJ, Faraone SV: Problems of diagnosis in family studies. J Psychiatr Res 21:391–399, 1987
58. Tsuang MT, Lyons ML, Faraone SV: The contribution of genetic research to diagnostic issues in schizophrenia, in Biological Perspectives of Schizophrenia. Edited by Helmchen H, Henn F. Chichester, England, John Wiley, 1987, pp 57–70

59. Tsuang MT, Lyons MJ and Faraone SV: Clinical phenotypes: problems in diagnosis. Münchener Genetikgesprachäche, Collegium Internationale Neuro-Psychopharmacologicum (CINP) President's Workshop: Genetic Research in Psychiatry. Munich, Germany, Springer-Verlag, 1991
60. Su Y, O'Neil A, Ni Nuallain M, et al: Linkage studies of schizophrenia in Irish pedigrees (abstract). Am J Hum Genet 47:A201, 1990
61. Coon H, Jensen S, Holik J, et al: A genomic scan for genes predisposing to schizophrenia. Am J Med Genet 54:59–71, 1994
62. Crowe RR, Black DW, Wesner R, et al: Lack of linkage to chromosome 5q11-q13 markers in six schizophrenia pedigrees. Arch Gen Psychiatry 48:357–361, 1991
63. Hallmayer J, Kennedy JL, Wetterberg L, et al: Exclusion of linkage between the serotonin$_2$ receptor and schizophrenia in a large Swedish kindred. Arch Gen Psychiatry 49:216–219, 1992
64. Macciardi F, Kennedy JL, Ruocco L, et al: A genetic linkage study of schizophrenia to chromosome 5 markers in a northern Italian population. Biol Psychiatry 31:720–728, 1992
65. Campion D, d'Amato T, Laklou H, et al: Failure to replicate linkage between chromosome 5q11-q13 markers and schizophrenia in 28 families. Psychiatr Res 44:171–179, 1993
66. Gill M, McGuffin P, Parfitt E, et al: A linkage study of schizophrenia with DNA markers from the long arm of chromosome 11. Psychol Med 23:27–44, 1993
67. Weise C, Lannfelt L, Kristbjarnarson H, et al: No evidence of linkage between schizophrenia and D_3 dopamine receptor gene locus in Icelandic pedigrees. Psychiatr Res 46:69–78, 1993
68. Goldin LR, Gershon ES: Power of the affected-sib-pair method for heterogeneous disorders. Genet Epidemiol 5:35–42, 1988
69. Chen WJ, Faraone SV, Tsuang MT: Linkage studies of schizophrenia: a simulation study of statistical power. Genet Epidemiol 9:123–139, 1992
70. Levinson DF: Power to detect linkage with heterogeneity in samples of small nuclear families. Am J Med Genet 48:94–102, 1993
71. Suarez BK, Hampe CL, Van Eerdewegh P: Problems of replicating linkage claims in psychiatry, in Genetic Approaches in Mental

Disorders. Edited by Gershon ES, Cloninger CR. Washington, DC, American Psychiatric Press, 1994, pp 23–46
72. Gottesman II: Schizophrenia Genesis: The Origin of Madness. New York, Freeman, 1991
73. American Psychiatric Association: Diagnostic and Statistical Manual of Mental Disorders, 4th Edition. Washington, DC, American Psychiatric Association, 1994
74. Baron M, Gruen R, Asnis L, et al: Familial relatedness of schizophrenia and schizotypal states. Am J Psychiatry 140:1437–1442, 1983
75. Baron M, Gruen R, Rainer JD, et al: A family study of schizophrenic and normal control probands: implications for the spectrum concept of schizophrenia. Am J Psychiatry 142:447–455, 1985
76. Kendler KS, Masterson CC, Ungaro R, et al: A family history study of schizophrenia-related personality disorders. Am J Psychiatry 141:424–427, 1984
77. Gunderson JG, Siever LJ, Spaulding E: The search for a schizotype: crossing the border again. Arch Gen Psychiatry 40:15–22, 1983
78. Kety SS: Schizophrenic illness in the families of schizophrenic adoptees: findings from the Danish national sample. Schizophr Bull 14:217–222, 1988
79. Siever LJ, Gunderson JG: Genetic determinants of borderline conditions. Schizophr Bull 5:59–86, 1979
80. Torgersen S: Relationship of schizotypal personality disorder to schizophrenia: genetics. Schizophr Bull 11:554–563, 1985
81. Coryell WH, Zimmerman M: Personality disorder in the families of depressed, schizophrenic, and never-ill probands. Am J Psychiatry 146:496–502, 1989
82. Squires-Wheeler E, Skodol AE, Bassett A, et al: DSM-III-R schizotypal personality traits in offspring of schizophrenic disorder, affective disorder, and normal control parents. J Psychiatr Res 23:229–239, 1989
83. Clementz BA, Grove WM, Katsanis J, et al: Psychometric detection of schizotypy: perceptual aberration and physical anhedonia in relatives of schizophrenics. J Abnorm Psychol 100:

607–612, 1991
84. Lenzenweger MF, Loranger AW: Detection of familial schizophrenia using a psychometric measure of schizotypy. Arch Gen Psychiatry 466:902–907, 1989
85. Kendler KS, Gruenberg AM, Strauss JS: An independent analysis of the Copenhagen sample of the Danish adoption study of schizophrenia, II: the relationship between schizotypal personality disorder and schizophrenia. Arch Gen Psychiatry 38:982–984, 1981
86. Rogers KL, Winokur G: The genetics of schizoaffective disorder and the schizophrenia spectrum, in Handbook of Schizophrenia, Vol 3: Nosology, Epidemiology, and Genetics. Edited by Tsuang MT, Simpson JC. New York, Elsevier, 1988, pp 481–500
87. Kendler KS, Gruenberg AM, Strauss JS: An independent analysis of the Copenhagen sample of the Danish adoption study of schizophrenia, II: the relationship between schizotypal personality disorder and schizophrenia. Arch Gen Psychiatry 38:982–984, 1981
88. Kendler KS, Hayes P: Paranoid psychosis (delusional disorder) and schizophrenia. Arch Gen Psychiatry 38:547–551, 1981
89. Winokur G: Familial psychopathology in delusional disorder. Compr Psychiatry 26:241–248, 1985
90. Kendler KS, Masterson CC, Davis KL: Psychiatric illness in first-degree relatives of patients with paranoid psychosis, schizophrenia, and medical illness. Br J Psychiatry 147:524–531, 1985
91. Kety SS, Rosenthal D, Wender PH, et al: Mental illness in the biological and adoptive families of adopted individuals who have become schizophrenic: a preliminary report based on psychiatric interviews, in Genetic Research in Psychiatry. Edited by Rieve RR, Rosenthal D, Brill H. Baltimore, MD, Johns Hopkins University Press, 1975, pp 147–165

CHAPTER

Postmortem Studies of Suicide Victims

J. John Mann, M.D.
Mark D. Underwood, Ph.D.
Victoria Arango, Ph.D.

Every year there are approximately 31,000 suicides in the United States.[1] Most of these suicides occur within the context of a major depressive episode. Schizophrenia, personality disorders, alcoholism, and substance abuse are other psychiatric disorders frequently associated with suicide. More than 90% of suicide victims have a psychiatric disorder, and it is uncommon for suicide to occur in an individual who is not psychiatrically ill. Conversely, many patients with psychiatric disorders may experience suicidal ideation but do not commit suicide. These observations raise an important question, namely, what distinguishes psychiatrically ill individuals who commit suicide from those who do not? A second related question is whether there is a common predisposing factor or set of factors across psychiatric diagnoses that

Support for this work was provided by Grants MH40210, AA09004, and MH46745 from the National Institutes of Health.

predispose individuals to commit suicide or whether there are other factors related to the risk of suicide in individuals with psychiatric disorders that are highly specific for each disorder.

In this chapter, we discuss the results of studies in postmortem brain tissue from suicide victims and how the findings of these studies address these questions. Relevant data from studies of psychiatric patients in vivo will also be addressed briefly.

In the literature describing postmortem studies of suicide victims, most of the work has concentrated on the serotonergic system and, to a lesser extent, on the noradrenergic system. Other neurotransmitters including γ-aminobutyric acid (GABA), acetylcholine, dopamine, and peptide modulators and transmitters, have been studied to a far lesser degree, thus preventing definite conclusions. This review is confined to the serotonergic and the noradrenergic systems, for which there is greatest information available. Transmitter turnover and receptor studies and their relationship to the type of suicidal behavior, namely, violent versus nonviolent, or the underlying psychiatric disorder are themes that guide this review.

The stability of measurements of brain chemistry is of particular importance in postmortem studies. To this end, neurotransmitter receptor proteins have been found to be more stable than the neurotransmitters themselves. Newer radiolabeled ligands afford the advantage of greater selectivity for the receptor of interest and provide quantitative measurements of receptor binding and receptor affinity. Quantitative autoradiography has provided further insights into the pathophysiology of suicide by providing a higher degree of anatomical resolution than studies of brain homogenates.

The Serotonergic System in Suicide Victims

Serotonin and 5-Hydroxyindoleacetic Acid

There have been approximately 14 studies of the concentration of serotonin, or 5-hydroxytryptamine (5-HT), and its major metabolite, 5-hydroxyindoleacetic acid (5-HIAA), in brain tissue from suicide victims (Table 8–1). Five of the seven studies of the brain stem of suicide victims found reductions in either 5-HT or 5-HIAA. In contrast, only three of eight studies of the prefrontal cortex found a reduction in 5-HIAA levels, and no study found a reduction in 5-HT. Four of six studies of other brain regions reported reductions in 5-HT or 5-HIAA. The evidence for a reduction in 5-HT or 5-HT turnover therefore appears most consistent in the brain stem. This may be a function of the sensitivity of the assay methodology, because the brain stem contains the 5-HT–synthesizing neurons and the highest concentrations of 5-HT and 5-HIAA. Alternatively, there may be a regional localization of changes in 5-HT levels or turnover, so that 5-HT and 5-HIAA in the terminal fields are altered in some areas and not others.

We previously reported that the degree of reduction in 5-HT or 5-HIAA in the brain stem of suicide victims reported in the literature has no relationship to diagnostic category.[2] The degree of re-

Table 8–1. 5-HT and 5-HIAA in brain tissue from suicide victims and control subjects

	Brain stem		Frontal cortex		Other regions	
Study	**5-HT**	**5-HIAA**	**5-HT**	**5-HIAA**	**5-HT**	**5-HIAA**
Shaw et al. 1967[52]	↓19%*	—	—	—	—	—
Bourne et al. 1968[29]	NC	↓28%*	—	—	—	—
Pare et al. 1969[53]	↓11%*	NC	—	—	—	—
Lloyd et al. 1974[54]	↓30%*	NC	—	—	NC	NC
Beskow et al. 1976[55]	NC	↓30%*	—	↓43%*	NC	↓18%*
Cochran et al. 1976[56]	NC	—	NC	—	NC	—
Owen et al. 1983[18]	—	—	—	↓71%	—	—
Crow et al. 1984[19]	—	—	—	↓25%	—	—
Korpi et al. 1986[57]	NC	NC	NC	NC	↓50%*	↓41%*
Owen et al. 1986[20]	—	—	—	—	—	↑27%*
Arato et al. 1987[58]	—	—	NC	NC	—	—
Cheetham et al. 1989[59]	—	—	NC	NC	↓23%*	NC
Ohmori et al. 1992[60]	—	—	—	NC	—	—
Lagattuta et al. 1992[61]	—	—	NC	NC	NC	NC

Note. NC = no change detected between groups.
*Statistically significant difference.

duction was similar in patients with depression, schizophrenia, personality disorders, and alcoholism. In patients with a major depressive illness versus other psychiatric diagnoses, the proportion of depressed suicide victims with decreased 5-HT or 5-HIAA was not different from suicide victims with other psychiatric disorders.[2] Similarly, violent suicide method was not associated with a greater degree of decrease in 5-HT or 5-HIAA than in nonviolent suicides.[3,4] Therefore, the method of suicide appears to be unrelated to the biochemical findings. These analyses, of course, did not extend to an examination of specific drugs that may have been used in a suicide attempt or the antemortem drug treatment history of the subjects. The time interval between death and brain collection (i.e., the postmortem delay) in studies that found a reduction in 5-HT or 5-HIAA did not differ significantly from postmortem delays in studies that did not make such a finding.[3] Therefore, although the length of the postmortem interval is considered critical in the quantification of indoleamines, differences in postmortem interval do not appear to be relevant in terms of explaining the discrepancies in the literature. This is probably because most of the decline in indoleamine levels occurs in the first 2 hours postmortem and virtually all cases have a longer postmortem delay.

In summary, there is evidence for a modest reduction in levels of 5-HT and 5-HIAA in the brain stem of suicide victims. It is an open question as to whether 5-HT and 5-HIAA are altered in the prefrontal cortex or other brain regions.

Serotonin Receptors

Transporter binding site. The serotonin binding site that has received the greatest attention in studies of suicidal behavior is the serotonin transporter. There have been at least 16 studies of serotonin transporter binding or of [^{3}H]imipramine binding in suicide victims (Table 8–2). Six of these studies reported a decrease in imipramine binding in suicide victims. In contrast, most of the studies that used ligands other than imipramine or used imipramine without using desipramine as the displacing agent did not find a reduc-

Table 8–2. 5-HT transporter binding studies in suicide victims

Study	Frontal cortex	Other regions	Ligand
Meyerson et al. 1982[62]	↑25%*	—	[^{3}H]imipramine
Stanley et al. 1982[63]	↓44%*	—	[^{3}H]imipramine
Paul et al. 1984[64]	—	↓30%*	[^{3}H]imipramine
Crow et al. 1984[19]	↓19%*	—	[^{3}H]imipramine
Owen et al. 1986[20]	NC	NC	[^{3}H]imipramine
Arato et al. 1987[58]	↓48%*	NC	[^{3}H]imipramine
Gross-Isseroff et al. 1989[65]	NC	↑* & ↓*	[^{3}H]imipramine
Arora and Meltzer 1989[66]	NC	—	[^{3}H]imipramine
Lawrence et al. 1990[9]	NC	NC	[^{3}H]paroxetine
Lawrence et al. 1990[6]	NC	NC & ↓*	[^{3}H]paroxetine
Arato et al. 1991[67]	↓53%*	—	[^{3}H]imipramine
Arora and Meltzer 1991[68]	NC	3	[^{3}H]imipramine
Andersson et al. 1992[8]	NC	NC	[^{3}H]paroxetine
Smith et al. 1992[7]	↓42%*	NC	[^{3}H]cyanoimipramine
Joyce et al. 1993[28]	—	↓*a	[^{3}H]cyanoimipramine
Laruelle et al. 1993[5]	↓31%*	NC	[^{3}H]paroxetine
Hrdina et al. 1993[23]	NC	NC	[^{3}H]paroxetine

Note. NC = no change detected between groups.
[a]Temporal and entorhinal cortex.
*Statistically significant difference.

tion in binding. Three studies, however, did find decreases in binding: Laruelle et al.,[5] who used [^{3}H]paroxetine combined with clomipramine as a displacing agent; Lawrence et al.,[6] who found a decrease in [^{3}H]paroxetine binding in the putamen; and a study from our laboratory[27] that examined [^{3}H]cyanoimipramine binding by autoradiography.

Some recent work in our laboratory (J. J. Mann, R. A. Henteleff, and V. Arango, unpublished data, 1994) using [^{3}H]paroxetine as the ligand and sertraline as the displacing agent suggests that [^{3}H]paroxetine binds with comparable high affinity to two binding sites. One site corresponds to the serotonin transporter, and the binding is sodium chloride dependent. Binding to the other site is sodium chloride independent and appears to be a related but nontransporter binding site. Binding to the sodium chloride-dependent serotonin transporter site was assayed in prefrontal cortex and found not to be lower in suicide victims than in control subjects.

Interestingly, this transporter binding site is the same site that is displaced by citalopram, the competition drug that was used in the studies by Andersson et al.[8] and Lawrence et al.,[6,9] who also found no change in serotonin transporter binding in the prefrontal cortex of suicide victims. In contrast, we found that the sodium-independent binding site, for which sertraline has low affinity, was lower in number in suicide victims than in control subjects, indicating that this site may account for previous reports of reduced [^{3}H]imipramine binding. Because [^{3}H]imipramine and [^{3}H]paroxetine bind with similar affinity to both the sodium chloride-dependent and the sodium chloride-independent binding sites, they fail to distinguish between the transporter and the nontransporter sites, and the competition drug must provide this selectivity. Thus, our findings suggest that the reductions reported in earlier studies may in fact have involved a binding site other than the physiologically relevant transporter site. The functional role of this nontransporter binding site is unclear; it is found in greater numbers than the transporter site itself, and further research is required to determine whether it has a physiological role.

Another factor to consider is the brain region that is being studied. For example, an autoradiography study of suicide victims by Gross-Isseroff et al.[65] found regions of unchanged, increased, and decreased [^{3}H]imipramine binding. Our own studies using autoradiography[11,12] found a reduction in [^{3}H]cyanoimipramine binding that was confined to the lateral and orbital prefrontal cortex. This suggests that, despite the problems of ligand specificity, there may indeed be a reduction in transporter binding, but the reduction appears to be localized to areas of the prefrontal cortex that are different from those previously studied. Our most current results suggest that transporter binding in the dorsal prefrontal cortex is not reduced in suicide victims. However, there may be fewer transporter sites in more lateral and ventral regions of the prefrontal cortex of suicide victims.

5-HT2 serotonin receptor. The postsynaptic 5-HT_2 receptor is one of the earliest identified serotonin receptors in cortical tissue. In 1983, we reported a 44% increase in [^{3}H]spiroperidol binding to the 5-HT_2 receptor as defined by mianserin in prefrontal cortex of suicide victims.[13] We replicated the result in 1986[14] and 1990[15] in two other series of brains. A study by Arango et al.[15] was carried out with ^{125}I-labeled lysergic acid diethylamide (LSD), using both membrane homogenates and autoradiography. That study not only confirmed the increase in binding in the prefrontal cortex but also demonstrated that the number of binding sites was increased with no difference in the binding affinity.

Since our first report, other investigators have replicated this finding, including Arora and Meltzer,[69] Laruelle et al.,[5] and Hrdina et al.[23] Of the five studies that have reported no alteration in 5-HT_2 binding,[18–22] four came from a single research group and the fifth was an autoradiography study by Gross-Isseroff et al.[22] Thus, there is evidence both for and against this finding (Table 8–3).

One of the reasons for discrepant results in the literature may relate to the ligand used. Most of the studies that failed to replicate this finding used [^{3}H]ketanserin, with the exception of Laruelle et al.[5] and Hrdina et al.,[23] who found increased binding in suicide victims. Although ketanserin has been reported to have considerable pharmacological specificity, it also binds with high affinity to the α_1-adrenergic receptor, the histamine receptor, and the tetrabenazine binding site.[24] Therefore, masking these non–5-HT_2 sites is clearly essential in order to determine whether there are meaningful changes in 5-HT_2 binding. For example, it is conceivable that a decrease in tetrabenazine or histamine binding sites could obscure an increase in 5-HT_2 receptor binding. α_1-Adrenergic binding has been reported to be increased or unaltered in suicide victims,[22,25] and therefore, because the changes are highly localized, it is unlikely that binding to α_1-adrenergic sites would significantly influence the detection of the possible increase in 5-HT_2 binding by [^{3}H]ketanserin. There has not been sufficient work performed in which the distribution of 5-HT_2 receptors is mapped throughout the prefrontal cortex in suicide victims with autoradiographic techniques in order to know

Table 8–3. 5-HT2 receptor binding studies in suicide victims

Study	Membranes: Frontal cortex	Membranes: Other regions	Autoradiography: Frontal cortex	Autoradiography: Other regions
Owen et al. 1983[18 a]	NC	—	—	—
Stanley and Mann 1983[13 b]	↑44%*	—	—	—
Crow et al. 1984[19 a]	NC	NC	—	—
Mann et al. 1986[14 b]	↑28%*	—	—	—
Owen et al. 1986[20 a]	NC	NC	—	—
Cheetham et al. 1988[21 a]	NC	↓23%*[c]	—	—
Arora and Meltzer 1989[69 b]	↑45%*	—	—	—
Arango et al. 1990[15 d]	↑57%*	NC	↑73%*	NC
Gross-Isseroff et al. 1990[22 a]	NC	NC	NC	NC
Henteleff et al. 1992[70 d]	—	↑91%*[c]	—	—
Laruelle et al. 1993[5 a]	↑25%*	NC	—	—
Hrdina et al. 1993[23 a]	↑67%*	↑97%*[e]	—	—

Note. NC = no change detected between groups.
[a][^{3}H]Ketanserin.
[b][^{3}H]Spiroperidol.
[c]Hippocampus.
[d][^{125}I]LSD.
[e]Amygdala.
*Statistically significant difference.

whether there is regional specificity to the changes. We have carried out autoradiography studies[15] comparing the temporal pole to the dorsal prefrontal cortex in control subjects and suicide victims and have found that the level of binding is greater in the temporal cortex than in the prefrontal cortex in both groups, suggesting that there are, in fact, regional differences. Moreover, the degree of difference between the suicide victims and the control subjects appears to be greater in prefrontal cortex than in temporal cortex, suggesting regional specificity of the suicide effect. Further work is needed to map the distribution of change in 5-HT$_2$ receptors in suicide victims throughout the prefrontal cortex, as well as in other cortical brain regions.

If one examines the effect of violent versus nonviolent suicide method, it becomes apparent that the six studies that found an increase in 5-HT_2 receptor binding in suicide victims had a higher proportion of subjects committing suicide by violent methods than the studies that did not find an increase in 5-HT_2 receptor binding. Yates et al.[26] reported that depressed subjects who had recently been treated with antidepressants had lower levels of 5-HT_2 receptor binding sites. Therefore, it is conceivable that those depressed subjects that kill themselves with nonviolent methods, which commonly involve an overdose of antidepressants or related psychotropics such as antipsychotics, may have had a reduction in 5-HT_2 receptor binding site number as a result of the psychotropic drugs that they had taken antemortem. Suicide victims who die by medication overdose most commonly take the drugs that they have been prescribed, and therefore this postulated relationship between negative findings and nonviolent suicide methodology has some merit. The presence or absence of a depressive illness may also be a relevant factor, but insufficient information is available in the published studies of 5-HT_2 receptors to determine whether this is so. It is therefore of considerable interest that the study by Yates et al.[26] found an increase in 5-HT_2 receptor number in depressed patients who died of causes other than suicide. This result suggests that there may be an additional or exclusive relationship of altered 5-HT_2 receptor number with the presence of a depressive illness even in suicide victims.

5-HT_{1A} serotonin receptors. There have been at least five published studies of 5-HT_{1A} receptors in suicide victims (Table 8–4). In prefrontal cortex, the 5-HT_{1A} receptor is predominantly postsynaptic. Of the five published studies, two reported an increase in suicide victims and three did not. One factor that may be relevant for explaining these discrepant results is that the two studies that found an increase in 5-HT_{1A} receptor binding, namely, those of Arango et al.[27] and Joyce et al.,[28] found this increase to be confined to very discrete brain regions. Thus, techniques such as autoradiography, which can map the regions that are likely to show receptor binding changes, are essential for detecting highly localized alterations.

Table 8–4. 5-HT_{1A} receptor binding in suicide victims

Study	Membranes		Autoradiography	
	Frontal cortex	Other regions	Frontal cortex	Other regions
Cheetham et al. 1990[71 a]	NC	NC & ↓*	—	—
Dillon et al. 1991[72]	—	NC	NC	NC
Arango et al. 1991[27]	—	—	↑28%*	NC
Matsubara et al. 1991[73]	NC	—	—	—
Joyce et al. 1993[28]	—	—	—	↑*b

Note. NC = no change detected between groups.
[a]Only depressed suicide victims were included in the study.
[b]Temporal and entorhinal cortex.
*Statistically significant difference.

Other serotonin receptor subtypes. Other receptor subtypes have barely begun to be investigated, and studies of 5-HT_{1C}, 5-HT_{1B}, and 5-HT_{1D} receptors in suicide victims are ongoing. Overall, the preponderance of data suggests that there are alterations in the serotonin system in suicide victims. The use of techniques such as autoradiography, coupled with gene expression studies, will help to clarify the range and extent of the receptor and transmitter changes, as well as identify where in the brain these changes are most pronounced. Such studies have obvious application, not only in understanding the pathogenesis of suicidal behavior, but also in terms of identifying regions in the brain that are accessible to functional brain imaging studies in high-risk suicidal patients in vivo.

The Noradrenergic System in Suicide Victims

Along with compromised serotonergic function in patients exhibiting suicidal behavior, a growing body of evidence has accumulated that implicates altered brain noradrenergic transmission. Authors of postmortem studies performed to date have sought to examine the noradrenergic system in brain by measuring the concentration of norepinephrine (NE) or its metabolites in brain tissue, performing morphometric studies of noradrenergic neurons, estimating the activity of tyrosine hydroxylase (the rate-limiting enzyme for NE synthesis), and assaying the various NE receptor subtypes. Each of these measures addresses a different aspect of noradrenergic function and has its own advantages and limitations, particularly in human postmortem brain. Studies of individuals who attempt suicide are by and large consistent with postmortem findings. Yet despite these varied approaches, methodological differences, and technical limitations, a picture of reduced noradrenergic neurotransmission in suicide victims is starting to emerge.

NE and Metabolites

Too few postmortem studies of cortical or brain stem NE concentrations have been carried out in suicide victims to draw firm conclusions (Table 8–5). For example, Bourne et al.[29] detected no differences in the brain stems of suicide victims and those of control subjects. We have studied the prefrontal and temporal cortex of suicide victims and matched control subjects and also performed receptor binding studies.[25] We found that suicide victims

Table 8–5. NE and MHPG in brain tissue from suicide victims versus control subjects

	Brain stem		Frontal cortex		Other regions	
Study	**NE**	**MHPG**	**NE**	**MHPG**	**NE**	**MHPG**
Bourne et al. 1968[29]	NC	—	—	—	—	—
Pare et al. 1969[53]	NC	—	—	—	—	—
Moses and Robins 1975[74]	NC[a]	—	NC	—	NC	—
Beskow et al. 1976[55]	—	—	—	—	↓73%*[b]	—
Crow et al. 1984[19]	—	—	—	NC	—	—
Arango et al. 1993[25]	—	—	NC[c]	—	↑143%*[d]	

Note. NC = no change detected between groups.
[a]NE was increased in 3 of 30 structures examined.
[b]Putamen.
[c]Of 13 suicide victims, 10 had higher NE than control subjects.
[d]Temporal cortex.
*Statistically significant difference.

had greater concentrations of NE than did matched control subjects, a finding that contrasts with the observed increase in both β- and α_1-adrenergic receptor binding (Tables 8–6 and 8–7). NE concentration did not correlate with either age or postmortem delay but was greater in males than in females. The observations of unaltered NE concentrations in the brain stem and of increased NE concentrations in the cerebral cortex provide little guide as to the amount of NE available for release or what the level of noradrenergic activity might be.

Other investigators have examined the cerebrospinal fluid of individuals who attempted suicide as a way of avoiding the postmortem degradation of neurotransmitter and obtaining an index of neuronal activity in vivo. In a minority of studies,[30,31] in contrast to the majority,[32–37] reduced concentrations of the principal NE metabolite 3-methoxy-4-hydroxyphenylglycol (MHPG) were found in the

Table 8–6. β-Adrenergic receptor binding studies in suicide victims

	Homogenates		Autoradiography	
Study	Frontal cortex	Other regions	Frontal cortex	Other regions
Meyerson et al. 1982[62 a]	NC	—	—	—
Crow et al. 1984[19 a]	NC	—	—	—
Mann et al. 1986[14 a]	↑73%*	—	—	—
Biegon and Israeli 1988[46 a,b]	↑49%*[a]	—	↑59%*[b]	↑36%*[c]
Arango et al. 1990[15 b]	↑32%*	NC[d]	↑38%*	↑27%*[d]
De Paermentier et al. 1990[47 e]	NC	↓18%*[d] & NC	—	—
De Paermentier et al. 1991[75 e]	NC	↓16%*[d] & NC[f]	—	—
Stockmeier and Meltzer 1991[48 a]	NC	—	—	—
Little et al. 1993[49 b,f]	↓15%*	—	—	—

Note. NC = no change detected between groups.
[a]$[^3H]$Dihydroalprenolol.
[b]$[^{125}I]$Iodopindolol.
[c]Cingulate gyrus.
[d]Temporal cortex.
[e]$[^3H]$CGP 12177.
[f]Alcohol-dependent individuals and/or subjects on antidepressants were included in these studies.
*Statistically significant difference.

Table 8–7. α_1- and α_2-Adrenergic receptor binding studies in suicide victims and control subjects

Study	Homogenates: Frontal cortex	Homogenates: Other regions	Autoradiography: Frontal cortex	Autoradiography: Other regions
Meana and Garcia-Sevilla 1987[50] [a]	↑72%*	—	—	—
Gross-Isseroff et al. 1990[51] [b]	—	—	↓36%–58%*	↓43%–52%*
Meana et al. 1992[76] [a]	↑45%*	↑91%*	—	—
Arango et al. 1993[25] [b]	—	—	↑37%*	NC
Arango et al. 1993[25] [a]	—	—	NC	NC

Note. NC = no change detected between groups.
[a]α_1-Adrenergic receptors.
[b]α_2-Adrenergic receptors.
*Statistically significant difference.

cerebrospinal fluid of suicide attempters. Excretion of MHPG is reduced in the urine of suicide attempters.[30,31]

We have recently begun to examine brain stem noradrenergic neurons directly, using quantitative morphometry. Noradrenergic innervation of the mammalian cerebral cortex arises almost exclusively from pigmented neurons of the locus ceruleus.[38–42] The colocalization of neuromelanin pigment and the norepinephrine biosynthetic enzymes tyrosine hydroxylase and dopamine-β-hydroxylase in immunocytochemical studies demonstrates that the pigmented neurons of the locus ceruleus are noradrenergic.[43,44] These neurons provide widespread innervation throughout the neuraxis, including the cerebral cortex and limbic system. In a preliminary study of 11 control subjects and 6 suicide victims,[45] we found that suicide victims had a 25% reduction in the number of pigmented locus ceruleus neurons. The reduction in neuron number was not widespread but was anatomically restricted to the rostral two-thirds of the locus ceruleus. Interestingly, evidence in rats and nonhuman primates suggests that the locus ceruleus is topographically organized, with rostral portions of the nucleus providing projections to forebrain regions and caudal locus ceruleus neurons supplying innervation to the hindbrain.

Taken together, these studies suggest a relationship between reduced noradrenergic neurotransmission and suicidal behavior. Our recent finding of anatomically restricted losses of locus ceruleus neurons in suicide victims may clarify several discrepancies in the literature. For example, differences in receptor binding studies (Tables 8–6 and 8–7) may be related to the presence of fewer locus ceruleus neurons that innervate prefrontal cortex. It will ultimately be of importance to determine whether fewer NE neurons represent a risk factor for a depressive disorder or for suicide, and whether such suicide victims were born with fewer noradrenergic neurons or experienced an accelerated loss during development. The application of molecular biological and other genetic methods will also be of importance in elucidating the role of NE in the pathophysiology of suicidal behavior and depression.

Adrenergic Receptors

β-Adrenergic receptors. Increased binding to β-adrenergic receptors in the cerebral cortex in suicide victims compared with control subjects has been reported by some investigators[14,15,46] but not by others.[47–49] (Table 8–6). Mann et al.[14] first reported increased binding to the β-adrenergic receptor in suicide victims in homogenates of prefrontal cortex and found a 73% increase in the total amount of binding. Biegon and Israeli[46] confirmed and extended these findings and reported a 50% increase in binding density but no change in affinity in homogenates of prefrontal cortex. They also found that the binding changes were largely confined to the β_1 subtype, although the β_2 subtype was increased to a lesser extent. They confirmed their observation using autoradiographic measures and found that the binding changes were anatomically confined to the cingulate and superior frontal gyrus but were not found in the inferior frontal gyrus, caudate, putamen, or white matter.

Arango et al.[15] combined quantitative autoradiographic methods with membrane homogenate assays and analyzed the prefrontal and temporal cortex for both β-adrenergic and 5-HT_2 receptors using [^{125}I]pindolol and [^{125}I]LSD. The study described the laminar cortical organization of these receptors in control subjects and suicide victims and found a 38% and 27% increase in β-adrenergic binding in prefrontal and temporal cortex, respectively, but no change in affinity. This study provided evidence that different receptor populations need not change in isolation but may reflect common regulation of functionally linked neurotransmitter systems.

Two other well-designed studies of β-adrenergic receptors failed to detect any difference in suicide victims and control subjects.[47,48] Interestingly, both studies were careful to match cases for postmortem delay, age, and sex and took precautions concerning possible drug use or pharmacological treatments, especially recent use. Despite these precautions and careful designs, however, such differences in findings among studies are not unusual when human postmortem material is studied and point out the necessity for continued parsing of the possible experimental variables and the need for replication studies.

α-Adrenergic receptors. Although few studies have examined the α-adrenergic receptor subtypes (Table 8–7), α_1-adrenergic and/or α_2-adrenergic receptor binding in cerebral cortex of suicide victims has been reported to be increased[25,50] or decreased.[51] Unlike β-adrenergic receptors, which are relatively homogeneously distributed across cortical layers, α-adrenergic receptors exhibit a marked laminar organization in cortex, outer layers having more binding than deep layers. Hence, it is critical to be aware of the anatomical heterogeneity of these receptor distributions when addressing the distribution of changes between groups. For this reason alone, quantitative autoradiographic methods have a great advantage over membrane homogenate techniques, in which tissue dissection cannot make such detailed discriminations.

Meana and Garcia-Sevilla[50] reported a 72% increase in α_2-adrenergic binding, but no change in affinity, in homogenates of frontal cortex of suicide victims. In a similar subregion of prefrontal cortex (Brodmann area 9), Arango et al.[25] used quantitative autoradiographic methods and were unable to find any differences in α_2-adrenergic binding, despite a detailed analysis of the five isodensity bands observed in that cortical area. They did, however, find a 37% increase in α_1-adrenergic binding, particularly in deeper cortical layers. Additional studies are warranted, particularly because different ligands were used by different studies to define the α_2-adrenergic receptor subtype.

Conclusions

In this review, we attempt to summarize studies spanning more than two decades regarding the status of the serotonergic and noradrenergic systems in the brains of suicide victims at the time of death. Given the discrepant findings reported in the literature, we have tried to point out critical aspects of the design of postmortem studies that may have contributed to the disparate results. As in any experiment, the data obtained are highly dependent on the methods employed. Moreover, many of the changes in receptor binding are anatomically discrete and not of large magnitude. Such changes can be detected only by using methods such as autoradiography, which have the capability of providing a significant degree of anatomical resolution. Other important methodological issues include careful characterization and matching of the experimental and control subjects based on data from a psychological autopsy and the use of pharmacologically selective ligands.

With these caveats in mind, a picture of reduced serotonergic and noradrenergic function in the brains of suicide victims is emerging (Figure 8–1). Most studies have focused on the cerebral cortex, and in particular the prefrontal cortex, because of its hypothesized role in behavioral restraint. It is in the prefrontal cortex that there is the greatest consensus regarding receptor binding changes in suicide victims.

With respect to the serotonergic system, postsynaptic serotonin 5-HT_2 and 5-HT_{1A} receptors are increased, and the 5-HT transporter binding (or a related binding site) is decreased. 5-HT_{1C} sites are present only in very low concentrations in prefrontal cortex and are more abundant, but appear unaltered, in the hippocampus of suicide victims. Because 5-HT_2 and 5-HT_{1A} receptors are located predominantly on local neurons in the cortex and the 5-HT transporter is located on the presynaptic axon terminal of serotonergic

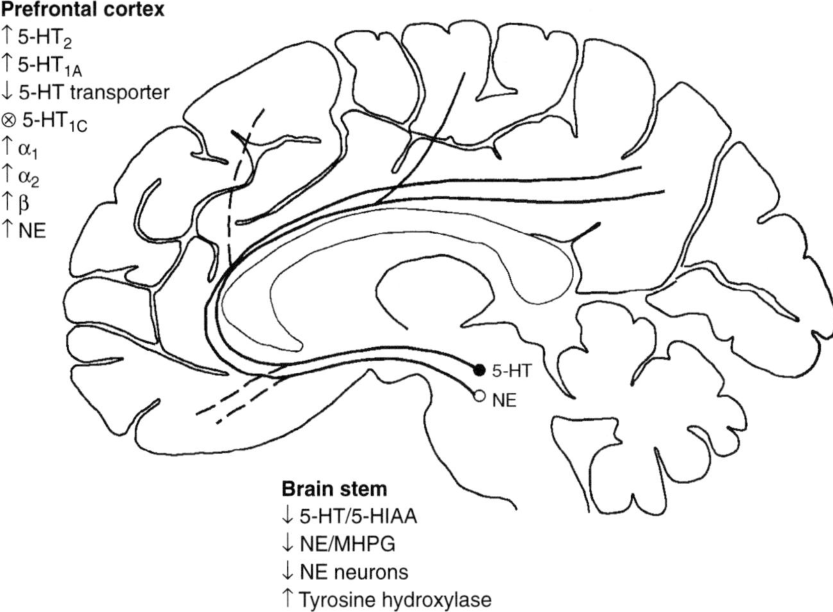

Figure 8–1. Schematic illustration summarizing studies of the serotonergic and noradrenergic systems in the postmortem brains of suicide victims. The text summarizes the predominant findings for receptors, neurotransmitter amounts, cell bodies, and enzyme activity in suicide victims and control subjects. Note that serotonergic and noradrenergic cell bodies in the brain stem provide widespread innervation throughout the cerebral cortex *(solid lines)* and that evidence suggests that the functional innervation of the prefrontal cortex is impaired in suicide victims *(dashed lines)*.

neurons that innervate the cortex, the most parsimonious conclusion is that there is reduced serotonergic innervation and a consequent upregulation of postsynaptic receptor sites in suicide victims. However, lesion studies in rodents have largely failed to demonstrate such upregulation, so the precise mechanism in suicide victims is unclear. In the brain stem of suicide victims, 5-HT and 5-HIAA levels appear to be lower. It remains to be determined whether this reduction is because of fewer serotonin-synthesizing neurons in the dorsal and median raphe that project to the cerebral cortex (and elsewhere) or whether there is reduced capacity for serotonin transmitter synthesis.

The picture for NE is less clear than for serotonin (Figure 8–1). In the cerebral cortex, α_1-adrenergic, α_2-adrenergic, and β-adrenergic receptors are altered, although there is not complete agreement. NE levels are reported to be increased in cortex, but there are insufficient data to determine whether MHPG is similarly changed, and as such it remains unclear whether suicide victims have altered NE turnover or activity. In the brain stem, NE and MHPG concentrations seem to be reduced, and there are fewer pigmented noradrenergic neurons. One study has reported the seemingly counterintuitive finding of increased activity of the NE biosynthetic enzyme tyrosine hydroxylase. Nevertheless, the conclusion that best fits the bulk of the findings is that there is reduced innervation of the cerebral cortex due to fewer noradrenergic neurons in the locus ceruleus. The finding of increased tyrosine hydroxylase may suggest that the remaining noradrenergic neurons have homeostatically compensated by increasing the amount or activity of the rate-limiting biosynthetic enzyme.

These findings represent a snapshot of brain function at the moment of suicide and therefore include the effects of genetics, development, and early life processes; the associated psychiatric disease and any treatment; environmental stresses; and the artifacts of postmortem delay. Age, sex, method of death, and drug use can be controlled for; use of a psychological autopsy method and psychiatric control subjects are needed to control for psychiatric illness and long-term treatment effects. Such studies have not yet been done. However, several other questions that will be critical to the interpretations of our existing knowledge can be asked and should serve to direct future studies. Are the serotonergic changes genetic in origin? Are the noradrenergic changes state dependent? Is there a highly specific and sensitive serotonergic trait marker that can identify the person at risk for suicide? Identification of the brain systems most affected, or predictive, of suicide may then provide the opportunity for effective pharmacological intervention. Much remains to be learned through further systematic postmortem neurochemical studies of tissue from individuals in whom clinical information is available.

References

1. Centers for Disease Control and Prevention: Advance report of final mortality statistics, 1990. Monthly Vital Statistics Report, Vol 41, 1993, pp 1–52
2. Mann JJ, Arango V, Marzuk PM, et al: Evidence for the 5-HT hypothesis of suicide: a review of post-mortem studies. Br J Psychiatry 155 (suppl 8):7–14, 1989
3. Arango V, Mann JJ: Relevance of serotonergic postmortem studies to suicidal behavior. International Review of Psychiatry 4:131–140, 1992
4. Mann JJ, Marzuk PM, Arango V, et al: Neurochemical studies of violent and nonviolent suicide. Psychopharmacol Bull 25:407–413, 1989
5. Laruelle M, Abi-Dargham A, Casanova MF, et al: Selective abnormalities of prefrontal serotonergic receptors in schizophrenia: a postmortem study. Arch Gen Psychiatry 50:810–818, 1993
6. Lawrence KM, De Paermentier F, Cheetham SC, et al: Brain 5-HT uptake sites, labelled with [^{3}H]paroxetine, in antidepressant-free depressed suicides. Brain Res 526:17–22, 1990
8. Andersson A, Eriksson A, Marcusson J: Unaltered number of brain serotonin uptake sites in suicide victims. J Psychopharmacol 6:509–513, 1992
9. Lawrence KM, De Paermentier F, Cheetham SC, et al: Symmetrical hemispheric distribution of ^{3}H-paroxetine binding sites in postmortem human brain from controls and suicides. Biol Psychiatry 28:544–546, 1990
10. Ikeda Y, Noda H, Sugita S: Olivocerebellar and cerebelloolivary connections of the oculomotor region of the fastigial nucleus in the macaque monkey. J Comp Neurol 284:463–488, 1989
11. Arango V, Miller ML, Smith RW, et al: Brain monoamine receptors in suicide. Paper presented at the 30th annual meeting of ACNP, San Juan, Puerto Rico, December 1991
12. Mann JJ: Integration of neurobiology and psychopathology in a unified model of suicidal behavior. Excerpta Medica International Congress Series 968 1:114–117, 1991

13. Stanley M, Mann JJ: Increased serotonin-2 binding sites in frontal cortex of suicide victims. Lancet 1:214–216, 1983
14. Mann JJ, Stanley M, McBride PA, et al: Increased serotonin$_2$ and β-adrenergic receptor binding in the frontal cortices of suicide victims. Arch Gen Psychiatry 43:954–959, 1986
15. Arango V, Ernsberger P, Marzuk PM, et al: Autoradiographic demonstration of increased serotonin 5-HT$_2$ and β-adrenergic receptor binding sites in the brain of suicide victims. Arch Gen Psychiatry 47:1038–1047, 1990
16. Schiavi RC, Theilgaard A, Owen DR, et al: Sex chromosome anomalies, hormones, and aggressivity. Arch Gen Psychiatry 41:93–99, 1984
17. Ikeda M, Mackay KB, Dewar D, et al: Differential alterations in adenosine A$_1$ and kappa$_1$ opioid receptors in the striatum in Alzheimer's disease. Brain Res 616:211–217, 1993
18. Owen F, Cross AJ, Crow TJ, et al: Brain 5-HT$_2$ receptors and suicide. Lancet 2:1256, 1983
19. Crow TJ, Cross AJ, Cooper SJ, et al: Neurotransmitter receptors and monoamine metabolites in the brains of patients with Alzheimer-type dementia and depression, and suicides. Neuropharmacology 23:1561–1569, 1984
20. Owen F, Chambers DR, Cooper SJ, et al: Serotonergic mechanisms in brains of suicide victims. Brain Res 362:185–188, 1986
21. Cheetham SC, Crompton MR, Katona CLE, et al: Brain 5-HT$_2$ receptor binding sites in depressed suicide victims. Brain Res 443:272–280, 1988
22. Gross-Isseroff R, Salama D, Israeli M, et al: Autoradiographic analysis of [^{3}H]ketanserin binding in the human brain postmortem: effect of suicide. Brain Res 507:208–215, 1990
23. Hrdina PD, Demeter E, Vu TB, et al: 5-HT uptake sites and 5-HT$_2$ receptors in brain of antidepressant-free suicide victims/depressives: increase in 5-HT$_2$ sites in cortex and amygdala. Brain Res 614:37–44, 1993
24. Hoyer D, Vos P, Closse A, et al: ^{3}H-ketanserin labels serotonin 5-HT$_2$ and α_1-adrenergic receptors in human brain cortex. J Cardiovasc Pharmacol 10 (suppl 3):S48–S50, 1987
25. Arango V, Ernsberger P, Sved AF, et al: Quantitative autoradiog-

raphy of α_1- and α_2-adrenergic receptors in the cerebral cortex of controls and suicide victims. Brain Res 630:271–282, 1993

26. Yates M, Leake A, Candy JM, et al: 5-HT_2 receptor changes in major depression. Biol Psychiatry 27:489–496, 1990
27. Arango V, Underwood MD, Gubbi AV, Mann JJ: Localized alterations in pre- and postsynaptic serotonin binding sites in the ventrolateral prefrontal cortex of suicide victims. Brain Res (in press)
28. Joyce JN, Shane A, Lexow N, et al: Serotonin uptake sites and serotonin receptors are altered in the limbic system of schizophrenics. Neuropsychopharmacology 8:315–336, 1993
29. Bourne HR, Bunney WE Jr, Colburn RW, et al: Noradrenaline, 5-hydroxytryptamine, and 5-hydroxyindoleacetic acid in hindbrains of suicidal patients. Lancet 2:805–808, 1968
30. Ågren H: Symptom patterns in unipolar and bipolar depression correlating with monoamine metabolites in the cerebrospinal fluid, II: suicide. Psychiatry Res 3:225–236, 1980
31. Ågren H. Depressive symptom patterns and urinary MHPG excretion. Psychiatry Res 6:185–196, 1982
32. Roy A, Pickar D, De Jong J, et al: Suicidal behavior in depression: relationship to noradrenergic function. Biol Psychiatry 25:341–350, 1989
33. Brown GL, Ebert MH, Goyer PF, et al: Aggression, suicide and serotonin: relationships to CSF amine metabolites. Am J Psychiatry 139:741–746, 1982
34. Pickar D, Roy A, Breier A, et al: Suicide and aggression in schizophrenia: neurobiologic correlates. Ann N Y Acad Sci 487:189–196, 1986
35. Roy A, Ninan PT, Mazonson A, et al: CSF monoamine metabolites in chronic schizophrenic patients who attempt suicide. Psychol Med 15:335–340, 1985
36. Secunda SK, Cross CK, Koslow S, et al: Biochemistry and suicidal behavior in depressed patients. Biol Psychiatry 21:756–767, 1986
37. Träskman L, Åsberg M, Bertilsson L, et al: Monoamine metabolites in CSF and suicidal behavior. Arch Gen Psychiatry 38:631–636, 1981

38. Dahlström A, Fuxe K: Evidence for the existence of monoamine-containing neurons in the central nervous system, I: demonstration of monoamines in the cell bodies of brain stem neurons. Acta Physiol Scand 62:1–55, 1964
39. Levitt P, Moore RY: Noradrenaline neuron innervation of the neocortex in the rat. Brain Res 139:219–231, 1978
40. Freedman R, Foote SL, Bloom FE: Histochemical characterization of a neocortical projection of the nucleus locus coeruleus in the squirrel monkey. J Comp Neurol 164:209–232, 1975
41. Jones BE, Moore RY: Ascending projections of the locus coeruleus in the rat, II: autoradiographic study. Brain Res 127:23–53, 1977
42. Porrino LJ, Goldman-Rakic PS: Brainstem innervation of prefrontal and anterior cingulate cortex in the rhesus monkey revealed by retrograde transport of HRP. J Comp Neurol 205:63–76, 1982
43. Iversen LL, Rossor MN, Reynolds GP, et al: Loss of pigmented dopamine-β-hydroxylase positive cells from locus coeruleus in senile dementia of Alzheimer's type. Neurosci Lett 39:95–100, 1983
44. German DC, Manaye KF, White CL III, et al: Disease-specific patterns of locus coeruleus cell loss. Ann Neurol 32:667–676, 1992
45. Arango V, Underwood MD, Mann JJ: Fewer pigmented locus coeruleus neurons in suicide victims. Biol Psychiatry, in press
46. Biegon A, Israeli M: Regionally selective increases in β-adrenergic receptor density in the brains of suicide victims. Brain Res 442:199–203, 1988
47. De Paermentier F, Cheetham SC, Crompton MR, et al: Brain β-adrenoceptor binding sites in antidepressant-free depressed suicide victims. Brain Res 525:71–77, 1990
48. Stockmeier CA, Meltzer HY: β-Adrenergic receptor binding in frontal cortex of suicide victims. Biol Psychiatry 29:183–191, 1991
49. Little KY, Clark TB, Ranc J, et al: β-Adrenergic receptor binding in frontal cortex from suicide victims. Biol Psychiatry 34:596–605, 1993
50. Meana JJ, Garcia-Sevilla JA: Increased α_2-adrenoceptor density

in the frontal cortex of depressed suicide victims. Journal of Neural Transmission 70:377–381, 1987

51. Gross-Isseroff R, Dillon KA, Fieldust SJ, et al: Autoradiographic analysis of α_1-noradrenergic receptors in the human brain postmortem. Arch Gen Psychiatry 47:1049–1053, 1990
52. Shaw DM, Camps FE, Eccleston EG: 5-Hydroxytryptamine in the hind-brain of depressive suicides. Br J Psychiatry 113:1407–1411, 1967
53. Pare CMB, Yeung DPH, Price K, et al: 5-Hydroxytryptamine, noradrenaline, and dopamine in brainstem, hypothalamus, and caudate nucleus of controls and of patients committing suicide by coal-gas poisoning. Lancet 2:133–135, 1969
54. Lloyd KG, Farley IJ, Deck JHN, et al: Serotonin and 5-hydroxyindoleacetic acid in discrete areas of the brainstem of suicide victims and control patients. Adv Biochem Psychopharmacol 11:387–397, 1974
55. Beskow J, Gottfries CG, Roos BE, et al: Determination of monoamine and monoamine metabolites in the human brain: post mortem studies in a group of suicides and in a control group. Acta Psychiatr Scand 53:7–20, 1976
56. Cochran E, Robins E, Grote S: Regional serotonin levels in brain: a comparison of depressive suicides and alcoholic suicides with controls. Biol Psychiatry 11:283–294, 1976
57. Korpi ER, Kleinman J, Goodman SI, et al: Serotonin and 5-hydroxyindoleacetic acid in brains of suicide victims: comparison in chronic schizophrenic patients with suicide as cause of death. Arch Gen Psychiatry 43:594–600, 1986
58. Arato M, Tekes K, Palkovits M, et al: Serotonergic split brain and suicide. Psychiatry Res 21:355–356, 1987
59. Cheetham SC, Crompton MR, Czudek C, et al: Serotonin concentrations and turnover in brains of depressed suicides. Brain Res 502:332–340, 1989
60. Ohmori T, Arora RC, Meltzer HY: Serotonergic measures in suicide brain: the concentration of 5-HIAA, HVA, and tryptophan in frontal cortex of suicide victims. Biol Psychiatry 32:57–71, 1992
61. Lagattuta TF, Henteleff RA, Arango V, et al: Reduction in cortical serotonin transporter site number in suicide victims in the ab-

sence of altered levels of serotonin, its precursors or metabolite. Proceedings of the 22nd Annual Meeting of the Society for Neuroscience, Vol 18, p 1598, October 1992

62. Meyerson LR, Wennogle LP, Abel MS, et al: Human brain receptor alterations in suicide victims. Pharmacol Biochem Behav 17:159–163, 1982
63. Stanley M, Virgilio J, Gershon S: Tritiated imipramine binding sites are decreased in the frontal cortex of suicides. Science 216:1337–1339, 1982
64. Paul SM, Rehavi M, Skolnick P, et al: High affinity binding of antidepressants to a biogenic amine transport site in human brain and platelet: studies in depression, in Neurobiology of Mood Disorders. Edited by Post RM, Bellinger CJ. Baltimore, MD, Williams & Wilkins, 1984, pp 846–853
65. Gross-Isseroff R, Israeli M, Biegon A: Autoradiographic analysis of tritiated imipramine binding in the human brain post mortem: effects of suicide. Arch Gen Psychiatry 46:237–241, 1989
66. Arora RC, Meltzer HY: ^{3}H-imipramine binding in the frontal cortex of suicides. Psychiatry Res 30:125–135, 1989
67. Arato M, Tekes K, Tothfalusi L, et al: Reversed hemispheric asymmetry of imipramine binding in suicide victims. Biol Psychiatry 29:699–702, 1991
68. Arora RC, Meltzer HY: Laterality and ^{3}H-imipramine binding: studies in the frontal cortex of normal controls and suicide victims. Biol Psychiatry 29:1016–1022, 1991
69. Arora RC, Meltzer HY: Serotonergic measures in the brains of suicide victims: 5-HT2 binding sites in the frontal cortex of suicide victims and control subjects. Am J Psychiatry 146:730–736, 1989
70. Henteleff RA, Arango V, Mann JJ: Serotonin 5-HT$_2$ but not 5-HT$_{1C}$ receptor number is increased in hippocampus of suicide victims. Proceedings of the 22nd Annual Meeting of the Society for Neuroscience, Vol 18, p 1598, October 1992
71. Cheetham SC, Crompton MR, Katona CLE, et al: Brain 5-HT$_1$ binding sites in depressed suicides. Psychopharmacology (Berl) 102:544–548, 1990
72. Dillon KA, Gross-Isseroff R, Israeli M, et al: Autoradiographic

analysis of serotonin 5-HT_{1A} receptor binding in the human brain postmortem: effects of age and alcohol. Brain Res 554:56–64, 1991

73. Matsubara S, Arora RC, Meltzer HY: Serotonergic measures in suicide brain: 5-HT_{1A} binding sites in frontal cortex of suicide victims. Journal of Neural Transmission 85:181–194, 1991
74. Moses SG, Robins E: Regional distribution of norepinephrine and dopamine in brains of depressive suicides and alcoholic suicides. Psychopharmacological Communications 1:327–337, 1975
75. De Paermentier F, Cheetham SC, Crompton MR, et al: Brain β-adrenoceptor binding sites in depressed suicide victims: effects of antidepressant treatment. Psychopharmacology (Berl) 105:283–288, 1991
76. Meana JJ, Barturen F, Garcia-Sevilla JA: α_2-Adrenoceptors in the brain of suicide victims: increased receptor density associated with major depression. Biol Psychiatry 31:471–490, 1992

CHAPTER

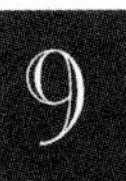

Schizophrenia: Postmortem Studies

Joel E. Kleinman, M.D., Ph.D.
Safia Nawroz, M.D.

Schizophrenia has been referred to as "the graveyard of neuropathology."[1] This quote, however, was never intended to discourage research in this area. On the contrary, it was suggested that success in this area would require new methods. Fortunately, advances in neuroimaging and neuropathology have made this suggestion a very realistic possibility. With the advent of computed axial tomographic (CAT) scans, magnetic resonance imaging (MRI) scans, positron-emission tomography (PET), and single photon emission computed tomography (SPECT), in vivo neuropathology became a reality. Moreover, postmortem studies benefitted from advances in autoradiography, neuronal morphometrics, and in situ hybridization.

One of the best examples of the impact of neuropathological research on a brain disease involved the discovery of reduced concentrations of dopamine in the striatum of patients with Parkinson's disease.[2] This discovery led to a successful replacement strategy, levodopa/carbidopa, which remains to this day the standard treatment of this disorder.[3] This example is relevant to the neuropathology of schizophrenia for two reasons. First, in order to make the initial discovery of reduced striatal dopamine, the researchers needed to know where in the brain to look, because the human brain has approximately 15–50 billion neurons. They were aided in this decision by the following two facts: 1) Parkinson's disease involves a loss of pigment from the pars compacta of the substantia nigra, and 2) dopaminergic neurons in the substantia nigra project to the striatum. These facts directed the investigators to measure dopamine in the striatum of patients with Parkinson's disease. Perhaps this is why the old joke about real estate applies to neuropathology as well, that is, there are only three things that matter in real estate (or neuropathology)—location, location, and location. This point is driven home still further by the second lesson from this research: although the etiology of most cases of Parkinson's disease is unknown, a successful treatment can be developed by understanding some of the anatomy and pathophysiology.

Can this strategy, then, be applied to schizophrenia? The first consideration involves the question of whether there are clues for schizophrenia, similar to those for Parkinson's disease, that tell us where in the brain to look. There are four widely accepted facts about schizophrenia, three of which may provide useful directions.

The first clue is that there is a genetic factor. This would indicate that the human genome should be looked at, a strategy that, although applicable to postmortem brain studies, has not as yet proved useful for neuroanatomy.

The second clue is that all drugs that are effective antipsychotics for schizophrenia block dopamine, subtype 2 (D_2), receptor and block D_2 receptor in proportion to their clinical efficacy.[4] An exception is clozapine, whose efficacy is relatively higher than its ability to block D_2 receptor.[5] This clue indicates that we should determine where the D_2 receptors are most numerous, namely, in the basal ganglia and nucleus accumbens, with decreasing numbers in the globus pallidus, cerebral cortex, and substantia nigra.[6]

The third clue is that there are structural abnormalities in the brains of schizophrenic patients, as seen on neuroimaging (CAT and MRI scans) and in postmortem studies. The most common abnormality seen with CAT scans involves ventriculomegaly,[7] which although important, does not indicate which brain structures should be examined. MRI, on the other hand, has directed studies to the hippocampus and temporal cortex,[8,9] a direction confirmed by postmortem studies that have highlighted the entorhinal cortex.[10–16]

Last, neuropsychological studies, especially when linked to blood flow, have implicated the dorsolateral prefrontal cortex as an important pathological site in patients with schizophrenia.[17] These clues implicate the basal ganglia with nucleus accumbens, the hippocampus-entorhinal cortex complex, and the dorsolateral prefrontal cortex. Other regions have been implicated, such as the brain stem, amygdala, cingulate cortex, and thalamus. In this chapter, we focus on the first three of these regions, which have been most consistently implicated by studies in neuropharmacology, neuroimaging, neuropathology, and neuropsychology.

The Basal Ganglia and the Nucleus Accumbens

One of the major reasons to study the basal ganglia and the nucleus accumbens is the dopamine hypothesis of schizophrenia. Because this hypothesis relates primarily to D_2 receptors, whose highest concentration is in these structures, it is no surprise that both postmortem studies and in vivo imaging have focused on this brain region. Probably the most replicable finding in postmortem neurochemical studies of schizophrenia is increased D_2 receptors in the caudate, putamen, and nucleus accumbens (Table 9–1).[18–37]

The major issue however, is whether these increases are primary to schizophrenia or are a result of neuroleptic treatment that blocks D_2 receptors, leading to dopamine supersensitivity and an increase in D_2 receptor numbers. Several studies with positive findings have had small numbers of drug-naive subjects,[18,20,36] supporting the notion that increases in D_2 are related to schizophrenia per se. At least two other studies have found that subjects who were drug free for 1 month or longer had no increases in D_2 receptors.[21,37] In these studies, only subjects receiving neuroleptics at the time of death or

Table 9–1. D2 receptors in postmortem studies of basal ganglia of schizophrenic patients

Study	Caudate	Putamen	Nucleus accumbens
Lee et al. 1978;[18] Lee and Seeman 1980[19]	+	+	+
Owen et al. 1978[20]	+	+	+
Mackay et al. 1980[21]	NC		NC
Reisine et al. 1980[22]	+	+	+
Reynolds et al. 1980[23]		NC	
Cross et al. 1981[24]	+		
Crow et al. 1981[25]	+	+	+
Kleinman et al. 1982[26]	+		
Mackay et al. 1982[27]	+		+
Cross et al. 1983[28]	+		
Seeman et al. 1984[29], 1987[30]	+	+	+
Pimoule et al. 1985[31]		+	
Mita et al. 1986[32]	+		
Mjörndal and Winblad 1986[33]	+	+	
Toru et al. 1988[34]		+	
Hess et al. 1987[35]	+		
Joyce et al. 1988[36]	+	+	+
Kornhuber et al. 1989[37]		NC	

Note. + = increase. NC = no change.

within 1 month of death had increased D_2 receptors, suggesting that the increases were related to treatment. Attempts to relate differences to psychotic symptoms[25] or to a subtype[29] have been advanced in support of the notion that D_2 receptor increases are related to the illness. These findings, however, can also be interpreted as being a result of treatment.

An alternative approach has been to study living drug-naive schizophrenic patients with D_2 receptor ligands by using PET scanning. These studies have had conflicting results. Using 11C-*N*-methylspiperone, which binds to D_2, D_3, and D_4 receptors, Wong et al.[38] reported increases in schizophrenic relative to control subjects in the striatum. Farde et al.,[39,40] using a more specific (D_2 and D_3)

but lower affinity compound, raclopride, found no difference between schizophrenic and control subjects. Two more recent studies in which 11C-raclopride and 76-bromospiperone were used found D_2 receptor numbers in the striatum to be normal in drug-naive schizophrenic patients.[41,42]

Two other intriguing postmortem findings related to D_2 and D_4 receptors have recently been reported by Seeman et al.[43,44] The first finding reports an abnormal linkage between D_1 and D_2 receptors in the striatum of schizophrenic patients.[43] The second finding involves increases in D_4 receptors in the putamen of schizophrenic patients as compared with control subjects.[44] Both of these findings will require replication in postmortem studies and in vivo imaging, but at the least they are promising new leads.

Although most of the findings in this area involve the caudate, putamen, and nucleus accumbens, the latter has somewhat greater appeal as a locus for psychosis. This emphasis on the nucleus accumbens derives from the fact that, unlike the caudate and putamen, it receives a substantial input from the limbic system, namely, the hippocampus, amygdala, and entorhinal cortex.

The Entorhinal Cortex

A second clue in the neuropathology of schizophrenia has come from neuroimaging of live subjects. The most replicable finding in this area has involved ventriculomegaly in the brains of schizophrenic versus control subjects.[7] Although CAT scans cannot show what specific brain areas are associated with these changes, these studies provide a number of findings about the nature of the neuropathology. Findings in psychotic patients argue against the possibility that this finding is a confounding factor of neuroleptic treatment.[45] Follow-up studies suggested that the changes are not progressive.[46–48] In addition, larger studies could not find meaningful subtypes based on ventricular size.[49] Taken together, these findings suggest that a static encephalopathology is present, at least at the onset of illness (not related to neuroleptic treatment), that is not progressive and that may involve, if not all, at least a large number of patients.

MRI studies have confirmed these results and have allowed the study of specific brain structures. Moreover, in an attempt to reduce variability, a cohort of identical twins who were discordant for schizophrenia were studied with MRI scans.[50] These studies yielded a number of useful findings with regard to the neuropathology of schizophrenia. First, they confirmed the finding of ventriculomegaly. They also showed that, even when ventricular size appeared to be normal in schizophrenic patients, there was enlargement relative to the nonschizophrenic control subject. Second, the results of these studies extended the structural abnormalities into the anterior hippocampus and temporal gray matter, both of which were reduced in size in the schizophrenic twin relative to the cotwin.

Postmortem studies have also found structural abnormalities in both the hippocampus and the entorhinal cortex (Table 9–2).[10–16,51–60] These studies may have found evidence for neurodevelopmental abnormalities with hippocampal disarray[51,53] and disruption of glomeruli in the second layer of the entorhinal cortex.[11,15] These changes have not been associated with gliosis, a hallmark of atrophy, suggesting that these findings may represent early developmental abnormalities. Not all groups have confirmed the hippocampal[10,54,59] or entorhinal findings,[58] but at least two other studies have used other immunocytochemical assays (reduced nicotinamide adenine dinucleotide phosphate [NADPH] diaphorase[61]) and microtubule-associated proteins (MAP-2 and MAP-5)[62] to support the notion of a developmental abnormality in the entorhinal cortex and hippocampus, respectively.

Postmortem neurochemical studies of the hippocampus and entorhinal cortex in schizophrenic patients have found a number of abnormalities that are consistent with a reduction in glutamate receptors.[63–66] Moreover, using in situ hybridization, Harrison et al.[67] reported reductions in messenger RNA (mRNA) kainic acid (glutamate) receptors in the hippocampus of schizophrenic patients relative to control subjects. Replications and further studies to rule out neuroleptic effects are necessary, but this is a potentially important group of findings.

Table 9–2. Neuropathological studies of the hippocampus and entorhinal cortex in patients with schizophrenia

Study	Hippocampus	Entorhinal cortex
Scheibel and Kovelman 1981[51]	+	
Kovelman and Scheibel 1984[52]	+	
Bogerts et al. 1985[12]	+	+
Brown et al. 1986[13]		+
Jakob and Beckmann 1986[14]		+
Colter et al. 1987[15]		+
Altshuler et al. 1987[53]	+	
Falkai et al. 1988[16]		+
Christison et al. 1989[54]	–	
Jeste and Lohr 1989[55]	+	
Jakob and Beckmann 1989[56]		+
Altshuler et al. 1990[10]	–	+/–
Bogerts et al. 1990[57]	+	
Heckers et al. 1990[58]		–
Arnold et al. 1991[11]		+
Benes et al. 1991[59]	+	
Conrad et al. 1991[60]	+	

Note. + = abnormal. – = normal. +/– = debatable.

The Dorsolateral Prefrontal Cortex

One of the hallmarks of schizophrenia has been the cognitive deficits that led Kraepelin to describe dementia praecox.[68] Through systematic study of these deficits with neuropsychological testing, a number of abnormalities, including low IQ, prolonged reaction times, decreased memory, and problems with planning and perseveration, have been identified. Some of the latter abnormalities appear to be referable to the prefrontal cortex. In a series of studies, Berman et al.[17] showed that patients with schizophrenia have difficulty with the Wisconsin Card Sorting Test,[69] a neuropsychological test that activates the dorsolateral prefrontal cortex. When subjects perform the test properly, they increase blood flow in the dorsolateral prefrontal cortex, as measured with SPECT scan. Many schizophrenic patients do poorly on the test and do not increase blood flow in the dorsolateral prefrontal cortex. Moreover, this test, when linked to blood flow, was one of the most reliable discriminators between schizophrenic patients and their healthier identical twins.[70]

Structural abnormalities in the prefrontal cortex have not been as numerous as the hippocampus or entorhinal cortex, but some have been intriguing and promising. In particular, Benes et al.[71] reported abnormalities in structural organization in this region. Moreover, there is evidence that NADPH diaphorase stains neurons in an abnormal distribution in the prefrontal cortex of schizophrenic patients.[72]

Although there have been a number of other neurochemical findings in the prefrontal cortex, one of the more replicated has involved a reduction in serotonin type 2 receptors[73–75] and serotonin reuptake sites.[75] Changes in glutamate receptors in prefrontal cortex have also been reported.[31,64,65,76] The significance of these findings remains to be determined.

Conclusions

A number of findings from neuropharmacology, neuropsychology, and neuroimaging support the notion that the neuropathology of schizophrenia involves the dorsolateral prefrontal cortex, the hippocampus, and the entorhinal cortex. Insofar as D_2 receptors in the nucleus accumbens are relevant to psychosis, it is not an unreasonable hypothesis that schizophrenia may involve an abnormality in a neural network including, but not necessarily restricted to, the dorsolateral prefrontal cortex, the hippocampus-entorhinal cortex, and the nucleus accumbens. Structural abnormalities in the hippocampus-entorhinal cortex may be connected to neurophysiological abnormalities in the dorsolateral prefrontal cortex, both of which contribute to disinhibition of the nucleus accumbens dopaminergic neurons. Whereas the former may explain some of the cognitive deficits in schizophrenia, the latter would be associated with the psychotic symptoms. It is hoped that further studies with autoradiography, in situ hybridization, and molecular biology will elucidate this neuropathology more clearly so that more effective treatments may follow.

References

1. Plum F: Prospects for research on schizophrenia, III: neuropsychology, neuropathological findings. Neurosciences Research Program Bulletin 10:384–388, 1972
2. Ehringer H, Hornykiewicz O: Verteilung von noradrenalin and dopamin (3-hydroxytyramin) im Gehim des Menschen und ihr veerhalten bei erkrankungen des extrapyramidalen systems. Wien Klin Wochenschr 72:1236–1239, 1960
3. Cotzias GC, Van Woert MH, Schiffer LM: Aromatic amino acids and modification of parkinsonism. N Engl J Med 276:374–397, 1967
4. Creese I, Burt DR, Snyder SH: Dopamine receptors binding predict clinical and pharmacological potencies of antischizophrenic drugs. Science 192:481–483, 1976
5. Seeman P: Dopamine receptors sequences: therapeutic levels of neuroleptics occupy D2 receptors, clozapine occupies D4. Neuropsychopharmacology 7:261–284, 1992
6. Hyde TM, Casanova MF, Kleinman JE, et al: Neuroanatomical and neurochemical pathology in schizophrenia, in American Psychiatric Press Review of Psychiatry, Vol 10. Edited by Tasman A, Goldfinger SM. Washington, DC, American Psychiatric Press, 1991, pp 7–23
7. Shelton RC, Weinberger DR: X-ray computerized tomography studies in schizophrenia: a review and synthesis, in Handbook of Schizophrenia, Vol 1: The Neurology of Schizophrenia. Edited by Nasrallah HA, Weinberger DR. Amsterdam, Elsevier North-Holland, 1986, pp 207–250
8. Suddath RL, Casanova MF, Goldberg TE, et al: Temporal lobe

pathology in schizophrenia: a quantitative magnetic resonance imaging study. Am J Psychiatry 146:462–472, 1989

9. DeLisi IE, Dauphinais ID, Gershon ES: Perinatal complications and reduced size of brain limbic structures in familial schizophrenia. Schizophr Bull 14:185–191, 1988
10. Altshuler LL, Casanova MF, Goldberg TE, et al: The hippocampus and parahippocampus in schizophrenic, suicide and control brains. Arch Gen Psychiatry 47:1029–1034, 1990
11. Arnold SE, Hyman BT, Van Hosen GW: Some cytoarchitectural abnormalities of the entorhinal cortex in schizophrenia. Arch Gen Psychiatry 48:625–632, 1991
12. Bogerts B, Meertz E, Schonfeld-Bausch R: Basal ganglia and limbic system pathology in schizophrenia. Arch Gen Psychiatry 42:784–791, 1985
13. Brown R, Colter N, Corsellis JA, et al: Postmortem evidence of structural brain changes in schizophrenia: differences in brain weight, temporal horn area, and parahippocampal gyrus compared with affective disorder. Arch Gen Psychiatry 43:36–42, 1986
14. Jakob H, Beckmann H: Prenatal developmental disturbance in schizophrenics. Journal of Neural Transmission 65:303–326, 1986
15. Colter N, Battal S, Crow TJ, et al: White matter reduction in the parahippocampal gyrus of patients with schizophrenia (letter). Arch Gen Psychiatry 44:1023, 1987
16. Falkai P, Bogerts B, Rozumek M: Limbic pathology in schizophrenia: the entorhinal region. Biol Psychiatry 24:515–521, 1988
17. Weinberger DR, Zec RF, Berman KF: Physiologic dysfunction of dorsolateral prefrontal cortex in schizophrenia, I: regional cerebral blood flow (rCBF evidence). Arch Gen Psychiatry 43:114–124, 1986
18. Lee T, Seeman P, Tourtelotte WW, et al: Binding of 3H-neuroleptics and 3H-apomorphine in schizophrenic brains. Nature 274:897–900, 1978
19. Lee T, Seeman P: Elevation of brain neuroleptic/dopamine receptors in schizophrenia. Am J Psychiatry 137:191–197, 1980
20. Owen F, Cross AJ, Crow TJ, et al: Increased dopamine-receptor

sensitivity in schizophrenia. Lancet 2:223–225, 1978

21. Mackay AVP, Bird O, Bird ED, et al: Dopamine receptors and schizophrenia: drug effect or illness? Lancet 2:915–916, 1980
22. Reisine TE, Rossor M, Spokes E, et al: Opiate and neuroleptic receptor alterations in human schizophrenic brain tissue, in Receptors for Neurotransmitter and Peptide Hormones. Edited by Pepeu G, Kuhar MJ, Enna SJ. New York, Raven, 1980, pp 443–450
23. Reynolds GP, Reynolds IM, Riederer P, et al: Dopamine receptors and schizophrenia: drug effect or illness? Lancet 2:1251, 1980
24. Cross AJ, Crow TJ, Owen F: 3H Flupenthixol binding in postmortem brains of schizophrenics: evidence for selective increase in dopamine D2 receptors. Psychopharmacology (Berl) 74:122–124, 1981
25. Crow TJ, Owen F, Cross AJ, et al: Neurotransmitter enzymes and receptors in postmortem brain in schizophrenia: evidence that an increase in D2 dopamine receptors is associated with type I syndrome, in Transmitter Biochemistry of Human Brain Tissue. Edited by Riederer P, Usdin E. London, Macmillan, 1981, pp 85–96
26. Kleinman JE, Karoum F, Rosenblatt JE, et al: Postmortem neurochemical studies in chronic schizophrenia, in Biological Markers in Psychiatry and Neurology. Edited by Usdin E, Hanin I. New York, Pergamon, 1982, pp 67–76
27. Mackay AVP, Iverson LL, Rossor M, et al: Increased brain dopamine and dopamine receptors in schizophrenia. Arch Gen Psychiatry 39:991–997, 1982
28. Cross AJ, Crow TJ, Ferrier IN, et al: Dopamine receptor changes in schizophrenia in relation to disease process and movement disorder. J Neural Transmission 18 (suppl):265–272, 1983
29. Seeman P, Ulpian C, Bergeron C, et al: Bimodal distribution of dopamine receptor densities in brains of schizophrenics. Science 225:728–731, 1984
30. Seeman P, Bzowej NH, Guan H-C, et al: Human brain D1 and D2 dopamine receptors in schizophrenia, Alzheimers, Parkinsons and Huntingtons disease. Neuropsychopharmacology 1:5–15, 1987

31. Pimoule C, Schoemaker H, Reynolds GP, et al: [3H]SCH23390 labeled D1 dopamine receptors are unchanged in schizophrenia and Parkinsons disease. Eur J Pharmacol 114:235–237, 1985
32. Mita T, Hanada S, Nishino N, et al: Decreased serotonin S2 and increased dopamine D2 receptors in chronic schizophrenics. Biol Psychiatry 21:1407–1414, 1986
33. Mjörndal T, Winblad B: Alteration of dopamine receptors in the caudate nucleus and the putamen in schizophrenic brain. Medical Biological 64:351–354, 1986
34. Toru M, Watanabe S, Shibuya H, et al: Neurotransmitters, receptors and neuropeptides in post-mortem brains of chronic schizophrenic patients. Acta Psychiatr Scand 78:121–137, 1988
35. Hess EJ, Bracha HS, Kleinman JE, et al: Dopamine receptor subtype imbalance in schizophrenia. Life Sci 40:1487–1497, 1987
36. Joyce JN, Lexow N, Bird E, et al: Organization of dopamine D1 and D2 receptors in human striatum: receptor autoradiographic studies in Huntingtons disease and schizophrenia. Synapse 2:546–557, 1988
37. Kornhuber J, Riederer P, Reynolds GP, et al: 3H-Spiperone binding sites in post-mortem brains from schizophrenic patients. Journal of Neural Transmission 75:1–10, 1989
38. Wong DF, Wagner HN, Tune LE, et al: Positron emission tomography reveals elevated D2 dopamine receptors in drug-naive schizophrenics. Science 234:1558–1563, 1986
39. Farde L, Wiesel FA, Hall H, et al: No D2 receptor increase in PET study of schizophrenia. Arch Gen Psychiatry 44:671–672, 1987
40. Farde L, Wiesel FA, Stone-Elander S, et al: D2 receptors in neuroleptic-naive schizophrenic patients. Arch Gen Psychiatry 47:213–219, 1990
41. Martinot J, Peron-Magnan P, Huret J, et al: Striatal D2 dopamine receptors assessed with positron emission tomography and [76 Br] bromospiperone in untreated schizophrenic patients. Am J Psychiatry 147:44–50, 1990
42. Hietala J, Syvalahti E, Vuorio K, et al: Striatal D2 dopamine receptor characteristics in neuroleptic-naive schizophrenic patients studied with positron emission tomography. Arch Gen Psychiatry 51:116–123, 1994

43. Seeman P, Guan H-C, Van Tol HH, et al: Dopamine D4 receptors elevated in schizophrenia. Nature 365:441–445, 1993
44. Seeman P, Niznik HB, Guan H-C et al: Link between D1 and D2 dopamine receptors is reduced in schizophrenia and Huntington diseased brain. Proc Natl Acad Sci U S A 86:10156–10160, 1989
45. Weinberger DR, DeLisi L, Perman GP, et al: Computed tomography in schizophreniform disorder and other psychiatry disorders. Arch Gen Psychiatry 39:778–793, 1982
46. Sponheim SR, Iacono WG, Beiser M: Stability of ventricular size after the onset of psychosis in schizophrenia. Psychiatr Res 40:21–29, 1991
47. Illowsky BK, Juliano DM, Bigelow LB, et al: Stability of CT finding in schizophrenia: result of an eight year follow-up study. J Neurol Neurosurg Psychiatry 51:209–213, 1988
48. Abi-Dargham A, Jaskiw G, Suddath R, et al: Evidence against progression of in vivo abnormalities in schizophrenia. Schizophr Res 5:210, 1991
49. Daniel DG, Goldberg TE, Weinberger DR: Lack of bimodal distribution of ventricular size in patients with schizophrenia. Biol Psychiatry 30:887–903, 1991
50. Suddath RL, Christison GW, Torrey EF, et al: Anatomical abnormalities in the brains of monozygotic twins discordant for schizophrenia. N Engl J Med 322:789–794, 1990
51. Scheibel AB, Kovelman JA: Disorientation of the hippocampal pyramidal cell and its process in the schizophrenic patient. Biol Psychiatry 16:101–102, 1981
52. Kovelman JA, Scheibel AB: A neurohistological correlate of schizophrenia. Biol Psychiatry 19:1601–1621, 1984
53. Altshuler LL, Conrad A, Kovelman JA, et al: Hippoccampal pyramidal cell orientation in schizophrenia: a controlled neurohistologic study of the Yakovlev collection. Arch Gen Psychiatry 44:1094–1098, 1987
54. Christison GW, Casanova MF, Weinberger DR, et al: A quantitative investigation of hippocampal orientation in schizophrenia. Arch Gen Psychiatry 46:1027–1037, 1989
55. Jeste DV, Lohr JB: Hippocampal pathological findings in schizo-

phrenia: a morphometric study. Arch Gen Psychiatry 46:1019–1024, 1989

56. Jakob H, Beckmann H: Gross and histological criteria for developmental disorders in brains of schizophrenics. J R Soc Med 82:466–469, 1989
57. Bogerts B, Falkai P, Haupts M, et al: Post-mortem volume measurements of limbic system and basal ganglia structure in chronic schizophrenics. Schizophr Res 3:295–301, 1990
58. Heckers S, Heinsen H, Heinsen Y, et al: Morphometry of the parahippocampal gyrus in schizophrenics and controls: some anatomical considerations. J Neural Transm Gen Sect 80:151–155, 1990
59. Benes FM, Sorenso I, Bird E: Reduced neuronal size in posterior hippocampus of schizophrenic patients. Schizophr Bull 17:597–608, 1991
60. Conrad AJ, Abebe T, Austin R, et al: Hippocampal pyramidal cell disarray in schizophrenia as a bilateral phenomenon. Arch Gen Psychiatry 48:413–417, 1991
61. Akbarian S, Vinuela A, Kim JJ, et al: Distorted distribution of nicotinamide-adenine dinucleotide phosphate-diaphorase neurons in temporal lobe of schizophrenics implies anomalous cortical development. Arch Gen Psychiatry 50:178–187, 1993
62. Arnold SE, Lee VM, Gur RE, et al: Abnormal expression of two microtubule-associated proteins (MAP2 and MAP5) in specific subfields of the hippocampal formulation in schizophrenia. Proc Natl Acad Sci U S A 88:10850–10854, 1991
63. Kerwin RW, Patel S, Meldrum BS, et al: Asymmetrical loss of glutamate receptor subtype in left hippocampus schizophrenia. Lancet 1:583–584, 1988
64. Deakin JF, Slater P, Simpson MB, et al: Frontal cortical and left temporal glutamatergic dysfunction in schizophrenia. J Neurochem 52:1781–1786, 1989
65. Kornhuber J, Mack-Burkhardt F, Riederer P, et al: [3H] MK-801 binding site in postmortem brain regions of schizophrenic patients. Journal of Neural Transmission 77:231–236, 1989
66. Kerwin R, Patel S, Meldrum B: Quantitative autoradiographic analysis of glutamate binding sites in the hippocampal forma-

tion in normal and schizophrenic brain postmortem. Neuroscience 39:25–32, 1990

67. Harrison PJ, McLaughlin D, Kerwin RW: Decreased hippocampal expression of a glutamate receptor gene in schizophrenia. Lancet 337:450–452, 1991
68. Kraeplin E: Dementia Praecox and Paraphrenia. Translated by Barclay RM, edited by Robertson GM. 1919 Facsimile edition. Huntington, NY, Krieger, 1971
69. Heaton R: Wisconsin Card Sorting Test. Odessa, TX, Psychological Assessment Resources, 1985
70. Weinberger DR, Berman KF, Suddath R, et al: Evidence for dysfunction of a prefrontal-limbic network in schizophrenia: an MRI and rCBF study of discordant monozygotic twins. Am J Psychiatry 149:890–897, 1992
71. Benes FM, Davidson J, Bird E: Quantitative cytoarchitectural studies of cerebral cortex of schizophrenics. Arch Gen Psychiatry 43:31–35, 1986
72. Akbarian S, Bunney WE, Potkin S, et al: Altered distribution of nicotinamide-adenine dinucleotide phosphate-diaphorase cells in frontal lobe of schizophrenics implies disturbance of cortical development. Arch Gen Psychiatry 50:169–177, 1993
73. Mita T, Hanada S, Nishino N, et al: Decreased serotonin S2 and increased dopamine D2 receptors in chronic schizophrenics. Biol Psychiatry 21:1407–1414, 1986
74. Arora RC, Meltzer HY: Serotonin 2(5HT2) receptor binding in the frontal cortex of schizophrenic patients. J Neural Transm Gen Sect 85:19–29, 1991
75. Laruelle M, Toti R, Abi-Dargham A, et al: Selective abnormalities of prefrontal serotonergic markers in schizophrenia: a postmortem study. Arch Gen Psychiatry 50:810–818, 1993
76. Nishikawa T, Takashima M, Toru M: Increased [3H] kainic acid binding in the prefrontal cortex in schizophrenia. Neurosci Lett 40:245–250, 1983

CHAPTER

10

Brain Circuits and Brain Function: Implications for Psychiatric Diseases

Marcus E. Raichle, M.D.
Wayne C. Drevets, M.D.

Relatively little is known about the functional anatomy of human emotional experience. This paucity of knowledge reflects the fact that research designed to inform us about the functional anatomy of human emotional experience must include research on humans. Until recently, tools did not exist that could accurately and safely reveal functional changes in the human brain associated with emotional experience. That changed in the early 1970s with the introduction of modern functional brain imaging techniques. Stimulated by the invention of X-ray computed tomography (CT), scientists developed positron emission tomography (PET) to permit classical tissue autoradiography to be performed safely in human subjects.[1]

PET, a nuclear medicine imaging technique in which radiopharmaceuticals are labeled with positron-emitting radionuclides,[1] has revolutionized scientists' ability to accurately study the biochemistry, metabolism, and circulatory physiology of the normal and diseased brain. Most important, because of the intimate relationship among neuronal activity, metabolism, and brain circulation,[2] this technique can reveal the changes within local circuits of the brain that accompany complex activities such as emotion, perception, remembering, learning, and speaking.[3–6] This ability has provided an obvious opportunity to study human emotional experience, an opportunity that has been exploited by a number of research groups.[7–15]

The Strategy of Functional Brain Imaging

The images of brain function that have been achieved with PET result from the ability of this technique to measure the local changes in blood flow and metabolism that accompany local changes in neuronal activity.[2] It is now estimated that, within several seconds of the onset of a change in neuronal activity in the human brain, there is an accompanying change in local blood flow and metabolism. Although the actual changes in neuronal activity occur much faster than the changes in blood flow and metabolism (e.g., on the order of a few milliseconds for neurons, as compared with a few hundred milliseconds for blood vessels and metabolism), these vascular and metabolic signals provide the basis for developing very reliable and detailed maps of those parts of the brain that collectively participate in specific types of cognitive activity. As such, these functional maps provide a description of the circuitry underlying specific mental operations.[6]

The studies from our laboratory described in this chapter were performed by using measurements of local blood flow in the brain with PET.[16,17] These measurements were accomplished by administering intravenously, as a bolus, a small quantity of saline containing water labeled with the cyclotron-produced, positron-emitting radionuclide ^{15}O. The actual measurement time was 40 seconds after the arrival of the intravenous bolus of $H_2{}^{15}O$ in the brain (approximately 20 seconds after injection). Because of the short (123 seconds) physical half-life of ^{15}O, the measurement of blood flow can be repeated every 10 minutes for a total of 10 measurements in a single experimental setting. A direct, linear correlation exists between the local quantity of radioactivity in the brain and brain blood flow when the measurement is made in the first minute after intravenous injection of the radiotracer;[16] it is therefore possible to achieve quite accurate brain mapping with PET and $H_2{}^{15}O$ by simply using radioactive counts. Doing so eliminates the need for arterial catheterization, improving the subject's comfort and acceptance of the procedure and simplifying the procedure itself.[18]

A critical feature of modern imaging strategies of human brain function is the notion of isolating specific mental operations or emotional states between a control state and an activated state.[5,6] This concept was first articulated in a study by the Dutch physiologist Donders in 1868,[19] in which he used the subject's reaction time to discern the components of mental operations. Today, by subtracting blood flow measurements made in a control state (e.g., viewing words) from those made in a task state (e.g., speaking the viewed words), it is possible to identify those areas of the brain concerned with the mental operations that are unique to the task state (i.e., motor programming and motor output).

This strategy is very different from that previously employed in many studies, in which particular regions of the brain were arbitrarily identified before the acquisition of data, based on preexisting hypotheses about the involvement of the area (e.g., the dorsolateral prefrontal cortex in schizophrenia). This latter strategy assumed a level of understanding of human cortical organization that, unfortunately, was often insufficient. With the current strategy, hypotheses are generated about cortical areas involved in particular tasks or emotional states. A variety of statistical strategies are then employed to determine which areas are significantly involved. One of the most challenging aspects of this work is the design of imaging paradigms that limit the number of mental operations under study in a particular blood flow subtraction pair.

One application of functional brain imaging with PET to the study of psychiatric disorders has been an extension of the strategy just described.[7,8] Functional imaging of experimentally manipulated cognitive states in psychiatrically normal individuals involves subtracting one state from another in the same individual.[6] Functional imaging of psychiatric disorders as we have employed it involves subtracting a single composite image composed of a group of individuals with a well-defined disorder (e.g., familial pure depressive disease [FPDD]) from a single composite image composed of a group of psychiatrically normal control subjects.[7] The study of FPDD conducted by our group[7,8] is a good example of how new insights can be gained with this approach.

Imaging Studies in Patients With FPDD

In 1992, we reported a study[7] in which,, using the PET image subtraction briefly described above, we measured the differences in regional cerebral blood flow between a group of patients with FPDD and a group of psychiatrically normal control subjects. The diagnosis of FPDD was based on a family history as well as symptoms and course. Using this strategy, we found increased blood flow in an area that extended from the left ventrolateral prefrontal cortex onto the medial prefrontal cortical surface (Figure 10–1). Based on the known connectivity between these portions of the prefrontal cortex and the amygdala, as well as evidence that the amygdala is involved in emotional modulation, activity was measured in the left amygdala and was found to be significantly increased in the depressed group. Additional findings included increased blood flow in the medial thalamus and reduced blood flow in the caudate nucleus.

From these data, along with other evidence from our imaging study,[7] we were able to suggest that a limbic-thalamo-cortical circuit and a limbic-striatal-pallidal-thalamic (LSPT) circuit (Figure 10–2) are involved in the functional anatomy of unipolar depression. In a separate group of individuals with FPDD who were in remission,[7] we attempted to determine whether any of these abnormalities were associated with the depressed state or with a trait difference that might underlie the tendency to become depressed. These data strongly suggested, although they did not prove, that changes in the amygdala were most likely to be associated with the trait to be depressed. The changes in other areas observed in the depressed state were absent in the remitted state.

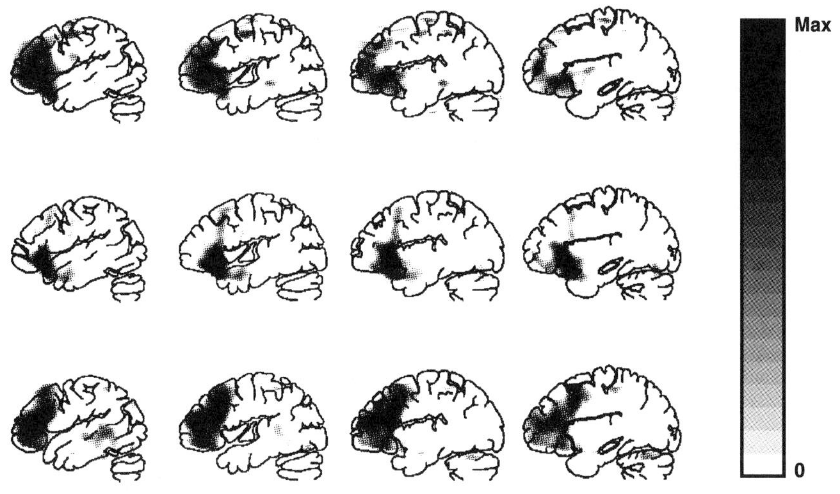

Figure 10–1. Sagittal PET images of differences in blood flow between patients with familial pure depressive disorder (FPDD) with major depression and control subjects *(top row)*; between a state of self-induced dysphoria and quiet rest in volunteers *(middle row)*; and between generating appropriate verbs for nouns read from a television monitor and simply reading the nouns aloud *(bottom row)*. Note that in each of these subtraction images there is increased blood flow in the dorsolateral and ventrolateral prefrontal cortex in the left hemisphere.

It was clear to us from these data that the clinical state of depression in patients with FPDD is the result of changes in neuronal activity within a group of cortical and subcortical areas that form a pair of interrelated functional circuits (Figure 10–2). It is not, as some might have suspected, due to a disorder in a single brain area. How are we to think about such circuits? How do they provide the basis for the observable behavior?

The hypothesis is that elementary operations form the basis of human behavior, and it is these elementary operations that are strictly localized in the brain and revealed by functional imaging studies in humans.[6] Many such operations are involved in any behavioral state or cognitive operation. A set of distributed brain areas, such as those observed in depression, must be orchestrated in the

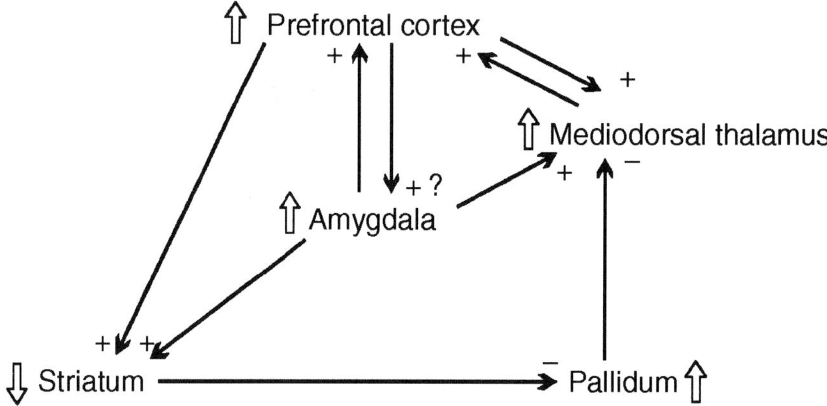

Figure 10–2. Neuroanatomical circuits hypothesized to participate in the functional anatomy of unipolar major depression, based on functional brain imaging studies with PET. Regions containing differences in blood flow are indicated by open arrows, which indicate the direction of change in flow in the patients with depression relative to control subjects. The regions' monosynaptic connections with each other are indicated by solid arrows. + = Excitatory projections. − = inhibitory projections. ? = experimental evidence is limited.

production of even a simple behavioral state. The behavior itself is not produced in any single area of the brain, but the operations that underlie the behavior are strictly localized. An appreciation of this type of functional brain organization can be enhanced by considering two other behavioral conditions that share some of the same circuitry with unipolar depression but differ in their manifested behavior. These include self-induced dysphoria[20] and a simple verbal response selection task.[21–23]

Imaging Studies in Subjects With Self-Induced Dysphoria

Dysphoria is a negative mood state manifested by feelings of sadness, sorrow, anguish, misery, and mental malaise. When severe and persistent, these symptoms characterize major depression. Although everyone has had vivid and personal experiences of at least transient dysphoria, the relationship between dysphoric mood and the persistent dysphoric affect seen in patients with major depression and other psychiatric diseases is unknown.

Several years ago, we thought it reasonable to test the hypothesis that acute, transient changes in mood reflect changes in the activity of discrete neuronal systems in the human brain. We tested this hypothesis by using PET to measure changes in blood flow[20] in psychiatrically normal young adults. The subjects were initially scanned while resting quietly with their eyes closed. They were then scanned a second time, during which they were asked to imagine or recall situations that would make them very sad. They had started to imagine such situations about 3 minutes before they were scanned. They were explicitly asked to experience sad feelings and to avoid feelings of anger or anxiety. Other studies[24,25] have found that similar procedures for inducing dysphoria produce characteristic covert facial electromyographic activity, as well as lacrimal flow. On completion of the PET scan, the subjects' moods were assessed by determination of tearing and by their self-rating of their emotional state on a visual analogue scale.

All subjects reported experiencing sadness during the active condition. Typical ruminations included imaging the death of a loved one or the loss of a pet. Tearing occurred in all three women studied and in two of the four men. The most striking area of activation for both the men and the women occurred in the left prefrontal and orbito-frontal cortices (Figure 10–1). This area of activation overlapped to some degree with the areas of left prefrontal cortex seen in the depressed patients with FPDD.

After the publication of our results on FPDD[7,8] and self-induced dysphoria,[20] we compared the results of these two studies in terms of the brain circuits revealed by our studies of FPDD (Figure 10–2). The results of this comparison are shown in Figure 10–3 (W. C. Drevets and M. E. Raichle, unpublished data, January 94). They suggest that both conditions share some areas in common (e.g., ventral lateral prefrontal cortex, medial orbital prefrontal cortex, and pregenual anterior cingulate cortex) but differ significantly in other areas. The areas of difference include the dorsal anterior cingulate,

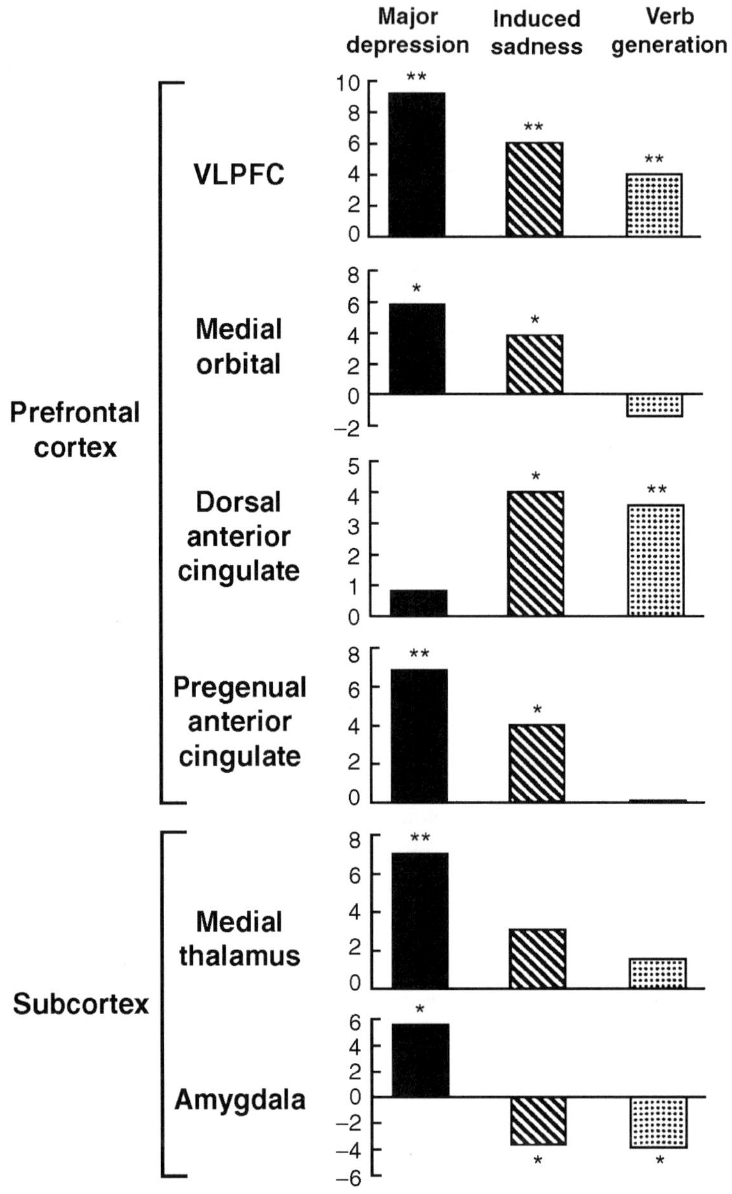

Figure 10–3. Changes in blood flow from the control state (see text) in three different conditions (major depression, self-induced sadness and generating verbs for visually presented nouns) within the areas of the circuit shown in Figure 10–2. VLPFC = Ventrolateral prefrontal cortex.
$^{*}P < .05$; $^{**}P < .01$.

where blood flow is significantly elevated in patients with self-induced dysphoria but not in those with the major depression of FPDD. In the amygdala, blood flow is significantly elevated in patients with the depression of FPDD but significantly reduced in those with the sadness of transient self-induced dysphoria. Not surprisingly, the negative mood states of transient self-induced dysphoria and the depression of FPDD share some of the same brain circuitry. Importantly, there are also significant differences that must reflect differences in the underlying mental operations, which have yet to be defined. Results of this type lend support to the hypothesis that functional imaging studies of emotional states and mood disorders will eventually permit a much more complete understanding of their underlying neurobiology.

Further insight into the task of unravelling the elementary mental operations represented in these circuits is revealed by the results of an additional PET study of verbal response selection.[21–23] Although behaviorally quite different from the results of imaging studies of transient self-induced dysphoria and major depression, PET functional imaging results from our study of verbal response selection revealed overlapping brain circuitry (Figures 10–1 and 10–3). Such an overlap immediately invites questions about possible shared, elementary mental operations.

Imaging Studies of Verbal Response Selection

The purpose of this work has been to explore the manner in which the normal human brain processes single words. The experiment we describe here was part of a much larger project[21–23] designed to explore processes ranging from the passive visual and auditory perception of words to reading, syntax, and semantics.

Subjects were asked to speak a verb for common English nouns presented at the rate of 40 words per minute on a television monitor. The control state for this task (hereafter referred to as the "verb generation task") was reading aloud the visually presented noun. Increases in blood flow were identified in four areas (anterior cingulate cortex, left prefrontal cortex, and left, posterior, middle temporal cortex, as well as the right cerebellar hemisphere). The increased blood flow in the left prefrontal cortex was remarkably similar in location and extent to the changes we observed in the left prefrontal cortex in the major depression associated with FPDD (Figure 10–1).

In addition to these increases in blood flow, significant decreases were observed in Sylvian-insular cortices. These decreases were bilateral but were greater on the right than on the left.[23] By decreases, we mean that these Sylvian-insular areas were active in the control task (i.e., reading aloud nouns) but were inactive during verb generation. Other areas of the motor system (i.e., primary motor cortex bilaterally, supplementary motor cortex, and paramedian regions of the cerebellum) were equally active during both noun reading and verb generation.

The results of the verb generation task caused us to consider the possibility that there existed two alternative routes for verbal response selection—an automatic route involving Sylvian-insular cortices bilaterally and a nonautomatic route involving anterior cingulate, left prefrontal and left temporal cortices, and the right cerebellar hemisphere. Behavioral studies of the verb generation task strengthened that hypothesis by demonstrating rapid learning of the task with the development of stereotyped responses when the same list of 40 nouns was used throughout. To test this hypothesis, we performed a PET imaging experiment in which subjects were tested on the verb generation task and then practiced on the same list of nouns for 15 minutes. At the end of the 15 minutes of practice, the PET measurements of blood flow were repeated. The results[23] indicated unequivocally that practice converted the functional anatomy seen with naive verb generation to that seen with simple noun repetition; that is, activity in anterior cingulate, left prefrontal and left temporal cortices, and cerebellum had disappeared and activity in Sylvian-insular cortices bilaterally had been restored.

Shared Circuits

Figure 10–3, which compares the selected subcortical and cortical areas active in the three conditions we consider in this chapter, provides some insight into the type of overlapping, spatially distributed functional organization underlying human behavior. For example, within the prefrontal cortex, areas outside the ventrolateral portion were activated in each of the three conditions. In the language task, blood flow increased in part of the left dorsolateral prefrontal cortex.[21–23] Blood flow was unchanged in this area in induced sadness and major depression. In contrast, blood flow was increased in the medial orbital cortex in the depressed phase of FPDD and the self-induced dysphoria task but not in the verb generation task (Figure 10–3).

Changes in blood flow in the anterior cingulate cortex also differed between the emotional and verb-generation conditions. During verb generation and self-induced dysphoria, blood flow increased in the portion of the anterior cingulate located dorsocaudal to the genu of the corpus callosum.[21–23] Blood flow was unchanged in this portion of the anterior cingulate in major depression but was increased in self-induced dysphoria. In contrast, blood flow was increased in the pregenual portion of the anterior cingulate cortex in both emotional states but not in the verb generation task.

In subcortical regions, all three conditions were associated with increased blood flow in the left medial thalamus. In the amygdala, however, blood flow was increased only in the depressed subjects with FPDD. In contrast, blood flow was significantly decreased in the amygdala during both the verb generation and the self-induced dysphoria tasks (Figure 10–3).

Data from these PET functional imaging studies indicate that these three different behavioral states must share in common at least some elementary mental operations. Each of these states is uniquely represented within a group of brain areas (Figure 10–3). Thus, clinically defined behavioral states such as major depression are neurobiologically defined by a unique, spatially distributed, functional network of brain areas acting together in a manner distinctive for that state (e.g., Figure 10–2). Major depression and, presumably, other psychiatric diseases are not neurobiologically defined by the abnormalities of a single brain area. None of the areas within such a network are necessarily unique, by themselves, to a particular behavioral state (e.g., see Figures 10–1 and 10–3).

Rather, each area within the network becomes a candidate for a specific, elementary mental operation.[6] These basic, elementary mental operations are likely to be the building blocks of a variety of behavioral states (Figure 10–3), much as the members of a great symphony orchestra are the building blocks of an infinite variety of musical experiences. We have tried to capture this concept in Figure 10–4. Our challenge is to continue to refine our analysis of both the mental state, in terms of its elementary mental operations, and its underlying neurobiology. Doing so will move us a step closer to an understanding of the relationship between the brain and the mind and provide a much more rational basis for the treatment of psychiatric diseases such as major depression.

Examining what we currently know about the brain circuits underlying major depression in patients with FPDD is useful in indicat-

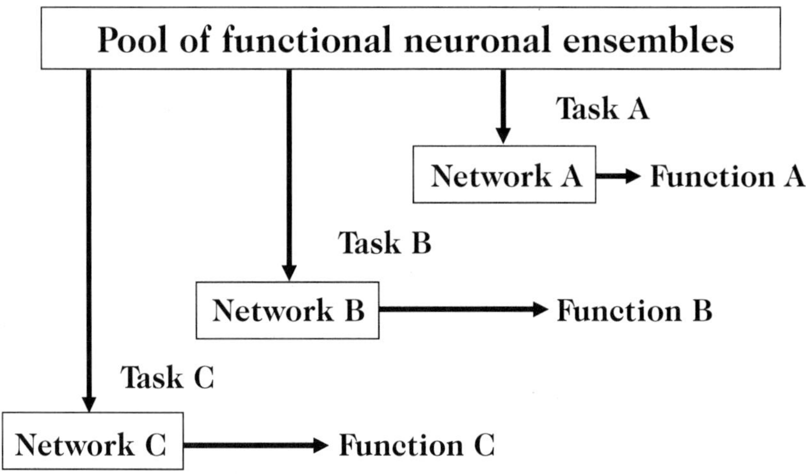

Figure 10–4. General concept of the manner in which the brain allocates a finite number of processing elements (each representing unique, elementary mental operations) into a potentially infinite number of circuits that represent the neurobiological instantiation of human behavior.

ing how such information can guide our thinking in the future. We next turn to a brief discussion of the neurobiology of these circuits.

The Anatomical Circuitry of FPDD

Our findings suggest that two interconnected circuits are involved in the pathophysiology of FPDD (Figure 10–2): a limbic-thalamo-cortical circuit involving the amygdala, the mediodorsal nucleus (MD) of the thalamus, and the ventrolateral and medial prefrontal cortex; and an LSPT circuit involving related parts of the striatum and the ventral pallidum, as well as the components of the other circuit. The first of these circuits can be conceptualized as an excitatory triangular circuit in which the amygdala and the prefrontal cortical regions are interconnected by excitatory projection with each other and with the MD.[26] Through these connections, the amygdala is in a position both to directly activate the prefrontal cortex and to modulate the reciprocal interaction between the prefrontal cortex and the MD.

The LSPT circuit constitutes a disinhibitory side loop between the amygdala or the prefrontal cortex and the MD. The amygdala and the prefrontal cortex send excitatory projections to overlapping parts of the ventromedial caudate and nucleus accumbens.[27] As with the more extensively studied dorsal striatal-pallidal pathway, this part of the striatum sends an inhibitory projection to the ventral pallidum,[28]which in turn sends γ-aminobutyric acid (GABA)-ergic, inhibitory fibers to the MD. Because the pallidal neurons have relatively high spontaneous firing rates,[29] activity in the prefrontal cortex or amygdala that activates the striatum and in turn inhibits the ventral pallidum would release MD from an inhibitory pallidal influence. Thus, if the amygdala is abnormally active in patients with major depression, it can potentially produce an episode of abnormal activity in the prefrontal cortex and MD, both directly and through the striatum and pallidum.

One of the major theories regarding the pathophysiology of major depression holds that stress-induced, long-term potentiation related to kindling or behavioral sensitization occurs in the amygdala and leads to recurrent spontaneous episodes of depression.[30] Because these phenomena represent permanent changes in neuronal sensitivity, this hypothesis appears to be compatible with our observation that activity in the amygdala is abnormally increased in remitted subjects with FPDD who are no longer taking antidepressant drugs.[9] More recently, we reported that antidepressant drug treatment profoundly decreased blood flow in the amygdala.[10] The amygdala had previously been implicated by preclinical data as a primary target of antidepressant drugs, which both ameliorate and prevent depressive episodes.[8] Our data are thus intriguing in light of Post's[30] hypothesis that long-term prophylactic treatment may be indicated to prevent abnormal amygdala activity from reemerging and inducing recurrences of major depression.

In a complementary hypothesis, Swerdlow and Koob[31] proposed a neural model of major depression involving the LSPT circuit. Their model is also compatible with our data and may additionally explain the observation of decreased blood flow in the caudate. Based in part on evidence of decreased dopaminergic activity in patients with depression, they hypothesized that decreased dopaminergic transmission into the ventromedial caudate and nucleus accumbens[32] enhances reentrant activity among the prefrontal cortex, amygdala, and MD. They proposed that this leads to the perseveration of a fixed set of cortical activity, manifested by the emotional, cognitive, and motor processes of depression. Dopaminergic projections from the substantia nigra and ventral tegmental area to the striatum, amygdala, and prefrontal cortex comprise an important inhibitory or modulatory input into these structures.[28] Thus, the effect of mesostriatal dopamine deficiency would be to increase striatal output, thereby inhibiting the pallidum and disinhibiting the MD. This, together with the decrease in direct dopamine effects in the amygdala and prefrontal cortex, would increase activity in the limbic-thalamo-cortical circuit, potentially yielding the blood flow increases we found (Figures 10–1 and 10–3). Moreover, if mesostriatal dopaminergic transmission is reduced, decreased synaptic activity at striatal dopamine receptors would probably appear as decreased blood flow in the caudate,[33] which is also consistent with our observations.

The LSPT Circuit and Other Depressive Subtypes

In humans, lesions that involve the parts of the prefrontal cortex that participate in these circuits (i.e., tumors and strokes) and diseases of the basal ganglia (e.g., Parkinson's disease and Huntington's disease) are associated with higher rates of major depression than are other, similarly debilitating conditions.[34–36] These associations suggest that dysfunction at multiple points within the LSPT circuit may give rise to major depressive syndrome. Moreover, because these conditions affect this system in different ways, it may also be suggested that the imbalances within these circuits, rather than overall increased or decreased activity within a particular area, may produce the major depressive syndrome.

If diverse types of modulatory dysfunction within the same circuit can result in mood disturbances, then different functional anatomical correlates reflected by distinct PET images could be associated with the major depressive syndrome. For example, in contrast to the PET findings in patients with primary unipolar depression, patients with bipolar depression generally display decreased blood flow and metabolism in the prefrontal cortex and normal caudate metabolism.[11–15] In our own investigations of patients with bipolar depression, blood flow was decreased in the medial orbital cortex, the prelimbic portion of the anterior cingulate gyrus, and the medial thalamus, areas where flow had been abnormally increased in the patients with unipolar depression with FPDD.[9] Moreover, discriminant analysis of the covariance of blood flow in the left prefrontal cortex, amygdala, caudate, and medial thalamus sensitively distinguished FPDD subjects from both control and bipolar subjects.[9] The observation that in the ventral prefrontal cortex both increased (in unipolar depression) and decreased (in bipolar depression) blood flow or metabolism are associated with major depression is consistent with the hypothesis that abnormal modulation within the LSPT circuit, rather than increased or decreased activity in any single structure, may produce the major depressive syndrome.

Distinct pathophysiologies within the LSPT circuit could also account for the clinical dissimilarities that distinguish unipolar and bipolar depression. This would again reflect the case in the motor circuit where opposite effects upon modulation at a given limb of the circuit yield distinct clinical movement disorders. For example, in Parkinson's disease, striatal-pallidal transmission is pathologically increased, and the resulting abnormal movements consist of tremor, bradykinesia, and cogwheel rigidity and the course of the induced depression is always unipolar. In contrast, in Huntington's disease, striatal-pallidal transmission is decreased, and the movements are choreiform and the course of the secondary mood disorder is frequently bipolar.[34]

Conclusions

In this brief review of functional brain imaging in patients with major depression, we attempt to reveal the current insights and future promise this approach offers. The data we present from studies by ourselves and others support the hypothesis that functional brain imaging will provide novel insights into the functional architecture of circuits of brain areas underlying the clinical state of major depression. These data strongly argue against the notion that the clinical manifestations of major depression are the result of an abnormality in a single brain area. Rather, major depression is the result of a group of spatially distinct brain areas acting together in a unique way. In all likelihood, other psychiatric diseases will also find their neurobiological instantiation in a similar manner. The unique circuitry underlying various forms of depression reinforce this idea and allow us to suggest that functional imaging studies of this type may provide a very important tool in classifying patients with major depression on the basis of the underlying neurobiology. Such an approach is likely to hasten our understanding of the most effective forms of therapy.

References

1. Raichle ME: Positron emission tomography. Annu Rev Neurosci 13:2–10, 1983
2. Raichle ME: Circulatory and metabolic correlates of brain function in normal humans, in Handbook of Physiology: The Nervous System V, Part 2. edited by Mountcastle VE, Plum F. Bethesda, MD, American Physiological Society, 1987, pp 643–674
3. Chadwick DJ, Whelan J (eds): Exploring Brain Functional Anatomy with Positron Emission Tomography. CIBA Foundation Symposium 163. New York, Wiley, 1991
4. Lassen NA, Ingvar DH, Raichle ME, et al (eds): Brain Work and Mental Activity. Alfred Benzon Symposium 31. Copenhagen, Munksgaard, 1991
5. Raichle ME: Visualizing the mind. Sci Am 270:58–64, 1994
6. Posner MI, Raichle ME: Images of Mind. New York, Freeman, 1994
7. Drevets W, Videen T, MacLeod A, et al: A functional study of unipolar depression. J Neurosci 12:3628–3641, 1992
8. Drevets WC, Raichle ME: Neuroanatomical circuits in depression: implications for treatment mechanisms. Psychopharm Bull 28:261–274, 1992
9. Drevets WC, Spitznagel EL, MacLeod AK, et al: Discriminatory capability of PET measurements of regional blood flow in familial pure depressive disease. Neuroscience Abstracts 1992
10. Drevets WC, Videen T, MacLeod A, et al: Regional blood flow changes during antidepressant treatment. Neuroscience Abstracts, 1993
11. Baxter LR, Phelps ME, Mazziotta JC, et al: Local cerebral glucose metabolic rates in obsessive-compulsive disorder: a comparison with rates in unipolar depression and in normal controls. Arch Gen Psychiatry 44:211–218, 1987
12. Baxter LR, Schwartz JM, Phelps ME, et al: Reduction of prefrontal cortex glucose metabolism common to three types of depression. Arch Gen Psychiatry 46:243–250, 1989
13. Buchsbaum MS, Wu J, DeLisi LE, et al: Frontal cortex and basal

ganglia metabolic rates assessed by positron emission tomography with [^{18}F]2-deoxyglucose in affective illness. J Affective Disord 10:137–152, 1986
14. Cohen RM, Semple WE, Gross MD, et al: Evidence for common alterations in cerebral glucose metabolism in major affective disorders and schizophrenia. Neuropsychopharmacology 2:241–254, 1989
15. Delvenne V, Delecluse F, Hubain PP, et al: Regional cerebral blood flow in patients with affective disorders. Br J Psychiatry 157:359–365, 1990
16. Herscovitch P, Markham J, Raichle ME: Brain blood flow measured with intravenous $H_2{}^{15}O$, I: theory and error analysis. J Nucl Med 24:782–789, 1983
17. Raichle ME, Martin WRW, Herscovitch P, et al: Brain blood flow measured with $H_2{}^{15}O$, II: implementation and validation. J Nucl Med 24:790–798, 1983
18. Fox PT, Mintun MA: Noninvasive functional brain mapping by change-distribution analysis of averaged PET images of $H_2{}^{15}O$ tissue activity. J Nucl Med 30:141–149, 1989
19. Donders FC: On the speed of mental processes (1868). Reprinted in Acta Psychol (Amst) 30:412–431, 1969
20. Pardo JV, Pardo PJ, Raichle ME: Neural correlates of self-induced dysphoria. Am J Psychiatry 150:713–719, 1993
21. Petersen SE, Fox PT, Posner MI, et al: Positron emission tomographic studies of the cortical anatomy of singly word processing. Nature 331:585–589, 1988
22. Petersen SE, Fox PT, Posner MI, et al: Positron emission tomographic studies of the processing of single words. Journal of Cognitive Neuroscience 1:153–170, 1989
23. Raichle ME, Fiez JA, Videen TO, et al: Practice-related changes in human brain functional anatomy during non-motor learning. Cereb Cortex 4:8–26, 1994
24. Schwartz GE, Fair PL, Salt P, et al: Facial muscle patterning to affective imagery in depressed and nondepressed subjects. Science 192:489–491, 1976
25. Delp MJ, Sackeim HA: Effects of mood on lacrimal flow: sex differences and asymmetry. Psychophysiology 24:550–556, 1987

26. Amaral DG, Price JL: Amygdalocortical projections in the monkey. J Comp Neurol 230:465–496, 1984
27. Fuller TA, Russchen FT, Price JL: Sources of presumptive glutaminergic/aspartergic afferents to the rat ventral striatopallidal region. J Comp Neurol 258:317–338, 1987
28. Graybiel AM: Neurotransmitters and neuromodulators in the basal ganglia. Trends Neurosci 13:244–254, 1990
29. DeLong MR: Activity of basal ganglia neurons during movement. Brain Res 40:127–135, 1972
30. Post RM: Transduction of psychosocial stress into the neurobiology of recurrent affective disorder. Am J Psychiatry 149:999–1010, 1992
31. Swerdlow NR, Koob GF: Dopamine, schizophrenia, mania and depression: toward a unified hypothesis of cortico-striato-pallido-thalamic function. Behavioral and Brain Sciences 10:197–245, 1987
32. Nauta WJH, Domesick V: Afferent and efferent relationships of the basal ganglia, in Function of the Basal Ganglia. CIBA Foundation Symposium 107. London, Pitman, 1984, pp 3–29
33. Brown LL, Wolfson LI: Apomorphine increases glucose utilization in the substantia nigra, subthalamic and corpus striatum of the rat. Brain Res 140:188–193, 1978
34. Mayeux R: Emotional changes associated with basal ganglia disorders, in Neuropsychology of Human Emotion. Edited by Heilman KM, Satz P. New York, Guilford, 1983, pp 144–164
35. Jeste DV, Lohr JB, Goodwin FK: Neuroanatomical studies of major affective disorders: a review and suggestions for further research. Br J Psychiatry 153:444–459, 1988
36. Starkstein SE, Robinson RG: Affective disorders and cerebral vascular disease. Br J Psychiatry 154:170–182, 1989

CHAPTER

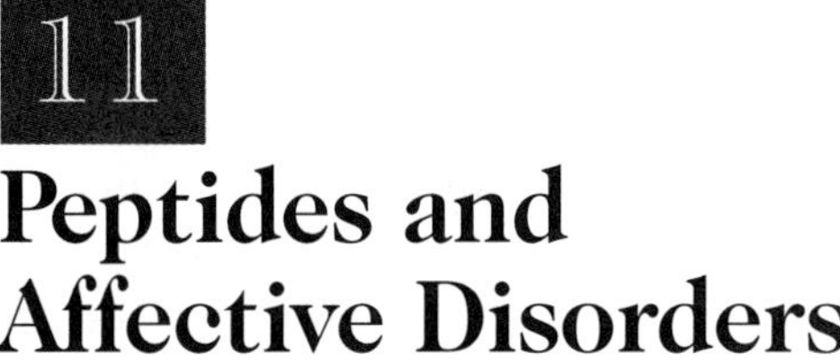

11 Peptides and Affective Disorders

Michael J. Owens, Ph.D.
Paul M. Plotsky, Ph.D.
Charles B. Nemeroff, M.D., Ph.D.

The past several decades have witnessed a veritable explosion of knowledge about the central nervous system (CNS), and in no area has this expansion been as impressive as in the field of peptide neurobiology. Dozens of peptide neurotransmitter candidates have been identified and characterized, their CNS distributions mapped, and their genes cloned. Dale's principle of "one neuron, one transmitter" has been convincingly refuted[1] with numerous demonstrations of neurons containing multiple peptides or combinations of peptide and nonpeptide neurotransmitters.[2]

In addition, the past 10 years have yielded an embarrassment of riches in the form of diversity of neurotransmitter receptors, receptor-effector coupling, and neurotransmitter transporters. These re-

---

This work was supported by Grants MH42088, MH40524, MH45216, and DK33093 from the National Institutes of Health.

cent discoveries have not yet been fully integrated into our concepts of normal or aberrant CNS function, although dysfunction at virtually any level could conceivably lead to neuropsychiatric deficits. Although a number of neuropeptide transmitters have been postulated to play a role in the pathophysiology of affective illness, we have chosen to focus on three neuropeptides in this chapter: corticotropin-releasing factor (CRF), somatostatin (SRIF), and thyrotropin-releasing hormone (TRH). These are arguably the three neuropeptides for which the best evidence exists for a preeminent role in the pathogenesis of affective illness.

Corticotropin-Releasing Factor

After a search spanning nearly three decades, corticotropin-releasing factor (CRF) was isolated and characterized in 1981 as a 41-amino acid peptide.[3] CRF is the primary and an obligatory hypothalamic adrenocorticotropic hormone (ACTH) secretagogue in most species.[4] It also functions as an extrahypothalamic neurotransmitter in a CNS network that apparently coordinates global responses to stressors.

CRF and its homologues represent an ancient family of peptides serving numerous functions. In higher organisms, including mammals, evidence supports the hypothesis that CRF plays a complex role in integrating endocrine, autonomic, immunological, and behavioral responses to stress.[5–7] The major focus in this chapter is the emerging evidence that implicates dysregulation of central CRF circuits in association with the affective disorders and anxiety disorders and, to a lesser extent, with anorexia nervosa and Alzheimer's disease, disorders also commonly associated with comorbid mood alterations.

Central administration of CRF to laboratory animals mimics many of the behavioral and autonomic aspects of the stress response.[5–8] Conversely, pretreatment with a specific CRF receptor antagonist or a CRF antiserum attenuates many of the behavioral and autonomic components of the stress response. This may be interpreted as support for the hypothesis that endogenous CRF acts on extrahypophysial targets to produce autonomic and behavioral components of stress responses. CRF acts centrally to induce two major classes of behavioral changes that can be dissociated: 1) increased locomotor activity in a familiar environment and 2) anxiogenic-like effects. Generally, in behavioral paradigms used as animal models of "anxiety" (i.e., paradigms considered sensitive to the effects of clinically efficacious anxiolytic drugs), CRF has an effect that is comparable to that of anxiogenic compounds and opposite to that of anxiolytics. In most but not all cases, these effects have been demonstrated to be independent of the effects of CRF on hypothalamic-pituitary-adrenal (HPA) function. Moreover, these effects are reversed by benzodiazepine treatment. The CRF receptor antagonist α-helical $CRF_{9\text{-}41}$ attenuates some but not all of the behavioral effects of various stressors.

One prevailing hypothesis for the anxiogenic actions of CRF are based on the known interactions between CRF and noradrenergic neurons in the locus ceruleus. Acute and chronic stressors elevate CRF concentrations in the locus ceruleus,[9] an effect opposite to that observed after acute or chronic benzodiazepine administration.[10,11] Butler et al.[12] demonstrated that infusion of very small doses of CRF into the locus ceruleus significantly increased nonambulatory spontaneous motor activity and anxiogenic activity. These results suggest that the behavioral activating effects of CRF in the locus ceruleus may be related to arousing or stress-related effects rather than to increased locomotor activity per se. These actions may be mediated by increased norepinephrine turnover in terminal fields of the locus ceruleus, as suggested by increases of 3,4-dihydroxyphenylglycol (a norepinephrine metabolite) concentrations in forebrain projection areas of the locus ceruleus after CRF infusion into the locus ceruleus.

Local CRF administration into the locus ceruleus region also increases the firing rate of locus ceruleus neurons,[13] an effect that is prevented by central administration of the CRF antagonist. Many stimuli activate locus ceruleus noradrenergic neurons, resulting in increased norepinephrine turnover throughout the CNS. Stressor-induced expression of tyrosine hydroxylase, the rate-limiting step in norepinephrine synthesis, in the locus ceruleus can be antagonized by α-helical $CRF_{9\text{-}41}$.[14]

These data, taken together, suggest that CRF produces its behavioral activating and anxiogenic effects, at least in part, by increasing the activity of locus ceruleus noradrenergic neurons. Furthermore, the connections between regions containing CRF neurons by both mono- and polysynaptic pathways provide an ideal network to ensure integration of diverse inputs corresponding to the physical and emotional status of the organism, thus resulting in coordinated behavioral, autonomic, and neuroendocrine responses. Thus, it appears that CRF may modulate the activity of the major CNS noradrenergic circuit that has long been implicated in the pathophysiology of stress, anxiety, and depression.

Hyperactivity of the HPA axis in patients with major depression remains one of the most consistent findings in biological psychiatry.[15] The reported HPA axis alterations in patients with major depression include hypercortisolemia, resistance to dexamethasone suppression of cortisol secretion, blunted ACTH responses to intravenous CRF challenge, and elevated CRF concentrations in cerebrospinal fluid (CSF). The exact pathological mechanism(s) underlying HPA axis dysregulation in patients with major depression and other affective disorders remains to be elucidated. It has been postulated that defects may exist at corticolimbic and/or hypothalamic loci, as reviewed in Sapolsky and Plotsky[16] and Owens and Nemeroff.[6]

Once the phenomenon of HPA axis hyperactivity in patients with major depression was established, many groups utilized various provocative neuroendocrine challenge tests as a window into the brain in attempts to elucidate pathophysiological mechanisms. In control subjects, the CRF stimulation test, in which either rat/human or ovine CRF is used, yields robust ACTH, β-endorphin, β-lipotropin, and cortisol responses after intravenous or subcutaneous administration.[6] However, in patients with major depression, blunting of ACTH or β-endorphin secretion with a normal cortisol response has been repeatedly reported.[17–22] Patients with posttraumatic stress disorder, 50% of whom also fulfill DSM-III[23] criteria for major depression, also show blunted ACTH secretion in response to a CRF challenge.[24] Importantly, Amsterdam et al.[25] reported normalization of the ACTH response to CRF after clinical recovery from depression, suggesting that the blunted ACTH response, like dexamethasone nonsuppression, may be a state marker for depression.

Mechanistically, two hypotheses have been advanced to account for the ACTH blunting observed after exogenous CRF administration. The first hypothesis suggests that downregulation of pituitary CRF receptors occurs as a result of hypothalamic CRF hypersecretion. The second hypothesis postulates altered sensitivity of the pituitary to glucocorticoid negative feedback. Substantial support has accumulated favoring the first hypothesis. This hypothesis, however, has not been directly tested in humans by measurement of hypothalamic CRF secretion, anterior pituitary CRF receptor density or function, or hypothalamic CRF messenger RNA (mRNA) concentrations in postmortem tissue. A series of studies by the Max Plank group[26] indicate that depressed patients show greater increases in post-CRF ACTH secretion than control subjects after dexamethasone pretreatment. These reports therefore suggest that ACTH blunting in depressed patients is not due primarily to hypercortisolemic negative feedback. In all of these studies, it should be kept in mind that neuroendocrine studies represent a secondary measure of CNS activity; the pituitary ACTH responses probably reflect the activity of hypothalamic CRF rather than that of the corticolimbic CRF circuits that are likely to be involved in the pathophysiology of depression.

A potentially more direct method for evaluation of extrahypothalamic CRF tone may be obtained from measurements of CRF in CSF. A marked dissociation between CSF and plasma neuropeptide concentrations has been described, indicating that neuropeptides are secreted directly into CSF from brain tissue rather than being derived from plasma-to-CSF transfer.[27] Evidence that CRF concentrations in CSF originate from nonhypophysiotropic CRF has been obtained from studies in which CRF concentrations in CSF were repeatedly measured over the course of the day. Both Garrick et al.[28] and Kalin[8] reported that CRF concentrations in CSF of rhesus monkeys are not entrained with pituitary-adrenal activity. The proximity of corticolimbic, brain stem, and spinal CRF neurons to the ventricular system suggests that these areas make substantial contributions to the CSF CRF pool. Furthermore, the report of diurnal alterations in regional CRF concentrations in CNS of laboratory animals supports an extrahypothalamic origin of CRF in CSF.[29]

In a series of studies, we demonstrated significant elevations of CRF concentrations in the CSF of drug-free patients with major depression or after suicide (Figure 11–1).[6] In our initial study, CRF concentrations were measured in the CSF of 10 control subjects, 23 patients with depression, 11 patients with schizophrenia, and 29 patients with dementia. CRF concentrations were higher in the CSF of depressed patients than in any of the other groups.[30] In a larger study of 54 depressed patients, 138 neurological control sub-

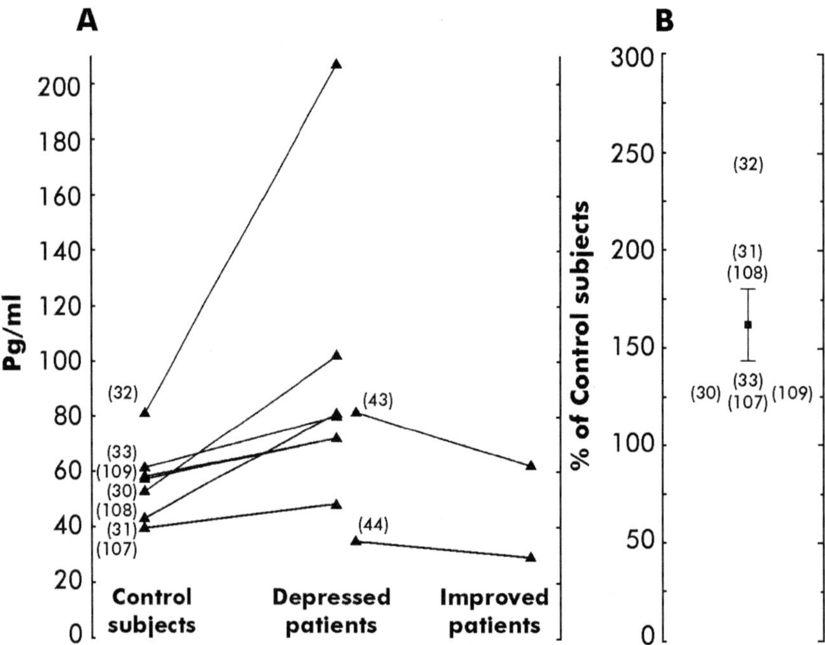

Figure 11–1. Summary of reports in which CRF concentrations were measured in CSF of depressed patients and suicide victims. *A:* Mean CRF concentrations in CSF of control subjects, depressed patients, or depressed patients after electroconvulsive therapy or fluoxetine treatment. *B:* Depressed patients exhibit 25%–150% increases in CRF concentrations in CSF as compared with control subjects. Numbers in parentheses represent individual references.

jects, 23 schizophrenic patients, and 6 manic patients, the depressed patients exhibited a marked twofold elevation in CRF concentrations in CSF.[31] Postmortem collection of CRF concentrations from the cisternal CSF of depressed suicide victims and sudden-death control subjects also revealed elevated CRF concentrations in the depressed group.[32]

Risch et al.[33] have confirmed these findings of elevated CRF concentrations in the CSF of depressed patients. In addition, the severity of depression appears to correlate significantly with CRF concentrations in CSF in patients with anorexia nervosa[34] and Huntington's disease.[35] Elevated CRF concentrations in the CSF of patients with anorexia nervosa[36] revert to the normal range as these patients approach normal body weight. No alterations of CRF concentrations in CSF have been reported in patients with other psychiatric disorders, including mania, panic disorder, and somatization disorders, as compared with control subjects.[37,38] In patients with Alzheimer's disease, increased,[39] decreased,[40,41] and unchanged[42] CRF concentrations in CSF have been reported; however, only limited numbers of patients were studied, and CRF levels in CSF may be correlated to the degree of cognitive impairment.[42]

Of particular interest is our demonstration that elevated CRF concentrations in the CSF of drug-free depressed patients are significantly decreased 24 hours after their final treatment with electroconvulsive therapy, indicating that CSF concentrations of CRF, like those of hypercortisolemia, represent a state rather than a trait marker.[43] Other recent studies have confirmed this normalization of CRF concentrations in CSF after successful treatment with fluoxetine.[44] Banki et al.[45] demonstrated a significant reduction of elevated CRF concentrations in the CSF of 15 female patients with major depression who remained depression free for at least 6 months after antidepressant treatment. In contrast, there was little significant treatment effect on CRF concentrations in the CSF of nine patients who relapsed during this 6-month period. The authors suggest that elevated or increasing CRF concentrations in CSF during antidepressant treatment may be the harbinger of a poor response in patients with major depression despite early symptomatic improvement. Of interest is that treatment of control subjects with desipramine[46] or, as noted above, of depressed subjects with fluoxetine[44] are associated with a reduction in CRF concentrations in CSF.

In laboratory models of CRF hypersecretion, evidence of CRF receptor downregulation is often apparent. Depression is a major determinant of suicide; more than 50% of completed suicides are accomplished by patients with major depression. Therefore, if CRF hypersecretion is a characteristic of depression, evidence of related CRF receptor downregulation should be evident in the CNS of depressed suicide victims. Indeed, we have reported that there is a marked (23%) decrease in the density of CRF receptors in the frontal cortex of suicide victims as compared with matched control samples (Figure 11–2).[47] Additional studies measuring regional CRF and CRF receptor heteronuclear RNA as an index of transcriptional activity and/or regional CRF and CRF receptor mRNA concentrations are needed.

In laboratory animal studies, increased central drive to the pituitary-adrenal axis is associated with an increase in the number and volume of adenohypophysial corticotrophs, as well as adrenal gland hypertrophy.[16,48] Recently, magnetic resonance imaging (MRI) and computed tomography (CT) have been used to measure human pituitary and adrenal gland volume in patients with affective disorders. Two studies reported enlargement of the pituitary gland in depressed patients as compared with age- and sex-matched control subjects (Figure 11–3).[49,50] Furthermore, a significant correlation existed between pituitary gland enlargement and post-dexamethasone cortisol concentrations. In a study of postmortem tissue, Zis and Zis[51] reported adrenal gland enlargement in suicide victims versus control subjects, a result confirmed in an early pilot CT study.[52] This result was confirmed in a study of adrenal volume by CT in depressed patients and age- and sex-matched control subjects.[53] Adrenal gland enlargement in depressed patients was confirmed by Rubin et al.[54] using MRI.

Because the adrenal cortex represents approximately 90% of the gland and is known to exhibit both hypertrophy and hyperplasia, it is presumed that the increased volume in depressed patients reflects changes in cortical rather than medullary mass. In our study, however, adrenal volume did not correlate with dexamethasone

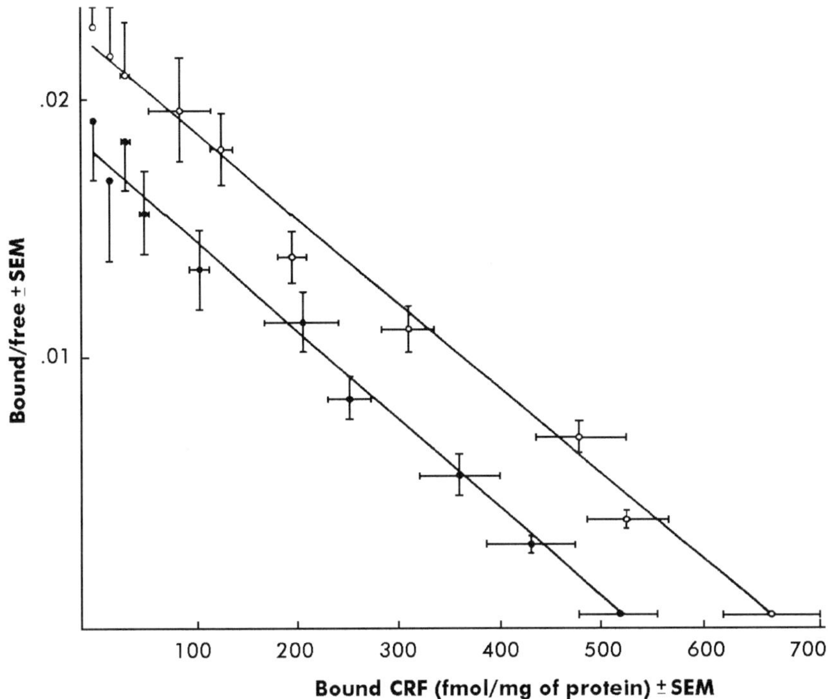

Figure 11–2. Scatchard analysis comparing frontal cortex CRF receptor binding from control subjects *(open circles)* and suicide victims *(solid circles)*. A significant reduction in B_{max} was observed in suicide victims as compared with control subjects ($P = .020$). For control subjects ($n = 29$), $K_d = 11.7 \pm 1.0$ nM; $B_{max} = 680 \pm 51$ fmol/mg of protein. For suicide victims ($n = 26$), $K_d = 10.2 \pm 0.7$ nM; $B_{max} = 521 \pm 43$ fmol/mg of protein. *Source.* Reprinted from Nemeroff CB, Owens MJ, Bissette G, et al.: "Reduced Corticotropin-Releasing Factor (CRF) Binding Sites in the Frontal Cortex of Suicides." *Archives of General Psychiatry* 45:577–579, 1988. Copyright 1988, American Medical Association.

suppression test results, patient age, or severity or duration of the depressive episode. Correlation of these depression-associated changes in pituitary and adrenal size with the results of CRF stimulation tests and measurements of CRF concentrations in CSF would be welcome.

In the relatively short span of a decade, the physiological role of CRF has expanded from that of a classical hypophysiotropic hor-

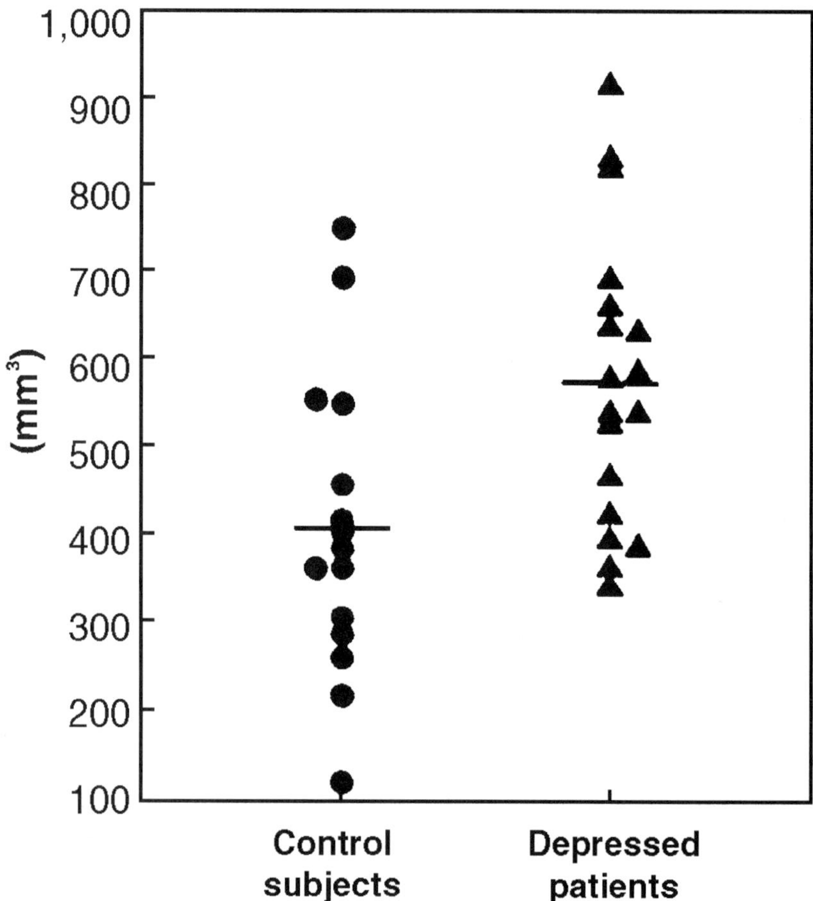

Figure 11–3. Pituitary gland volumes, estimated from area and width, in depressed patients and control subjects. Depressed patients had significantly larger pituitary gland volumes (t = 2.85; df = 31; P = .007) than age- and sex-matched control subjects. The two-tailed t test was used to evaluate significant differences between groups.
Source. Reprinted from Krishnan KRR, Doraiswamy PM, Lurie SN, et al.: "Pituitary Size in Depression." *Journal of Clinical Endocrinology and Metabolism* 72:256–259, 1991. Copyright 1991, The Endocrine Society.

mone that regulates the activity of the pituitary-adrenal axis to that of a central neurotransmitter that is implicated in the organization of counterregulatory responses to a variety of stressors. This expanded role was first suggested by immunohistochemical mapping studies that identified a unique extrahypothalamic distribution of CRF and was further supported by the results of electrophysiological, pharmacological, and behavioral studies conducted first in animals and, subsequently, in clinical studies.

Functional alterations in the HPA axis and central CRF systems have been studied most extensively in patients with major depression. The concatenation of available evidence has led to the hypothesis that CRF hypersecretion of hypothalamic and/or extrahypothalamic origin occurs in patients with depression. Evidence of CRF hypersecretion in patients with depression may be inferred from basic and clinical observations of downregulation of CRF receptors in the frontal cortex and, possibly, the adenohypophysis; increased CRF concentrations in CSF; a blunted ACTH response to a standard CRF stimulation test; and enlargement of the pituitary and adrenal glands. Many, if not all, of these abnormalities revert to normal after successful treatment of depression. Therefore, in major depression, the CRF/HPA axis serves as a "window into the brain," and abnormalities reflect a state rather than a trait marker of depression.

Interpretation of the cerebrocortical reductions in CRF concentration in the brains of patients with Alzheimer's disease is unclear. Increased receptor numbers in these same brain areas support the hypothesis of reduced CRF secretion; however, no direct demonstration of degeneration of CRF-containing neurons in this disorder has yet been reported.[6] Furthermore, as in depression, little work has been performed at the molecular level. Although extrahypothalamic CRF circuits are increasingly accepted as participating in cognitive processes, it is unclear which, if any, symptoms of Alzheimer's disease are secondary to the pathological involvement of CRF neurons in patients with this disease.

Many important research avenues remain unexplored with respect to the role of CRF in the pathophysiology of depression. Postmortem studies of CNS tissue from these patients at the molecular level are in progress in our and others' laboratories. It is of paramount importance, however, to examine tissue from age- and sex-matched, "disease-free" control groups as well as from populations of patients with other neuropsychiatric disorders. The recent cloning of the CRF-binding protein and the CRF receptor provides new tools, both specific molecular probes and antisera, for assessing changes in these critical entities in various disease states. On the basis of the considerable pharmacological and behavioral work cited previously, it is clear that one of the most exciting areas will be the development of long-acting, CNS-active, CRF antagonist or CRF-binding protein analogues for the treatment of depression and/or anxiety disorders. Perhaps the recent cloning of the CRF-binding protein and the CRF receptor will aid in the elucidation of the active portion of the peptide or the active site on the receptor. It is hoped that these discoveries will lead to the rational design of lipophilic drugs with clinical utility. Neuronal cell culture systems are available to study the genetic regulation of CRF, CRF-binding protein, and CRF receptor expression (i.e., second-messenger response elements, steroidal sites of interaction, transcriptional factors, etc.). Elucidation of the flanking sequences could conceivably lead to the use of antisense oligonucleotides as a form of pharmacotherapy. In addition, the use of antisense oligonucleotides directed against the initiation site of the CRF or CRF receptor genes could conceivably inhibit translation and could also be utilized therapeutically. Finally, design of appropriate ligands for positron-emission tomography (PET) scanning would permit evaluation of CRF receptor binding during the course of these diseases.

Somatostatin

Somatostatin (somatotropin release-inhibiting factor [SRIF]), like a number of other neuropeptides, was serendipitously discovered during attempts to purify growth hormone-releasing factor. As the name implies, somatostatin inhibits growth hormone release from the anterior pituitary. Since its structural identification 20 years ago, SRIF has been unequivocally shown to be the major inhibitory influence on growth hormone secretion. Additionally, and perhaps of equal interest, SRIF fulfills a number of criteria for neurotransmitter status within the CNS. The acceptance of somatostatin's role as a neurotransmitter has led to its investigation in a number of psychiatric and neurological diseases. As discussed below, nonhypophysiotropic SRIF-containing neurons may play a role in a number of illnesses including, but not limited to, depression, various forms of dementia, and epilepsy.

Before discussing the role of SRIF in affective illness, we briefly review several aspects of basic SRIF neurobiology. A more detailed review of SRIF can be found in the work by Rubinow et al.[55]

Radioimmunoassay and immunocytochemical studies have revealed that SRIF-containing neurons are heterogeneously distributed throughout the CNS. High concentrations of the tetradecapeptide are found in the hypothalamus and median eminence, amygdala, hippocampus, cerebral cortex, medial preoptic area, and nucleus accumbens. Cell bodies are most numerous in the preoptic and periventricular nuclei of the hypothalamus, although they are also present in significant numbers in cortical and limbic regions. As noted above, like many neurotransmitter systems, SRIF is colocalized within a number of other monoamine- or neuropeptide-containing neurons. Moreover, like many neuropeptide systems, the distribution of SRIF-containing neurons in humans is similar to, but not identical with, that observed in rodents. Of the two major native forms of SRIF, $SRIF1_{14}$ and $SRIF1_{28}$, the former is the major form found in brain (70%–80%).

Recent studies have indicated that pharmacologically distinct SRIF receptor subtypes exist in the CNS with different affinities for somatostatin analogues, a differential localization, a differential coupling to second-messenger systems, and differing functional responses. These subtypes have been termed $SRIF_1$ and $SRIF_2$ receptors; the $SRIF_1$ subtype is predominant. Recently, four distinct somatostatin receptors ($SSTR_1$ through $SSTR_4$) have been cloned. The receptor sequences appear to be highly conserved across species and are members of the G protein-coupled family of receptors.

Electrophysiological experiments have revealed both excitatory and inhibitory actions of SRIF. In addition, central administration of SRIF has been observed to alter cholinergic, dopaminergic, noradrenergic, and serotonergic neurotransmission. Moreover, SRIF not only regulates the release of growth hormone from the anterior pituitary, but also inhibits the secretion of a number of other hormones, particularly thyroid-stimulating hormone (TSH) and CRF-stimulated ACTH.

Like many other neuropeptide transmitters, central administration of SRIF produces a variety of behavioral and physiological effects. In brief, the peptide produces a non-opioid-mediated analgesia in animals and humans. Changes in sleep patterns, food consumption, locomotor activity, and memory processes are also altered by central SRIF administration. This wide spectrum of effects of SRIF led to the investigation of its involvement in a number of psychiatric and neurologic disorders. Of particular interest is that the above changes in sleep, eating, psychomotor activity, and anterior pituitary hormone secretion are all altered in depressed patients.

The greatest number of clinical studies of SRIF have focused on its putative involvement in neuropsychiatric disorders. Consistent decreases in SRIF concentrations in tissue and CSF are observed in patients with senile dementia, Alzheimer's disease, Parkinson's disease, and multiple sclerosis during relapse, as well as in patients with depression (vide infra). SRIF-containing neurons have also been found to be a source of the observed plaques and tangles associated with the pathology of Alzheimer's disease. In contrast to the decrements in central SRIF measures in patients with these disorders, elevated SRIF concentrations in CSF, presumably reflecting leakage due to neuronal damage, are observed in patients with a number of inflammatory or destructive neurologic disorders, including spinal cord compression, meningitis, and metabolic encephalopathy.

Based on preclinical studies of the behavioral effects of SRIF, investigation of its role in affective illness was of interest. The clearest evidence for the involvement of SRIF in psychiatric illness has come from studies of major depression. A consistent decrease has been reported in SRIF concentrations in the CSF of drug-free depressed patients (Figure 11–4). SRIF concentrations in CSF have been reported to undergo circadian variation in primates; concentrations vary by 10% over 24 hours, and the highest concentrations

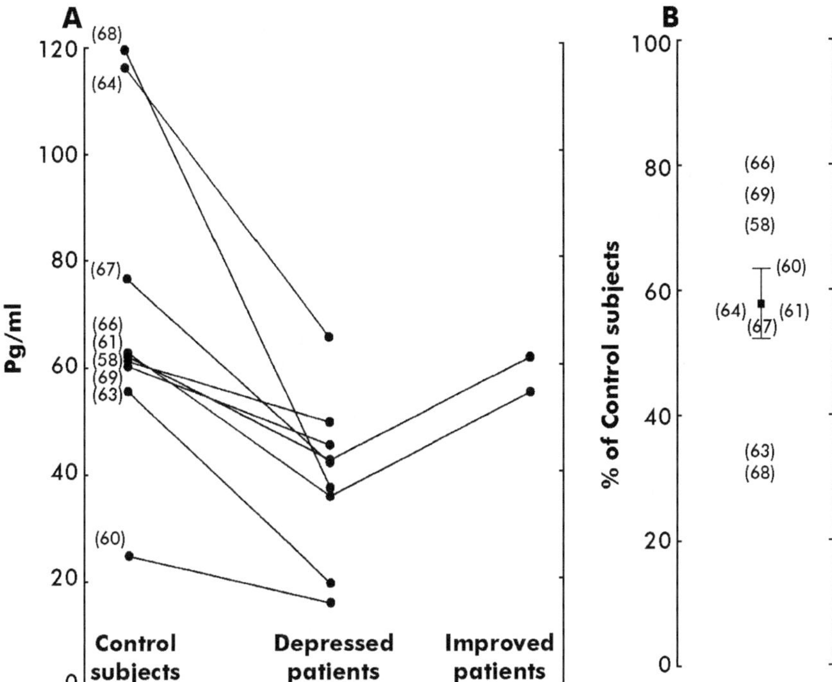

Figure 11–4. Summary of reports to date in which SRIF concentrations were examined in the CSF of depressed patients. *A:* Mean SRIF concentrations in CSF of control subjects, depressed patients, and depressed patients after clinical improvement. *B:* Depressed patients exhibited >40% lower SRIF concentrations in CSF as compared with control subjects. Numbers in parentheses represent individual references.

are observed at night.[56,57]

Although the reported differences between depressed and control subjects are substantially greater than this, it highlights the importance for CSF sampling at uniform times. Although Rubinow[58] found no differences in SRIF concentrations in CSF according to the time of day samples were collected, he did note large differences (increases and decreases) in subjects who were sampled in both morning and evening. Research over the past 15 years on a number of neuropeptides found in CSF have revealed that they are almost exclusively of central origin, although the actual sites of production remain obscure.[27,59] Decreases in SRIF concentrations in CSF are proposed to be the result of decreased neuronal synthesis and release. Whether this is a primary or a secondary effect of the illness is unknown (see below).

Gerner and Yamada[60] first measured SRIF concentrations in the CSF of psychiatric patients. In their study, medication-free patients with either depression or anorexia nervosa had lower SRIF concentrations than did either control subjects or healthy young women, respectively. This result was replicated shortly thereafter in a large study by Rubinow et al.[61] SRIF concentrations in CSF were significantly decreased in both unipolar and bipolar depressed patients. Moreover, although SRIF levels in CSF did not correlate with severity of depression, clinically improved patients exhibited increases in CSF SRIF that approached "normal" concentrations. In nine bipolar patients followed longitudinally, SRIF concentrations in CSF were significantly lower during the depressed state than during improved or manic states. SRIF concentrations in CSF were similar in men and women and among different age groups in this study.

After adding a number of patients to his original study, Rubinow[58] again reported lower SRIF concentrations in the CSF of depressed patients than in control subjects and in patients with improved depression, mania, dysthymia, and schizophrenia. No correlations between SRIF concentrations and age, severity of depression, or time of day were observed.

In a large study lacking control subjects, Ågren and Lundqvist[62] reported significant correlations between severity of depression and SRIF concentrations in CSF. Moreover, SRIF concentrations were significantly lower in the CSF of patients studied during their worst week of depression than in those studied more than 2 months after their most severe week of depression. Black et al.[63] also reported that SRIF concentrations in ventricular CSF from medicated depressed patients who had been referred for cingulotomy were lower than SRIF concentrations in lumbar CSF from control subjects.

Bissette et al.[64] also observed decreased SRIF concentrations in CSF of depressed patients. As in the study of Ågren and Lundqvist,[62] SRIF concentrations in CSF were not correlated with cortisol concentrations after treatment with dexamethasone. In contrast to this finding, Doran et al.[65] reported a significant negative correlation between cortisol concentrations in plasma after dexamethasone treatment and SRIF concentrations in CSF in depressed patients. Kling et al.[66] also reported decreased SRIF concentrations in CSF of depressed patients. Rather than finding a simple linear relationship, these investigators observed an inverted U-shaped relationship between cortisol concentrations in plasma after dexamethasone treatment and SRIF concentrations in CSF in depressed patients. This result suggested a complicated relationship between SRIF-containing neurons and hypothalamic CRF neurons. Sunderland et al.[67] also reported decreases in SRIF concentrations in CSF in elderly depressed patients, with no correlation between CSF concentrations and severity of depression.

Davis et al.[68] also observed decreased SRIF concentrations in CSF of geriatric patients with depression when compared with elderly control subjects. Molchan et al.[69] confirmed and extended these findings in elderly depressed and control populations. Moreover, SRIF concentrations in CSF of depressed patients with Alzheimer's disease were significantly lower than the already low concentrations in the nondepressed Alzheimer's disease population. Although 5-hydroxyindoleacetic acid (5-HIAA) concentrations in CSF did not differ among diagnostic groups, SRIF and 5-HIAA concentrations in CSF were positively correlated among both Alzheimer's disease and non-Alzheimer's disease depressed groups (i.e., the lower the 5-HIAA concentrations, the lower the SRIF concentrations).

As Gold and Rubinow[70] stated several years ago, "although the evidence in support of depression-related reductions of CSF SRIF is increasingly convincing, the meaning of this finding is at present unclear and requires further knowledge of the source and regulation of CSF SRIF" (p. 624). Unfortunately, at present this statement remains true.

SRIF concentrations in CSF have also been measured in patients with several other psychiatric disorders. Kaye et al.[34] found no differences in anorexic patients but observed a small increase in SRIF concentrations in CSF of bulimic patients of normal weight when they stopped bingeing. Berrettini et al.[71] found no differences in SRIF concentrations in CSF among control subjects, unmedicated euthymic bipolar patients, and lithium-treated bipolar patients. Altemus et al.[72] reported significantly higher SRIF concentrations in CSF of patients with obsessive-compulsive disorder than in control subjects. Although a control group was lacking in their study, Kruesi et al.[73] also reported that SRIF levels in the CSF of a small group of children with obsessive-compulsive disorder were higher than those in a group of children with conduct disorder.

Few postmortem studies of SRIF in CNS of depressed patients have been reported to date. Charlton et al.[74] found no differences in SRIF concentrations or in SRIF receptor affinity or number in the temporal or occipital cortices of a small group of control subjects ($n = 7$) and a group of depressed patients who died of coincidental physical illness while inpatients at a psychiatric hospital ($n = 9$). In another study of 7 depressed patients and 12 control subjects, Bowen et al.[75] measured SRIF concentrations in the pars opercularis and orbital gyrus of the frontal lobe, the parahippocampal gyrus and pole of the temporal lobe, and the postcentral gyrus and superior lobule of the parietal lobe. Significant decreases (30%) in SRIF concentrations were observed only in the pole of the temporal lobe. Although these studies are complicated by wide ranges in the length of delay postmortem until sampling and freezing of the tissue, and further by the finding that SRIF concentrations decrease within the first 6 hours after death,[76] studies of this nature are exceptionally useful and sorely needed.

Preclinical studies clearly show that a variety of neurotransmitter systems can alter the activity of SRIF neurons in the CNS. One group of clinically useful psychotropic drugs, the serotonin-selective uptake inhibitors, increase SRIF concentrations in rat brain.[77] In one study,[78] carbamazepine was found to produce a significant decrease in SRIF concentrations in the CSF of a group of depressed patients. In the same study, it was found that the selective 5-hydroxytryptamine uptake inhibitor zimelidine significantly increased SRIF concentrations in the CSF of five of five patients. In a small group of patients, neither desipramine nor lithium had any effect on CSF SRIF concentrations. The further reductions in SRIF concentrations in CSF that are produced by carbamazepine were not correlated to worsening or improvement of symptoms. This finding suggests that SRIF may be implicated in the anticonvulsant mechanism of action of carbamazepine and that, together with the neurological disorders that are characterized by decreased SRIF concentrations in CSF but not necessarily accompanied by concomitant changes in mood, decreases in SRIF concentrations in CSF are not responsible for the changes in affect seen in patients with depression.

Although the data are still relatively limited, an overview of the extant literature suggests that decreases in SRIF concentrations in CSF are a consistent state-dependent finding in patients with depression. Indeed, secondary to the hypercortisolemia associated with depression, this is one of the more consistent findings in biological psychiatry. The finding has no apparent diagnostic usefulness, however, because similar changes are observed in a number of neurological disorders without psychiatric comorbidity. However, reductions in SRIF concentrations in CSF appear to be associated with impairment in cognitive function. The decrease in SRIF concentrations in CSF may be related to the overactivity of the HPA axis that is commonly found in patients with depression. Whether one is responsible for the other or whether both are responses to dysregulation of other neurotransmitter systems associated with depression is unknown. Finally, SRIF-active drugs may not have therapeutic utility because changes in SRIF concentrations in CSF are apparently without effect on mood. Nevertheless, rational design of peptide or non-peptide-based drugs that are selectively active at different SRIF receptor subtypes will certainly aid in understanding its role in behavior and may ultimately lead to therapeutic benefits.

Thyrotropin-Releasing Hormone

The early availability of adequate tools (i.e., assays and synthetic peptides), coupled with observations that primary hypothyroidism is associated with depressive symptomatology, ensured extensive investigation of the involvement of the hypothalamic-pituitary-thyroid (HPT) axis in affective disorders. Indeed, thyrotropin-releasing hormone (TRH), a pyroglutamylhistidylprolinamide tripeptide, was the first of the hypothalamic-releasing hormones to be isolated and characterized.[79,80] In its role as a hypophysiotropic factor, TRH is released from hypothalamic nerve endings in the median eminence into the primary capillary plexus of the hypophysial-portal circulatory system, where it is transported to thyrotropes in the adenohypophysis. TRH then diffuses out of these capillaries and binds to specific TRH membrane receptors to facilitate the release and synthesis of TSH. Circulating TSH acts at the thyroid gland to evoke the release of triiodothyronine (T_3) and thyroxine (T_4).

Early studies established the hypothalamic and extrahypothalamic distribution of TRH.[81] This extensive extrahypothalamic presence of TRH quickly led to speculation that TRH might function as a neurotransmitter or neuromodulator. Subsequent studies established the necessary foundation required to seriously consider TRH in such a role. Indeed, a large body of evidence supports the involvement of TRH as a neurotransmitter or neuromodulator. A detailed review of the neurobiology of TRH may be found in the recent report by Mason et al.[82]

Administration of exogenous TRH is associated with a variety of physiological and behavioral effects, including alterations in cardiovascular function, respiratory rate, body temperature, gastric secretion, colonic motility, and electroencephalographic activity.[81,82] Interest in putative CNS actions of TRH were stimulated by studies of the thyroid axis and depression by Prange et al.[83] Utilizing the levodopa potentiation test to screen for putative antidepressant effects in mice, Plotnikoff et al.[84] found that TRH produced enhancement of motor activity, a behavioral marker of compounds possessing putative antidepressant efficacy. Indeed, the effects of TRH in this test were similar to those observed in imipramine-treated mice, suggesting that TRH might act as an antidepressant compound. Of importance is the finding that TRH was equally effective in intact and hypophysectomized mice, indicating that the observed effects were not dependent on activation of the HPT axis but rather reflected a direct action of TRH on the CNS.

Profound increases in CNS activity evoked by electroconvulsive shock administered on an alternate-day schedule for 5 days[85] or kainic acid-induced limbic seizures[86] produced pronounced increases in TRH concentration in limbic regions, including the amygdala and hippocampus. Neither administration of a single electroconvulsive shock treatment nor administration of a subconvulsant electrical current altered TRH concentrations in any region assayed, indicating that the induction of a seizure was essential to produce effects on TRH. Other observations suggest that the efficacy of TRH or analogues in the treatment of seizure disorders is an area ripe for further evaluation.

In summary, these animal studies have highlighted the wide range of physiological and behavioral effects exerted by TRH. One may speculate on the possibility that TRH-containing circuits in the limbic system may in part mediate the antidepressant actions of electroconvulsive therapy and may be involved in the pathophysiological mechanisms of seizure disorders. The potential clinical implications of these studies include the possible utility of TRH in treating sedative-hypnotic overdose and certain forms of epilepsy.

Learned helplessness, an animal model of depression, can be reversed by many clinically effective antidepressants and by electroconvulsive therapy. Interestingly, when animals are rendered hypothyroid, they exhibit resistance to the effects of tricyclic antidepressants, and treatment with thyroid hormone reverses the antidepressant resistance. Over a decade ago, Whybrow and Prange[87] hypothesized that thyroid function was integral to the pathogenesis of and recovery from affective disorders, due to the copious interactions among thyroid hormones, catecholamines, and adrenergic receptors in the CNS. Overall, these studies suggest a role for thyroid dysfunction in refractory depression and are consonant with the results of clinical studies suggesting the existence of an increased rate of hypothyroidism among patients with refractory depression. Furthermore, animal and clinical studies suggest that depressive symptoms in hypothyroid patients may in part be determined by thyroid function before the onset of depression.[88]

The use of TRH as a provocative agent for assessment of thyroid axis function evolved rapidly after its isolation and synthesis. A relatively standard protocol involves the measurement of basal plasma TSH concentrations, followed by intravenous administration of exogenous TRH (200–500 μg) and subsequent measurement of plasma TSH concentrations at 30-minute intervals for a period of

2–3 hours.[89] Clinical use of the TRH stimulation test to assess HPT axis function revealed blunting of the TSH response in approximately 25% of euthyroid patients with major depression, as reviewed by Loosen,[90] Nemeroff,[91] and Howland.[88] These data have been widely confirmed.

It has been proposed that decreased nocturnal plasma TSH concentration may be a sensitive marker of depression.[92] Using a modified TRH stimulation test in which 200 μg of the peptide is administered intravenously at 8 A.M. and at 11 P.M., Duval et al.[93] claimed a diagnostic specificity of 95% and a diagnostic sensitivity of 89%. The difference between the TSH responses obtained from the 11-P.M. and the 8-A.M. tests (δδTSH) appeared to be markedly lower in depressed patients than in control subjects.

Recently, Shelton et al.[94] reported that, among outpatients with major depression, 26% exhibited some abnormality of thyroid hormone concentrations; most of these effects were normalized by antidepressant treatment. Although antidepressants did not exhibit a statistically significant effect on thyroid hormone concentrations when tested across the whole group, it must be noted that patients in this study did not exhibit a high frequency of TSH blunting to TRH. Overall, the results of this study imply that subpopulations of more severely depressed patients may be more likely to exhibit TSH blunting and elevations of T_4 before therapy. The relevance of TRH to psychiatric disorders has been reviewed by Nemeroff.[91]

The observed blunting of TSH in depressed patients does not appear to be the result of either excessive negative feedback due to hypersecretion of thyroid hormone or to SRIF hypersecretion. In fact, as noted previously in detail, depressed patients exhibit reduced CSF concentrations of SRIF. It is possible that TSH blunting is a reflection of pituitary TRH receptor downregulation as a result of hypersecretion of endogenous TRH by the median eminence.[27] The observation that TRH concentrations in lumbar CSF are higher in depressed patients than in control subjects supports a hypothesis of TRH hypersecretion but does not elucidate the origin of this tripeptide.[95,96]

Banki et al.[96] studied 16 control subjects (12 patients diagnosed as having only peripheral neurological disease and four patients with a DSM-III diagnosis of somatization disorder) and 17 patients with major depression. None of the subjects had been treated with psychotropic medications for at least 2 weeks before the start of the study. The mean TRH concentration in CSF for the combined control group was 4.4 ± 1.8 pg/ml, and the concentration in the depressed group was 12.8 ± 5.7 pg/ml.

In a more recent study conducted in severely depressed patients at the National Institute of Mental Health, we did not confirm this finding.[97] In animal models, chronic administration of TRH for 2–3 weeks results in blunting of the TSH response to TRH and decreased circulating concentrations of TSH, T_3, and T_4.[81] Furthermore, repeated administration of TRH in humans also produces a blunted TSH response to TRH.[98] Finally, these elevations of TRH concentrations in CSF may be relatively specific to depression, as no such alteration has been reported in patients with Alzheimer's disease, anxiety disorders, or alcoholism.[99,100] Clearly, further studies are needed in which TRH concentrations in CSF are measured.

Although most depressed patients respond readily to treatment with antidepressants, approximately 15%–30% are refractory to treatment.[101] Approximately 15% of depressed patients display grade III hypothyroidism, characterized by normal T_3, T_4, and TSH concentrations and an exaggerated TSH response to TRH; almost 60% of these patients have detectable antimicrosomal and/or antithyroglobulin antibodies.[102] Of interest is that approximately 50% of depressed patients who are dexamethasone suppression test nonsuppressors exhibit increases in TSH concentrations.[103] Overall, the rate of asymptomatic autoimmune thyroiditis in depressed patients is greater than would be expected in the general population.[88,91] It may be postulated that the development of autoimmune thyroiditis gives rise to hypersecretion of hypothalamic TRH as a compensatory mechanism to maintain normal plasma T_3 and T_4 concentrations. There is a considerable body of literature, recently reviewed by Joffe et al.,[104] on the interactions between the HPT axis and affective disorders.

Preclinical studies have added to our current understanding of the physiological and behavioral effects exerted by TRH. Clinical studies of TRH in patients with depression, however, have yielded mixed results and have indicated no definitive role for TRH in the pathophysiology or treatment of any psychiatric disorder. Thus, despite the initial promise offered by early preclinical and clinical studies of TRH, many subsequent investigations have yielded equivocal results.

At present, the diagnostic utility of the TRH stimulation test remains open to question with respect to depression. Several investigators, however, have suggested that this test has prognostic value in predicting treatment responses. For instance, Langer et al.[105] presented evidence to suggest that a change in the TSH response from blunted to normal predicts a positive response to antidepressant therapy, and Kirkegaard[106] suggested that the TSH response to TRH challenge appears to be of value in predicting long-term clinical outcome (remission or relapse). Obviously, additional studies are required to clarify the potential clinical utility of the TRH stimulation test in the diagnosis and treatment of depression.

Thus, despite years of study, considerable gaps in our knowledge remain. Many avenues for future experimentation are available. A concerted effort should be made to perform postmortem measurements of regional brain TRH concentrations, TRH mRNA levels, pituitary and brain TRH receptor kinetics, and TRH receptor mRNA concentrations, as well as postreceptor signal transduction in tissues obtained from depressed suicide victims and well-matched control subjects. Furthermore, studies of TRH concentrations and rhythms in CSF should be performed in populations of patients with depression, those with autoimmune thyroiditis, and well-matched control subjects. Finally, the synthesis of a long-acting TRH analogue, as well as development of a lipophilic TRH radioligand permitting PET/SPECT visualization of TRH receptor density in the CNS and pituitary, would be of great utility in assessing the importance of the HPT axis in the development of affective disorders.

Future Directions

Although significant progress has been made over the past decade, many new tools have now entered the armamentarium of basic and clinical scientists. Application of the ribonuclease (RNase) protection assay and of in situ hybridization will permit detection and mapping of specific mRNAs in the CNS of laboratory animals and in human postmortem tissue. Widespread use of these methods will provide a picture of the concentrations and distributions of CRF and TRH mRNA and their receptor mRNAs in populations of control subjects and patients with affective disorders and other disorders. For those mRNAs of particularly low abundance, in situ hybridization or RNase protection assays may be preceded with polymerase chain reaction amplification of the target mRNA. Studies to assess postmortem stability of the mRNAs of interest will be necessary and might be most easily accomplished by using CNS tissue removed during neurosurgical procedures and then subjected to controlled processing delays. A more accurate determination of transcriptional activity may be derived by measurement of heteronuclear RNA (hnRNA), using intronic antisense hybridization probes in RNase protection or in situ hybridization protocols. However, the rapid turnover time and small pool size of nuclear hnRNA will necessitate rigid control of the postmortem delay and studies of hnRNA stability after death.

With our advancing knowledge of potential peptidergic circuit or peptide receptor dysfunction contributing to the pathophysiology of affective disorders, the development of animal models will assume increasingly greater importance. This may be most readily accomplished by the use of transgenic overexpression or "knockout" models or by the use of stereotaxic microinjection of sense or antisense DNA, either directly or carried by adenovirus or modified herpes virus vectors. With these models, the consequences of hypo- or hyperactivity of each of these neuropeptides or receptor systems may be assessed at the neurobiological and behavioral levels, and potential therapeutic approaches may be developed.

Another exciting development is the ability to image CNS tissue with MRI, PET, and variants of these methods. It is becoming more likely that we will be able to monitor the activity of CNS neuronal circuits in healthy and diseased CNS tissue by using metabolic markers and to assess receptor distribution by using labeled ligands. As these techniques are refined and increase in sensitivity and resolution, they should have a major impact on both basic and clinical studies of the CNS mechanisms underlying affective disorders.

References

1. Eccles J: Chemical transmission and Dales principle, in Progress in Brain Research. Edited by Hökfelt T, Fuxe K, Pernow B. Amsterdam, Elsevier North-Holland, 1986, pp 3–13
2. Hökfelt T: Neuropeptides in perspective: the last ten years. Neuron 7:867–879. 1991
3. Vale W, Spiess J, Rivier C, et al: Characterization of a 41 residue ovine hypothalamic peptide that stimulates secretion of corticotropin and β-endorphin. Science 213:1394–1397, 1981
4. Plotsky PM: Pathways to the secretion of ACTH: a view from the portal. J Neuroendocrinol 3:1–9, 1991
5. Owens MJ, Nemeroff CB: The physiology and pharmacology of corticotropin releasing factor. Pharmacol Rev 43:425–473, 1991
6. Owens MJ, Nemeroff CB: The role of CRF in the pathophysiology of affective disorders: laboratory and clinical studies, in Corticotropin-Releasing Factor. CIBA Foundation Symposium 172. Edited by Chadwick DJ, Marsh J, Ackrill K. New York, Wiley, 1993, pp 296–316
7. Koob GF, Heinrichs SC, Pich EM, et al: The role of CRF in behavioral responses to stress, in Corticotropin-Releasing Factor. CIBA Foundation Symposium 172. Edited by Chadwick DJ, Marsh J, Ackrill K. New York, Wiley, 1993, pp 277–295
8. Kalin NH: Behavioral and endocrine studies of corticotropin-releasing hormone in primates, in Corticotropin-Releasing Factor: Basic and Clinical Studies of a Neuropeptide. Edited by De Souza EB, Nemeroff CB. Boca Raton, FL, CRC Press, 1990, pp 275–289
9. Chappell PB, Smith MA, Kilts CD, et al: Alterations in CRF-like immunoreactivity in discrete rat brain regions after acute and chronic stress. J Neurosci 6:2908–2914, 1986

10. Owens MJ, Bissette G, Nemeroff CB: Acute effects of alprazolam and adinazolam on the concentrations of corticotropin-releasing factor in the rat brain. Synapse 4:196–202, 1989
11. Owens MJ, Vargas MA, Knight DL, et al: The effects of alprazolam on corticotropin-releasing factor neurons in the rat brain: acute time course, chronic treatment and abrupt withdrawal. J Pharmacol Exp Ther 258:349–356, 1991
12. Butler PD, Weiss JM, Stout JC, et al: Corticotropin-releasing factor produces fear-enhancing and behavioral activating effects following infusion into the locus coeruleus. J Neurosci 10:176–183, 1990
13. Weiss JM, Stout J, Aaron M, et al: Experimental studies of depression and anxiety: role of locus coeruleus and corticotropin-releasing factor. Brain Res Bull 35:561–572, 1994
14. Melia KR, Duman RS: Involvement of corticotropin-releasing factor in chronic stress regulation of the brain noradrenergic system. Proc Natl Acad Sci U S A 88:8382–8386, 1991
15. Plotsky PM, Owens MJ, Nemeroff CB: Neuropeptide alterations in affective disorders, in Psychopharmacology: The Fourth Generation of Progress. Edited by Bloom FE, Kupfer DJ. New York, Raven, 1995, pp 971–981
16. Sapolsky RM, Plotsky PM: Hypercortisolism and its possible neural basis. Biol Psychiatry 27:937–952, 1990
17. Gold PW, Loriaux DL, Roy A, et al: Responses to corticotropin-releasing hormone in the hypercortisolism of depression and Cushing's disease: pathophysiologic and diagnostic implications. N Engl J Med 314:1329–1335, 1986
18. Gold PW, Gwirtsman HE, Avgerinos PC, et al: Abnormal hypothalamic-pituitary-adrenal function in anorexia nervosa. N Engl J Med 314:1335–1342, 1986
19. Holsboer F, Muller OA, Doerr HG, et al: ACTH and multisteroid responses to corticotropin-releasing factor in depressive illness: relationship to multisteroid responses after ACTH stimulation and dexamethasone suppression. Psychoneuroendocrinology 4:147–160, 1984
20. Holsboer F, Gerken A, Stalla GK, et al: Blunted aldosterone and ACTH release after human corticotropin-releasing factor ad-

ministration in depressed patients. Am J Psychiatry 144:229–231, 1987

21. Krishnan KRR, Rayasam K, Reed DR, et al: The corticotropin-releasing factor stimulation test in patients with major depression: relationship to dexamethasone suppression test results. Depression 1:133–136, 1993
22. Young EA, Watson SJ, Kotun J, et al: β-Lipotropin/β-endorphin response to low-dose ovine corticotropin releasing factor in endogenous depression. Arch Gen Psychiatry 47:449–457, 1990
23. American Psychiatric Association: Diagnostic and Statistical Manual of Mental Disorders, 3rd Edition. Washington, DC, American Psychiatric Association, 1980
24. Smith MA, Davidson J, Ritchie JC, et al: The corticotropin-releasing hormone test in patients with post-traumatic stress disorder. Biol Psychiatry 26:349–355, 1989
25. Amsterdam JD, Maislin G, Winokur A, et al: The oCRH test before and after clinical recovery from depression. J Affective Disord 14:213–222, 1988
26. von Bardeleben U, Holsboer F: Cortisol response to a combined dexamethasone-h-CRH challenge in patients with depression. J Neuroendocrinol 1:485–488, 1989
27. Post RM, Gold P, Rubinow DR, et al: Peptides in cerebrospinal fluid of neuropsychiatric patients: an approach to central nervous system peptide function. Life Sci 31:1–15, 1982
28. Garrick NA, Hill JL, Szele FG, et al: Corticotropin-releasing factor: a marked circadian rhythm in primate cerebrospinal fluid peaks in the evening and is inversely related to the cortisol circadian rhythm. Endocrinology 121:1329–1334, 1987
29. Owens MJ, Bartolome J, Schanberg SM, et al: Corticotropin-releasing factor concentrations exhibit an apparent diurnal rhythm in hypothalamic and extrahypothalamic brain regions: differential sensitivity to corticosterone. Neuroendocrinology 52:626–631, 1990
30. Nemeroff CB, Widerlov E, Bissette G, et al: Elevated concentrations of CSF corticotropin-releasing factor-like immunoreactivity in depressed patients. Science 226:1342–1344, 1984
31. Banki CM, Bissette G, Arato M, et al: CSF corticotropin-releasing

factor-like immunoreactivity in depression and schizophrenia. Am J Psychiatry 144:873–877, 1987
32. Arato M, Banki CM, Bissette G, et al: Elevated CSF CRF in suicide victims. Biol Psychiatry 25:355–359, 1989
33. Risch SC, Lewine RJ, Jewart RD, et al: Relationship between cerebrospinal fluid peptides and neurotransmitters in depression, in Central Nervous System Peptide Mechanisms in Stress and Depression. Edited by Risch SC. Washington, DC, American Psychiatric Press, 1991, pp 93–103
34. Kaye WH, Rubinow D, Gwirtsman HE, et al: CSF somatostatin in anorexia nervosa and bulimia: relationship to the hypothalamic pituitary-adrenal cortical axis. Psychoneuroendocrinology 13: 265–272, 1988
35. Kurlan R, Caine E, Rubin A, et al: Cerebrospinal fluid correlates of depression in Huntington's disease. Arch Neurol 45:881–883, 1988
36. Kaye WH, Gwirtsman HE, George DT, et al: Elevated cerebrospinal fluid levels of immunoreactive corticotropin-releasing hormone in anorexia nervosa: relation to state of nutrition, adrenal function, and intensity of depression. J Clin Endocrinol Metab 64:203–208, 1987
37. Banki CM, Karmacsi L, Bissette G, et al: Cerebrospinal fluid neuropeptides in mood disorder and dementia. J Affective Disord 25:39–45, 1992
38. Jolkkonen J, Lepola U, Bissette G, et al: CSF corticotropin-releasing factor is not affected in panic disorder. Biol Psychiatry 33:136–138, 1993
39. Martignoni E, Petraglia F, Costa A, et al: Cerebrospinal fluid corticotropin-releasing factor levels and stimulation test in dementia of the Alzheimer type. J Clin Lab Anal 4:5–8, 1990
40. May C, Rapoport SI, Tomai TP, et al: Cerebrospinal fluid concentrations of corticotropin-releasing hormone (CRH) and corticotropin (ACTH) are reduced in patients with Alzheimer's disease. Neurology 37:535–538, 1987
41. Mouradian MM, Farah JMJ, Mohr E, et al: Spinal fluid CRF reduction in Alzheimers disease. Neuropeptides 8:393–400, 1986
42. Pomara N, Singh RR, Deptula D, et al: CSF corticotropin-releas-

ing factor (CRF) in Alzheimers disease: its relationship to severity of dementia and monoamine metabolites. Biol Psychiatry 26:500–504, 1989
43. Nemeroff CB, Bissette G, Akil H, et al: Neuropeptide concentrations in the cerebrospinal fluid of depressed patients treated with electroconvulsive therapy: corticotropin-releasing factor, β-endorphin and somatostatin. Br J Psychiatry 158:59–63, 1991
44. DeBellis MD, Gold PW, Geracioti TD, et al: Fluoxetine significantly reduces CSF CRH and AVP concentrations in patients with major depression. Am J Psychiatry 150:656–657, 1993
45. Banki CM, Karmacsi L, Bissette G, et al: CSF corticotropin-releasing hormone and somatostatin in major depression: response to antidepressant treatment and relapse. Eur Neuropsychopharmacol 2:107–113, 1992
46. Veith RC, Lewis N, Langohr JI, et al: Effect of desipramine on cerebrospinal fluid concentrations of corticotropin-releasing factor in human subjects. Psychiatr Res 46:1–8, 1992
47. Nemeroff CB, Owens MJ, Bissette G, et al: Reduced corticotropin-releasing factor (CRF) binding sites in the frontal cortex of suicides. Arch Gen Psychiatry 45:577–579, 1988
48. Gertz BJ, Cantreras LN, McComb DJ, et al: Chronic administration of corticotropin-releasing factor increases pituitary corticotroph number. Endocrinology 120:381–388, 1987
49. Axelson DA, Doraiswamy PM, Boyko OB, et al: In vivo assessment of pituitary volume with magnetic resonance imaging and systematic stereology: relationship to dexamethasone suppression test results in patients. Psychiatr Res 46:63–70, 1992
50. Krishnan KRR, Doraiswamy PM, Lurie SN, et al: Pituitary size in depression. J Clin Endocrinol Metab 72:256–259, 1991
51. Zis KD, Zis A: Increased adrenal weight in victims of violent suicide. Am J Psychiatry 144:1214–1215, 1987
52. Amsterdam JD, Marinelli DL, Arger P, et al: Assessment of adrenal gland volume by computed tomography in depressed patients and healthy volunteers: a pilot study. Psychiatr Res 21:189–197, 1987
53. Nemeroff CB, Krishnan KRR, Reed D, et al: Adrenal gland enlargement in major depression: a computed tomography study.

Arch Gen Psychiatry 49:384–387, 1992
54. Rubin RT, Phillips JJ, Sadow TF, et al: Adrenal gland volume in major depression: increase during the depressive episode and decrease with successful treatment. American College of Neuropsychopharmacology Abstracts 31:90, 1992
55. Rubinow DR, Davis CL, Post RM: Somatostatin, in Psychopharmacology: The Fourth Generation of Progress. Edited by Bloom FE, Kupfer DJ. New York, Raven, 1995, pp 553–562
56. Arnold MA, Reppert SM, Rorstad OP, et al: Temporal patterns of somatostatin immunoreactivity in the cerebrospinal fluid of the rhesus monkey: effect of environmental lighting. J Neurosci 2:674–680, 1982
57. Berelowitz M, Perlow MJ, Hoffman HJ, et al: The diurnal variation of immunoreactive thyrotropin-releasing hormone and somatostatin in the cerebrospinal fluid of the rhesus monkey. Endocrinology 109:2102–2109, 1981
58. Rubinow DR: Cerebrospinal fluid somatostatin and psychiatric illness. Biol Psychiatry 21:341–365, 1986
59. Post RM, Weiss SRB: Endogenous biochemical abnormalities in affective illness: therapeutic versus pathogenic. Biol Psychiatry 32:469–484, 1992
60. Gerner RH, Yamada T: Altered neuropeptide concentrations in cerebrospinal fluid of psychiatric patients. Brain Res 238:298–302, 1982
61. Rubinow DR, Gold PW, Post RM: CSF somatostatin in affective illness. Arch Gen Psychiatry 40:409–412, 1983
62. Ågren H, Lundqvist G: Low levels of somatostatin in human CSF mark depressive episodes. Psychoneuroendocrinology 9:233–248, 1984
63. Black PMcL, Ballantine HT Jr, Carr DB, et al: Beta-endorphin and somatostatin concentrations in the ventricular cerebrospinal fluid of patients with affective disorder. Biol Psychiatry 21:1075–1077, 1986
64. Bissette G, Widerlöv E, Walléus H, et al: Alterations in cerebrospinal fluid concentrations of somatostatinlike immunoreactivity in neuropsychiatric disorders. Arch Gen Psychiatry 43:1148–1151, 1986

65. Doran AR, Rubinow DR, Roy A, et al: CSF somatostatin and abnormal response to dexamethasone administration in schizophrenic and depressed patients. Arch Gen Psychiatry 43: 365–369, 1986
66. Kling MA, Rubinow DR, Doran AR, et al: Cerebrospinal fluid immunoreactive somatostatin concentrations in patients with Cushings disease and major depression: relationship to indices of corticotropin-releasing hormone and cortisol secretion. Neuroendocrinology 57:79–88, 1993
67. Sunderland T, Rubinow DR, Tariot PN, et al: CSF somatostatin in patients with Alzheimer's disease, older depressed patients, and age-matched control subjects. Am J Psychiatry 144:1313–1316, 1987
68. Davis KL, Davidson M, Yang R-K, et al: CSF somatostatin in Alzheimers disease, depressed patients, and control subjects. Biol Psychiatry 24:710–712, 1988
69. Molchan SE, Lawlor BA, Hill JL, et al: CSF monoamine metabolites and somatostatin in Alzheimers disease and major depression. Biol Psychiatry 29:1110–1118, 1991
70. Gold PW, Rubinow DR: Neuropeptide function in affective illness: corticotropin-releasing hormone and somatostatin as model systems, in Psychopharmacology: The Third Generation of Progress. Edited by Meltzer HY. New York, Raven, 1987, pp 617–627
71. Berrettini WH, Nurnberger JL Jr, Zerbe RL, et al: CSF neuropeptides in euthymic bipolar patients and controls. Br J Psychiatry 150:208–212, 1987
72. Altemus M, Pigott T, L'Heureux F, et al: CSF somatostatin in obsessive-compulsive disorder. Am J Psychiatry 150:460–464, 1993
73. Kruesi MJP, Swedo S, Leonard H, et al: CSF somatostatin in childhood psychiatric disorders: a preliminary investigation. Psychiatr Res 33:277–284, 1990
74. Charlton BG, Leake A, Wright C, et al: Somatostatin content and receptors in the cerebral cortex of depressed and control subjects. J Neurol Neurosurg Psychiatry 51:719–721, 1988
75. Bowen DM, Najlerahim A, Procter AW, et al: Circumscribed

changes of the cerebral cortex in neuropsychiatric disorders of later life. Proc Natl Acad Sci U S A 86:9504–9508, 1989
76. Sorensen KV: Rapid post-mortem decomposition of the somatostatin cells in human brain: an immunohistochemical examination. Biomed Pharmacother 38:458–461, 1984
77. Kakigi T, Maeda K, Kaneda H, et al: Repeated administration of antidepressant drugs reduces regional somatostatin concentrations in rat brain. J Affective Disord 25:215–220, 1992
78. Rubinow DR, Post RM, Gold PW, et al: Effects of carbamazepine on cerebrospinal somatostatin. Psychopharmacology 85:210–213, 1985
79. Bowers CY, Schally AV, Schalch DS, et al: Activity and specificity of synthetic thyrotropin-releasing hormone in man. Biochem Biophys Res Commun 39:352–355, 1970
80. Burgus R, Dunn TE, Desideris D, et al: Characterization of ovine hypothalamic hypophysiotropic TSH-releasing factor. Nature 226:321–325, 1970
81. Nemeroff CB, Bissette G, Martin JB, et al: Effect of chronic treatment with thyrotropin-releasing hormone (TRH) or an analog of TRH (linear β-alanine TRH) on the hypothalamic-pituitary-thyroid axis. Neuroendocrinology 30:193–199, 1980
82. Mason GA, Garbutt JC, Prange AJ Jr: Thyrotropin-releasing hormone: focus on basic neurobiology, in Psychopharmacology: The Fourth Generation of Progress. Edited by Bloom FE, Kupfer DJ. New York, Raven, 1995, pp 493–503
83. Prange AJ Jr, Breese GR, Cott JM, et al: Thyrotropin-releasing hormone: antagonism of pentobarbital in rodents. Life Sci 14:447–455, 1974
84. Plotnikoff NP, Prange AJ Jr, Breese GR, et al: Thyrotropin releasing hormone: enhancement of DOPA activity by a hypothalamic hormone. Science 178:417–418, 1972
85. Kubek MJ, Sattin A: Effect of electroconvulsive shock on the content of thyrotropin-releasing hormone in rat brain. Life Sci 34:1149–1152, 1984
86. Kreider MS, Wolfinger BL, Winokur A: Effect of systemic kainic acid on regional TRH concentrations in rat central nervous system. Society for Neuroscience Abstracts 13:1656, 1987

87. Whybrow PC, Prange AJ: A hypothesis of thyroid-catecholamine receptor interaction. Arch Gen Psychiatry 38:106–113, 1981
88. Howland RH: Thyroid dysfunction in refractory depression: implications for pathophysiology and treatment. J Clin Psychiatry 54:47–54, 1993
89. Schlesser MA, Rush AJ, Fairchild C, et al: The thyrotropin-releasing hormone stimulation test: a methodological study. Psychiatr Res 9:59–67, 1983
90. Loosen PT: Pituitary-thyroid axis in affective disorders, in Psychopharmacology: The Third Generation of Progress. Edited by Meltzer HY. New York, Raven, 1987, pp 629–636
91. Nemeroff CB: The relevance of thyrotropin-releasing hormone to psychiatric disorders, in Neuropeptides and Psychiatric Disease. Edited by Nemeroff CB. Washington, DC, American Psychiatric Press, 1990, pp 15–28
92. Bartalena L, Placidi GF, Martino E, et al: Nocturnal serum thyrotropin (TSH) surge and the TSH response to TSH-releasing hormone: dissociated behavior in untreated depressives. J Clin Endocrinol Metab 71:650–655, 1990
93. Duval F, Macher JP, Mokrani MC: Difference between evening and morning thyrotropin response to protirelin in major depressive episode. Arch Gen Psychiatry 47:443–448, 1990
94. Shelton RC, Winn S, Ekhatore N, et al: The effects of antidepressants on the thyroid axis in depression. Biol Psychiatry 33:120–126, 1993
95. Kirkegaard C, Faber J, Hummer L, et al: Increased levels of TRH in cerebrospinal fluid from patients with endogenous depression. Psychoneuroendocrinology 4:227–235, 1979
96. Banki CM, Bissette G, Arato M, et al: Elevation of immunoreactive CSF TRH in depressed patients. Am J Psychiatry 145:1526–1531, 1988
97. Roy A, Wolkowitz OM, Bissette G, et al: Differences in CSF concentrations of thyrotropin-releasing hormone in depressed patients and normal subjects: negative findings. Am J Psychiatry 151:600–602, 1994
98. Maeda K, Yoshimoto Y, Yamadori A: Blunted TSH and unaltered PRL responses to TRH following repeated administration of TRH

in neurologic patients: a replication of neuroendocrine features of major depression. Biol Psychiatry 33:277–283, 1993

99. Fossey MD, Lydiarel RB, Larara MT, et al: CSF thyrotropin-releasing hormone in patients with anxiety disorders. Biol Psychiatry 27 (suppl):167A, 1990
100. Roy A, Bissette G, Nemeroff CB: Cerebrospinal fluid thyrotropin-releasing hormone concentrations in alcoholics and normal controls. Biol Psychiatry 28:767–772, 1990
101. Russ MJ, Ackerman SH: Antidepressant treatment response in depressed hypothyroid patients. Hosp Community Psychiatry 40:954–956, 1989
102. Gold MS, Pottash AL, Extein I: Hypothyroidism and depression: evidence from complete thyroid function evaluation. JAMA 245: 919–922, 1981
103. Haggarty JJ Jr, Garbutt JC, Evans DL, et al: Subclinical hypothyroidism: a review of neuropsychiatric aspects. Int J Psychiatry Med 20:193–208, 1990
104. Joffe RT, Sokolov STH: Thyroid hormones, the brain and affective disorders. Crit Rev Neurobiol 8:45–63, 1994
105. Langer G, Koinig G, Hatzinger R, et al: Response of thyrotropin to thyrotropin-releasing hormone as predictor of treatment outcome. Arch Gen Psychiatry 43:861–868, 1986
106. Kirkegaard C: The thyrotropin response to thyrotropin-releasing hormone in endogenous depression. Psychoneuroendocrinology 6:189–212, 1981
107. Arato M, Banki CM, Nemeroff CB, et al: Hypothalamic-pituitary-adrenal axis and suicide, in Psychobiology of Suicidal Behavior. Edited by Mann JJ, Stanley M. New York, New York Academy of Science, 1986, pp 263–270
108. France RD, Urban B, Krishnan KRR, et al: CSF corticotropin-releasing factor-like immunoreactivity in chronic pain patients with and without major depression. Biol Psychiatry 23:86–88, 1988
109. Widerlov E, Bissette G, Nemeroff CB: Monoamine metabolites, corticotropin releasing factor and somatostatin as CSF markers in depressed patients. J Affective Disord 14:99–107, 1988

CHAPTER

12

Mechanism of Action of Antidepressants: Monoamine Hypotheses and Beyond

Robert M. Berman, M.D.
John H. Krystal, M.D.
Dennis S. Charney, M.D.

Current biological theories of depression have largely unfolded from studies on the mechanism of action of antidepressants. In 1965, classic papers by Schildkraut[1] and Bunney and Davis[2] set forth the catecholamine deficiency hypothesis of depression. This hypothesis was based on the observations that antidepressants increased synaptic norepinephrine (NE) concentrations, whereas reserpine induced depressive symptoms and diminished synaptic NE concentrations. A short time later, Coppen[3] and Lapin[4] presented the indoleamine deficiency hypothesis of depression, based on observations that drugs that relieved depressive

We thank Lisa Roach and Evalyn Testa for their excellent help in the preparation of the manuscript, and Ron Duman, Ph.D., for reviewing parts of this chapter.

symptoms, including monoamine oxidase inhibitors (MAOI) as well as the serotonin (5-HT) precursors 5-hydroxytryptophan (5-HTP) and L-tryptophan (TRP), increased synaptic concentrations of 5-HT.

In this chapter, we review the evolution of selected neurotransmitter and neuropeptide hypotheses of antidepressant action and their current explanatory limitations. In addition, we focus on the evidence for and against a common mechanism of action of antidepressant treatments, the brain regions involved in antidepressant action, and the future development of novel antidepressant treatments.

5-HT Function and the Mechanism of Action of Antidepressants

A growing body of evidence implicates the 5-HT system in regulating mood (Table 12–1). The original indoleamine deficiency hypothesis asserted that depression resulted from decreased 5-HT activity and that antidepressants work by increasing 5-HT activity. This hypothesis, however, did not explain several important clinical phenomena. First, the onset of action of antidepressants typically lags 2 or more weeks behind its initial synaptic effects. Second, monoamine metabolites are not consistently shown to be lower in depressed patients than in nondepressed subjects. Third, drugs that markedly and acutely enhance 5-HT release do not alter mood. In fact, concurrent administration of TRP and MAOIs more consistently resulted in nausea and involuntary clonic movements rather than an elevation of mood in one study.[5]

Several groups have advanced a hypothesis of antidepressant action based on enhanced 5-HT neurotransmission.[6–8] This hypothesis asserts that chronic administration of antidepressants enhances 5-HT neurotransmission, possibly via an alteration of receptor sensitivity, receptor density, or neural firing characteristics. Over the past several years, there has been an extensive growth of research evaluating this perspective on the neurobiology and pharmacotherapy of depression.

Table 12–1. Findings implicating serotonergic function in mood regulation at various neuropharmacologic levels of action

Level of action	Findings	Replicability
Precursor availability	Plasma TRP is lower in subgroups of depressed patients.	+/–
	Depletion of plasma TRP results in depressive relapse in antidepressant-treated patients.	++
	Oral TRP augments MAOI but not TCA efficacy.	++
	Low brain uptake of L-[^{11}C]5-HT is seen in depressed patients.	+
Neurotransmitter synthesis	PCPA, inhibitor of TRP hydroxylase, results in depressive relapse in antidepressant-treated patients.	+
	Tetrahydrobiopterin, cofactor of both TRP and tyrosine hydroxylases, may have antidepressant properties.	+
Neurotransmitter storage	Long-term treatment with reserpine, which depletes monoamine stores, results in depressive symptoms in patients with a history of depression.	++
Neurotransmitter release	Fenfluramine and MDMA, which increase 5-HT release, may produce a mild sense of well-being.	+
	Lithium, which enhances 5-HT release, augments many antidepressants.	+++
5-HT autoreceptor function	5-HT$_{1A}$ agonists (e.g., gepirone, buspirone) may have antidepressant properties.	++

(continued)

Table 12–1. Findings implicating serotonergic function in mood regulation at various neuropharmacologic levels of action *(continued)*

Level of action	Findings	Replicability
Neurotransmitter reuptake	Decreased imipramine binding is seen in postmortem brain regions of depressed patients.	+/–
	Decreased platelet reuptake sites have been found.	+++
	5-HT reuptake inhibitors are effective antidepressants.	+++
Neurotransmitter metabolism	MAOIs are effective antidepressants.	+++
	Low 5-HT metabolites have been found in subgroups of depressed patients.	+/–
	Low 5-HT metabolites have been found in CSF of patients prone to violent suicide.	+++
Neurotransmitter postsynaptic binding	5-HT_2 antagonists such as ritanserin may improve mood of dysthymic patients.	+
	Increased 5-HT_2 receptor density has been found in postmortem brains of depressed patients.	+

Note. TRP = L-tryptophan. MAOI = monoamine oxidase inhibitor. TCA = tricyclic antidepressant. 5-HT = 5-hydroxytryptamine (serotonin). PCPA = parachlorophenylalanine. MDMA = 3,4-methylenedioxymethamphetamine ("Ecstasy"). CSF = cerebrospinal fluid.

Replication key: + = no or one replicated study. ++ = several replication studies. +++ = highly replicated by more than two research groups. +/– = mixed or inconsistent results.

Preclinical Studies

Receptor binding. Largely based on molecular biology studies (Table 12–2), there have been major advances in the discovery of the 5-HT receptor subtypes that may mediate the actions of antidepressant drugs.[9] The 5-HT receptors consist of at least three distinct types of molecular structures: guanine nucleotide-binding, G protein–coupled receptors; ligand-gated ion channels; and transporters. The G protein–coupled 5-HT receptors have been divided into 5-HT_1 (5-HT_{1A}, 5-HT_{1B}, 5-HT_{1D}, 5-HT_{1E}, and 5-HT_{1F}) and 5-HT_2 (5-HT_{2A}, 5-HT_{2B}, and 5-HT_{2C}, formerly 5-HT_{1C}) receptor families. Thus far, at least seven distinct classes of 5-HT receptors have been identified in the brain of mammals.

High densities of 5-HT_{1A} receptors are found on the cell bodies of 5-HT neurons in the raphe and postsynaptic locations in hippocampus, lateral septum, entorhinal cortex and amygdala.[10] Antidepressant administration has inconsistent effects on 5-HT_{1A} receptor density. Most[11–15] but not all[11,16,17] studies have shown that antidepressant treatment does not alter hippocampal 5-HT_{1A} receptor densities. 5-HT_{1A} receptor densities in the dorsal raphe nucleus have been shown to be decreased[11,16] or unaltered.[16] 5-HT_{1A} densities in the frontal cortex have been shown to be increased[17,18] as well as decreased.[14–16] These markedly divergent results vary among antidepressant categories and among different laboratories.

5-HT_{1B} receptors are rich in the globus pallidus, substantia nigra pars reticulatum, striatum, hypothalamus, amygdala, and neocortex in the rodent brain.[19,20] 5-HT_{1B} receptors are not found in the human brain, but their distribution and coupling mechanism suggest that they may function analogously to the 5-HT_{1D} receptor.[21] The effects of chronic antidepressant treatment on 5-HT_{1B} receptor density have not been well studied. One study suggests that chronic treatment with chlorimipramine, tianeptine, or iprindole does not affect the density of 5-HT_{1B} receptors in the frontal cortex.[22] In another preliminary report, long-term administration of tianeptine significantly increased receptor binding in the dorsomedial nucleus of the hypothalamus and the sensory region of the parietal cortex.[23] The same study confirmed findings that long-term administration of flu-

Table 12–2. Effects of chronic antidepressant treatment on serotonergic

	Receptor binding					
Antidepressant category	**5-HT$_{1A}$ raphe nucleus**	**5-HT$_{1A}$ hippocampus**	**5-HT$_{1A}$ cortex**	**5-HT$_2$ cortex**	**Brain reuptake sites**	**Platelet 5-HT reuptake site**
NE reuptake inhibitors	—	0	↓↑	↓	0	↓0
Mixed reuptake inhibitors[a]	↓0	0↑	0↑↓	↓0	0	↓0
5-HT reuptake inhibitors	↓	0	0	↑↓0	0↓	↑0↓
MAOIs	—	—	—	↓	0	↑0
ECT	—	0	↓	↑	0	↓0
Other antidepressants						
Trazodone	—	—	↑	↓	—	—
Bupropion	—	—	—	0	—	—
Mianserin	—	—	↑	↓	—	0

Note. 5-HT = 5-hydroxytryptamine (serotonin). TRP = L-tryptophan. NE = norepinephrine. MAOIs = monoamine oxidase inhibitors. ECT = electroconvulsive therapy.
↑ = increased responsiveness. ↓ = decreased responsiveness. 0 = no change.
— = not tested. Multiple symbols indicate mixed results.
[a]Mixed reuptake inhibitors include antidepressants that exhibit both norepinephrine and 5-HT reuptake inhibition, such as amitriptyline and imipramine.
[b]Robust response.

oxetine does not alter 5-HT$_{1B}$ receptor densities.[23]

The highest density of 5-HT$_{1D}$ receptors are in the globus pallidus and the substantia nigra; to a lesser extent, they also are found in the caudate-putamen, nucleus accumbens, and frontal cortex.[24] The 5-HT$_{1D}$ receptors function as nerve terminal autoreceptors, regulating the release of 5-HT.[25] Presynaptic autoreceptors control 5-HT release from serotonergic terminals in the cerebral cortex of the human brain.[26] To date, no studies have evaluated the effects of antidepressant treatment on the 5-HT$_{1D}$ receptor.

The 5-HT$_2$ receptor family includes the 5-HT$_{2A}$, 5-HT$_{2B}$, and 5-HT$_{2C}$ receptors. 5-HT$_2$ receptors are coupled by G proteins to phospholipases that hydrolyze phosphoinositides and mobilize intracellular calcium.[27,28] High densities of 5-HT$_{2A}$ and 5-HT$_{2B}$ receptors are located in the claustrum, olfactory tubercle, neocortex, anterior olfactory nucleus, piriform cortex, caudate-putamen, and nucleus accumbens. Low densities are found in the thalamus, hip-

function in laboratory animals

Neurochemical sensitivity				Electrophysiologic sensitivity				Behavioral sensitivity				
TRP hydroxylase		Hippocampal 2nd-messenger responsiveness		Presynaptic		Post-synaptic	Overall trans-mission	Synaptic 5-HT_{1A}				
Activity	mRNA	5-HT_{1A}	$5\text{-HT}_{2/1C}$	5-HT_{1A}	5-HT_{1B}	5-HT_{1A}		Post	Pre	5-HT_{1B}	5-HT_{1C}	5-HT_{2}
—	—	↑0	↓	—	—	↑	↑	↓0↑	↓0	—	—	↓↑0
↑0	—	—	↓0	—	0↓	↑	↑	↓0↑	↓0	—	—	↓↑0
↑↓	↑	↑0	0	↓	↓	0	↑[b]	↓0	↓0	↑↓	↓	↓
—	0	↑0	—	↓	0	0	↑[b]	↓0	↓	↓	—	↓
—	—	↑0	—	0	0	↑	↑[b]	↓	↓	—	—	↑
—	—	—	—	—	—	—	—	0	0	—	—	0↑
—	—	—	—	—	—	—	—	—	—	—	—	—
—	—	—	↓	—	—	↑	↑	0↑	↓	—	—	0↑

pocampus, brain stem, cerebellum, and spinal cord.[29]

Preclinical studies indicate that chronic but not acute antidepressant administration reduces 5-HT_2 density and 5-HT_2 messenger RNA (mRNA). Notable exceptions include the administration of electroconvulsive therapy, which may increase 5-HT_2 receptor density,[30] and 5-HT reuptake inhibitors (SSRIs), which do not alter 5-HT_2 receptor density.[31] Mianserin decreases 5-HT_2 receptor density after only several doses; however, it requires several weeks of administration for antidepressant efficacy.[32] Changes in 5-HT_2 receptor density are not directly correlated with mRNA expression. Chronic electroconvulsive therapy leads to increased 5-HT_2 receptor binding and mRNA levels; however, chronic administration of imipramine, mianserin, and tranylcypromine leads to decreased 5-HT_2 receptor binding but not decreased mRNA levels.[31]

The mechanism by which many antidepressants reduce 5-HT_2 receptor binding has not been clearly established. The regulation of 5-HT_2 receptors does not require intact 5-HT nerve terminals,[33,34] suggesting a direct action at the 5-HT_2 receptor site. In support of this assertion, many, if not most, antidepressants are antagonists with a high affinity for the 5-HT_2 receptor.[35,36] Administration of both 5-HT_2 agonists and antagonists decrease 5-HT receptor binding.[37,38] Thus, the ability of antidepressants to decrease 5-HT_2 receptor binding may be a combined consequence of reuptake blockade and receptor antagonism on intracellular processes, including post-transcriptional regulation.

The greatest density of 5-HT_{2C} receptors is found in the choroid plexus, but significant levels are also found in the cerebral cortex, hippocampus, basal ganglia, hypothalamus, and thalamic nuclei.[39] Typical antidepressants, such as nortriptyline, amoxapine, and amitriptyline, have high affinities for the 5-HT_{2C} receptors. Sertraline and fluoxetine have weak affinities for cloned 5-HT_{2C} receptors.[40] 5-HT_{2C} receptors may be regulated in a manner similar to that of other 5-HT_2 subtypes, that is, with chronic antidepressant treatment probably leading to downregulation.[31] In rodent spinal cord, downregulation of 5-HT_{2C} receptors highly correlates with the potency of either agonist or antagonist affinity at the 5-HT_{2C} receptor.[41] In one study to date, chronic imipramine dosing led to decreased 5-HT_{2C} receptor densities in the frontal cortex, hippocampus, and choroid plexus.[16] Further studies are needed to assess 5-HT_{2C} activity.

5-HT_1 and 5-HT_2 receptor families interact. For example, the 5-HT_{1A} receptor serves as an autoregulatory receptor that leads to subsequent decreased release of 5-HT.[42] Recent behavioral and iontophoretic studies[43,44] have demonstrated that 5-HT_{1A} activation inhibits 5-HT_2-mediated head twitching and glutamate-induced locomotor activation, respectively. Therefore, discriminating independent treatment effects on specific receptor types may be indeterminable.

Several other receptor subtypes are only beginning to be fully characterized. Effects of antidepressant treatment on receptors 5-HT_3 through 5-HT_7 have not been studied. 5-HT_3 receptors are found in the nucleus tractus solitarius.[45,46] A lower density is apparent in the hippocampus, amygdala, and entorhinal cortex.[47] 5-HT_4 distribution has not yet been studied; however, there is preliminary evidence that it is involved in anxiety regulation.[48,49] The 5-HT_5 receptor has recently been cloned, although its function remains to be characterized.[50] The 5-HT_6 receptor has been localized predominantly in the striatum but also in limbic and cortical regions.[51] Tricyclic and antipsychotic drugs, including clozapine, amoxapine, clomipramine, and amitriptyline, have high affinities for this receptor.[49,52] The 5-HT_7 receptors are distributed throughout limbic brain structures such as the thalamus, hypothalamus, and hippocampus.[53] This receptor has been hypothesized to be involved in circadian rhythms and other functions such as learning, mood, and neuroendocrine regulation.[54]

The density of 5-HT reuptake sites, also known as 5-HT transporters, is generally unaltered by antidepressant treatment. Chronic treatment has not been associated with altered binding by radiolabeled paroxetine or imipramine. A possible exception is chronic dosing with the SSRIs, for which some studies[23,55–57] have indicated decreased receptor density. Furthermore, SSRIs, in contrast to MAOIs, have been shown to decrease the concentration of mRNA coding for the 5-HT reuptake site after chronic antidepressant administration.[58] Measurement of 5-HT reuptake sites in human platelets shows less consistent results but demonstrate a general trend toward increased density after long-term antidepressant treatment.[59–68]

Neurochemical sensitivity. The effects of antidepressant administration on 5-HT_{1A} receptor-mediated inhibition of forskolin-stimulated adenylate cyclase activity in the rat hippocampus have recently been examined. Results from two laboratories[69–72] demonstrated a consistently decreased inhibition with all antidepressants tested except iprindole, whereas another group[73] demonstrated only a mild (approximately 5%) decrease in inhibition for electroconvulsive therapy and MAOIs and no decrease for specific 5-HT or NE reuptake inhibitors.

Second-messenger responsiveness of 5-HT_2 receptor-mediated cellular events have been studied. Findings show that repeated antidepressant dosing decreases the 5-HT_2-mediated inositol monophosphate accumulation in rodent hippocampus and cortex.[74–76]

Electrophysiologic sensitivity. In studies of electrophysiologic sensitivity, single-unit intracranial probes are used in laboratory animals to assess neuronal potentials in brain regions that are rich in either presynaptic 5-HT receptors (e.g., dorsal raphe nucleus) or postsynaptic receptors (e.g., cortex and hippocampus).[77–80]

Chronic antidepressant administration influences the various receptor subtypes that are responsible for the modulation of 5-HT neurotransmission.[77] The firing rate of dorsal raphe 5-HT neurons is regulated by 5-HT_{1A} autoreceptors. The 5-HT release from neuronal terminals is regulated by terminal autoreceptors—5-HT_{1B} in rodents and 5-HT_{1D} in other animals. Postsynaptic responsiveness in the hippocampus is regulated by 5-HT_{1A} receptors. The pre- and postsynaptic 5-HT_{1A} receptors, despite having similar radioligand binding profiles, functionally respond differently to 5-HT agonists.[81,82]

Electrophysiologic studies have consistently shown that antidepressant treatments enhance 5-HT neurotransmission by facilitating 5-HT release or increasing postsynaptic responsivity. The net increase in 5-HT neurotransmission is much more robust after chronic dosing with MAOIs and SSRIs than with the NE reuptake inhibitors.[80] Chronic administration of SSRIs results in a desensitization of the somatodendritic and terminal 5-HT autoreceptors.[8,78,79] Chronic administration of MAOIs results in desensitization of somatodendritic, but not terminal, autoreceptors.[78] Chronic administration of the tricyclic NE and mixed reuptake inhibitors does not affect autoreceptor function but enhances postsynaptic 5-HT_{1A} responsivity.[8,78,79] Repeated electroconvulsive therapy also enhances postsynaptic 5-HT_{1A} responsivity while not affecting 5-HT autoreceptors.[78,83] Similarly, short-term lithium treatment may exert its effects on postsynaptic 5-HT_{1A} receptors while not affecting autoreceptor function.[84]

Behavioral sensitivity. Behavioral assays in laboratory animals have examined the role of 5-HT in the modulation of motor function and thermoregulation.[6,7,12,40,85–88] The most studied paradigm, 5-HT agonist-induced head-shaking behavior in rodents and dogs, assesses 5-HT_2 receptor-mediated function.[85,89] The 5-HT behavioral syndrome, characterized by forepaw treading, hind limb abduction, and head weaving, assesses postsynaptic 5-HT_{1A} receptor-mediated function. The 5-HT_{1A} agonist-induced hypothermia is thought to be a function of presynaptic 5-HT_{1A} responsiveness;[89] however, a recent study[90] suggests that it may conversely indicate postsynaptic function. The behavior mediated by the 5-HT_{2C} receptor is assessed by *m*-chlorophenylpiperazine (m-CPP)–induced exploratory hypoactivity in mice.[91,92] 5-HT_{1B} receptor-mediated activity is measured by m-CPP–induced hypothermia in mice[91,94] and a recently described isolation-induced social behavioral deficit model.[93,94] In general, chronic antidepressant dosing has been associated with decreased behavioral activity at 5-HT_{1A} (presynaptic and postsynaptic) and 5-HT_2 receptors. Early studies also suggest possible decreased activity in 5-HT_{1B} and 5-HT_{2C} function.

These behavioral studies are limited by their ability to assess brain regions that are likely to be involved in antidepressant action. For example, the 5-HT_2-mediated head-twitching response does not involve serotonergic transmission in the frontal cortex.[95]

Summary. The preclinical studies reviewed here suggest that, through a combination of pre- and postsynaptic mechanisms, chronic antidepressant administration enhances the function of 5-HT systems in the brain. These studies are limited by the uncertain clinical relevance of the regions assessed, their generalizability to human brain function, and the inconsistency of the results themselves. Furthermore, since the time that many of the studies were performed more 5-HT receptor subtypes have been characterized, each one of which has potentially discriminate actions. In addition, that most preclinical studies have been performed on rodents limits their generalizability to primates. Known differences across animal classes include the presence of 5-HT_{1B} versus 5-HT_{1D} terminal autoreceptors, as well as differential receptor and second-messenger responsiveness after chronic antidepressant treatment.[96]

Clinical Studies

In summary, clinical studies to date have predominantly focused on neuroendocrine responses to pharmacologic probes (Table 12–3). The most consistently demonstrated neuroendocrine abnormality in depressed patients is a blunted prolactin (PRL) response to tryp-

Table 12–3. Effects of chronic antidepressant treatment on serotonergic function as measured by clinical studies

Antidepressant category	PRL response: TRP challenge	PRL response: FEN challenge	Hypothermic response to ipsapirone	Cortisol response to 5-HTP challenge	Platelet reuptake site	Depressive relapse during TRP depletion
NE reuptake inhibitors	↑	—	—	↓	↑ 0	Rare
Mixed reuptake inhibitors[a]	↑	↑	↓	↓	↑ ↓	Common
5-HT reuptake inhibitors	↑[b]	↑	↓[c]	—	↑ ↓	Common
MAOIs	↑[b]	—	—	↑	0	Common
ECT	—	↑	—	—	↑	—
Other antidepressants						
Trazodone	0	—	—	—	—	—
Bupropion	—	—	—	—	—	Rare
Mianserin	0	—	—	—	0	—

Note. PRL = prolactin. TRP = L-tryptophan. FEN = fenfluramine. 5-HTP = 5-hydroxytryptophan. NE = norepinephrine. 5-HT = 5-hydroxytryptamine (serotonin). MAOIs = monoamine oxidase inhibitors. ECT = electroconvulsive therapy.
↑ = increased responsiveness. ↓ = decreased responsiveness. 0 = no change. — = not tested. Multiple symbols indicate mixed results.
[a]Mixed reuptake inhibitors include antidepressants that exhibit both norepinephrine and 5-HT reuptake inhibition, such as amitriptyline and imipramine.
[b]Robust response.
[c]Demonstrated after chronic fluoxetine treatment in patients with obsessive-compulsive disorder.

tophan challenge. After chronic antidepressant treatment, patients show an increased PRL response to TRP infusion.[5,97–99] Notable exceptions[101] include mianserin and trazodone, which have no measured effects on PRL response, possibly secondary to their 5-HT antagonist properties. Also notable is that the degree of enhancement of PRL responsiveness produced by antidepressant administration is not predictive of clinical outcome.

Another neuroendocrine measure of 5-HT function is the PRL response to fenfluramine challenge, a 5-HT–releasing agent and reuptake inhibitor. To date, studies have consistently shown a blunted response in patients with depression. In humans, this response has been shown to be significantly blocked by the 5-HT_{1A} antagonist pindolol.[102] Antidepressant treatment has consistently been shown to enhance this response.[101,103–107] Addition of lithium to clomipramine treatment slightly decreased this response.[108]

Another clinical paradigm is the hypothermic response to the challenge of 5-HT_{1A} agonists, such as flesinoxan and ipsapirone.[109,110] Patients with unipolar depression demonstrate decreased ipsapirone-induced hypothermia as compared with healthy control subjects.[111,112] Chronic treatment with amitriptyline blunts this response further in depressed patients,[112] and chronic treatment with fluoxetine blunts this response in patients with obsessive-compulsive disorder.[113] A limitation of the neuroendocrine and body temperature studies is that they measure brain 5-HT function in regions and systems that may not be relevant to mood regulation.

A novel clinical paradigm, TRP depletion, studies the effects of a rapid reduction of plasma TRP on mood and behavior.[114–117] In these studies, a diet low in TRP, followed by ingestion of a TRP-free amino acid drink, resulted in an 80% reduction of plasma TRP. Low plasma TRP has been associated with decreased 5-HT in primate brains, as well as decreased levels of 5-HT metabolites in human cerebrospinal fluid (CSF). This method of TRP depletion is therefore likely to lower brain 5-HT content in humans. TRP depletion of drug-free depressed patients reveals variable but usually mild responses in mood. Patients whose depression remitted on medication, however, commonly demonstrated a relapse of their depressive symptoms that temporally correlated with the nadir of plasma TRP levels. Patients whose depression remitted on 5-HT reuptake inhibitors or MAOIs were much more likely to relapse than were those treated with tricyclic antidepressants. These results suggest that the mechanism of action of the SSRIs and MAOIs is dependent on intact 5-HT transmission.

Clinical studies of fenfluramine and TRP challenges suggest that antidepressant treatment enhances 5-HT activity, at least partially, at postsynaptic 5-HT_{1A} sites. Ipsapirone challenge studies, however, suggest attenuated 5-HT_{1A}-mediated activity. The latter finding parallels findings of decreased 5-HT_{1A} responsiveness in preclinical studies of second-messenger responsiveness and behavioral sensitivity. Differences in clinical studies of 5-HT responsiveness may depend on pre- versus postsynaptic receptor site of action. 5-HT_2 responsiveness, as measured by cortisol response to 5-HTP challenge, parallels preclinical findings of 5-HT_2 receptor binding density and behavioral studies: electroconvulsive therapy increases 5-HT_2 receptor-mediated binding and behavioral activity, whereas most other selected antidepressants decrease these indices of 5-HT_2 function.

Therapeutic Studies

As predicted by the 5-HT hypothesis of depression, agents that functionally enhance 5-HT transmission would be expected to have antidepressant activity. Numerous studies have demonstrated the efficacy of lithium augmentation in antidepressant treatment,[118–136] with upwards of a 70% response rate.[137] Although the mechanism of action of this response to lithium is not well elucidated itself, one of its overall effects is to enhance 5-HT function, as evidenced by the ability of lithium in humans to increase levels of 5-hydroxyindoleacetic acid in CSF, increase platelet 5-HT uptake, and increase the neuroendocrine responses of 5-HT agonists.[138] Poor response to antidepressants may be associated with no or minimal enhancement of 5-HT function as measured by prolactin response to TRP challenge.[133] Although the addition of lithium in this context tends to enhance neuroendocrine function, enhancement is not directly proportional to clinical response. Another tested augmentation strategy based on enhancing 5-HT function is the addition of fenfluramine to an antidepressant regimen. In one double-blind study, a 2-week course of fenfluramine augmentation of tricyclic treatment in refractory patients did not lead to clinical improvement.[139]

Summary

That antidepressants may work by enhancing 5-HT neurotransmission is supported by results from electrophysiological, behavioral, and neuroendocrine studies. The antidepressants that most directly affect 5-HT systems, the SSRIs and MAOIs, have been shown in electrophysiologic studies to enhance 5-HT neurotransmission more prominently than do other antidepressants. Furthermore, these agents similarly enhance neurotransmission via decreased autoreceptor sensitivity. Conversely, compromise of 5-HT transmission by TRP depletion acutely reverses the antidepressant effects of MAOIs and SSRIs much more commonly than in other classes of antidepressants.

Although many data suggest that most antidepressants enhance 5-HT neurotransmission, the specific potency of an antidepressant in enhancing neurotransmission is not directly proportional to its clinical efficacy. 5-HT function plays a complex role in the mechanism of antidepressant action. In this context, the role of the newly discovered 5-HT receptor subtypes in the pathophysiology of depression and the mechanism of action of antidepressant treatments should be the focus of investigation.

NE Function and the Mechanism of Action of Antidepressants

A large body of evidence implicates the role of NE function in depression and in the mechanism of action of antidepressants. Explaining early findings, the catecholamine deficiency hypothesis asserted that depression was a result of diminished catecholamine activity and that antidepressants work by increasing catecholamine activity. This hypothesis is limited by its inability to account for the time lag between the initial reuptake inhibition and clinical outcome, paradoxical findings of increased NE metabolites in depressed patients, and the efficacy of SSRIs.

Preclinical Studies

Tyrosine hydroxylase activity. Tyrosine hydroxylase (TH) is the rate-limiting enzyme in the biosynthesis of NE. Chronic administration of multiple antidepressants reduces the expression of this protein as measured by immunoblot assays (Table 12–4).[140,141] Chronic administration of desipramine, imipramine, clorgyline, and milnacipram, but not citalopram, decreased TH activity as measured by NE precursor accumulation in response to TH inhibition.[142] TH mRNA levels in response to chronic administration of antidepressants have shown variable results. Interestingly, one study showed that locus ceruleus cyclic adenosine monophosphate (cAMP)-dependent protein kinase activity in cytosolic fractions correlated with TH mRNA expression and locus ceruleus cell firing rate[143] in response to stress, NE depletion, and imipramine. Although fluoxetine and phenelzine have been shown to increase TH mRNA,[144] immunoblot assays demonstrate decreased protein expression.[140,141] Further studies are needed to assess the effects of other classes of antidepressants on cAMP kinase activity, TH mRNA, and locus ceruleus cell firing.

NE uptake sites. Repeated antidepressant dosing has demonstrated mixed results on NE uptake site density as measured by tritiated desipramine.[145–149] In a recent study in which labeled nisoxetine, a potent and relatively specific ligand for the NE uptake site, was used, significantly decreased binding was demonstrated in multiple brain regions, including the hippocampus, thalamus, and amygdala,[150] after repeated administration of desipramine or electroconvulsive therapy.

β-Adrenergic function. The most consistent preclinical findings concern β-adrenergic receptor function. Long-term, but not short-term, administration of most antidepressants decreases β-receptor binding.[6,151] Weak or no effects on binding have been reported after long-term administration of mianserin, bupropion, nomifensine, citalopram, trazodone, and maprotiline.[152–157]

Most[158] but not all[156] antidepressants downregulate β-adrenergic receptor function as assessed by β-adrenergic receptor–stimulated cAMP accumulation. This phenomenon may occur via the uncoupling of β-adrenergic receptors from second messengers.[159] Supporting this view, chronic administration of antidepressants

Table 12–4. Effects of chronic antidepressant treatment on noradrenergic function in laboratory animals

Antidepressant category	Receptor binding				Neurobiochemical sensitivity					Electrophysiologic sensitivity			Behavioral sensitivity		
	NE reuptake site				Tyrosine hydroxylase										
		β[a]	α_2	α_1	Activity	mRNA	β[a]	α_2	α_1	β	α_2	α_1	β	α_2	α_1
NE reuptake inhibitors	0	↓	0 ↓ ↑	0 ↑	↓	—	↓	—	0	↓ 0	↓	↑	↓	↓	↑ 0
Mixed reuptake inhibitors[b]	—	↓	0 ↓ ↑	0 ↑	↓ ↑	↓	↓	↓	—	↓ 0	↓ 0	↑	↓	↓ 0	↑ 0
5-HT reuptake inhibitors	—	↓ 0	0	0 ↑	↓ 0	↑	0 ↓	↓	0 ↑	0	↓	—	↓	—	↑ 0
MAOIs	—	↓	↓	0 ↑	↓	↑	↓	—	0	↓	0	—	↓	↓	↑ 0
ECT	↓ 0	↓	↓ 0	↑	↓	—	↓	—	—	0	—	—	↓	↓	↑ 0
Other antidepressants															
Trazodone	—	↓	—	—	—	—	—	↓	—	—	—	—	—	—	—
Bupropion	—	0 ↓	0	↑	↓	—	0 ↓	—	—	—	—	—	—	—	—
Mianserin	—	0 ↓	0 ↑	↑	—	—	0 ↓	↓	—	—	0	—	↓	0	↓ ↑

Note. NE = norepinephrine. 5-HT = 5-hydroxytryptamine (serotonin). MAOIs = monoamine oxidase inhibitors. ECT = electroconvulsive therapy.
↑ = increased responsiveness. ↓ = decreased responsiveness. 0 = no change. — = not tested. Multiple symbols indicate mixed results.
[a]Robust and generally consistent findings.
[b]Mixed reuptake inhibitors include antidepressants that exhibit both norepinephrine and 5-HT reuptake inhibition, such as amitriptyline and imipramine.

commonly shifts β-adrenergic receptors from high- to low-affinity states.[160] The effects of antidepressants on β-adrenergic receptor sensitivity are modulated by 5-HT systems; for example, antidepressant-induced β-adrenergic receptor downregulation may be prevented by depletion or lesions of the 5-HT system.[159]

In electrophysiologic studies, repeated desipramine dosing resulted in decreased β-adrenergic receptor responsiveness in the cingulate cortex, cerebellar neurons, and hippocampus.[161–163] Behavioral studies reliably demonstrate that chronic antidepressant administration decreases the motor suppressant effect of salbutomol, a β-adrenergic receptor agonist.[164,165] Overall, the findings for β-adrenergic receptor function consistently, but not universally, demonstrate an antidepressant-induced decrease in β-adrenergic system responsiveness.

α_2-Adrenergic function. Preclinical assessment of α_2-adrenergic function yields less reliable results. Generally, α_2-adrenergic receptor binding, mediated behaviors, and electrophysiologically measured activity are decreased by chronic antidepressant administration.[166] Ligand binding studies of receptor density after repeated antidepressant dosing show variable results.[167] In biochemical studies, α_2-adrenergic agonist enhancement of cAMP accumulation is decreased after long-term administration of imipramine, trazodone, mianserin, citalopram, and fluoxetine.[168] Electrophysiologic studies generally demonstrate a decreased α_2-adrenergic responsiveness after chronic antidepressant treatment. In a recent study,[161] chronic desipramine dosing attenuated responsiveness of α_2-adrenergic terminal autoreceptors in rat hippocampus, whereas cell body α_2-adrenergic autoreceptor and α_2-adrenergic postsynaptic receptor function were unchanged. Another study,[169] however, demonstrated that antidepressant administration increased postsynaptic α_2-adrenergic receptor responsiveness in amygdala neurons. Chronic administration of desipramine, imipramine, and zimelidine, but not clomipramine, mianserin, or iprindole, decreased the responsiveness of locus ceruleus neurons to iontophoretically applied clonidine.[170] Behavioral paradigms designed to assess α_2-adrenergic autoreceptor function include clonidine suppression of spontaneous locomotor activity,[168,171–175] inhibition of the acoustic startle reflex,[176] and clonidine-induced hypothermia.[177] Generally, long-term but not short-term administration of most but not all antidepressants led to decreased behavioral responsiveness. The discordance between receptor binding studies versus behavioral, neurophysiologic, and biochemical studies may reflect an inability of ligand to distinguish α_2-adrenergic receptor subtypes or pre- versus postsynaptic receptors, as well as the confusion between α_2-adrenergic and imidazoline receptors when ligands such as clonidine and idazoxan are used.

α_1-Adrenergic function. Chronic antidepressant dosing generally enhanced the behaviorally and electrophysiologically assessed α_1-adrenergic receptor responsivity.[178–181] Receptor binding studies of antidepressant effects have not yielded consistent results. In electrophysiologic studies, chronic antidepressant treatment has been shown to increase α_1-adrenergic responsiveness in dorsolateral geniculate and facial nuclei.[182,183] In the hippocampus, however, α_1-adrenergic receptor responsiveness was increased under the neurophysiologic conditions associated with arousal states.[161] In two biochemical studies of α_1-adrenergic–mediated second-messenger responsiveness as measured by monoinositol phosphate accumulation, long-term administration of antidepressants resulted in either increased[156] or unchanged[184] accumulation. The α_1-adrenergic antagonist properties of many antidepressants may contribute to the changes described previously.[185]

Clinical Studies

Numerous studies have examined the neuroendocrine effects of specific adrenergic probes (Table 12–5). Studies in which the α_2-adrenergic agonist clonidine and the antagonist yohimbine were used yielded consistent results. Clonidine infusion results in decreased plasma 3-methoxy-4-hydroxyphenylglycol (MHPG), decreased cortisol, increased growth hormone, decreased blood pressure, and increased sedation in both healthy subjects and depressed patients. The only highly replicated abnormality identified

Table 12–5. Effects of long-term antidepressant treatment on noradrenergic function as measured by clinical studies

Antidepressant category	Blood pressure and MHPG response to clonidine α_2 pre-synaptic	Growth hormone response to clonidine α_2 post-synaptic	Iris dilatation α_1	Cortisol response to amphetamine α_1 post-synaptic	Melatonin levels β	Cardiovascular responsiveness β_1	Cardiovascular responsiveness β_2	Platelet α_2	Depressive relapse during AMPT catecholamine depletion
NE reuptake inhibitors	↓	0 ↓	↓	0	↑	↓[a]	0[a]	—	Common
Mixed reuptake inhibitors[b]	↓	0	—	0	—	↓[a]	0[a]	↓ 0	—
5-HT reuptake inhibitors	—	—	—	—	—	—	—	↓	Rare
MAOIs	↓	0	↑	—	↑	—	—	—	—
ECT	—	—	—	0	—	—	—	—	—
Other antidepressants									
Trazodone	0	0	—	—	—	—	—	—	—
Bupropion	—	—	—	—	—	—	—	—	—
Mianserin	0	0	0	—	—	—	—	—	—

Note. MHPG = 3-methoxy-4-hydroxyphenylglycol. AMPT = α-methyl-*p*-tyrosine. NE = norepinephrine. 5-HT = 5-hydroxytryptamine (serotonin). MAOIs = monoamine oxidase inhibitors. ECT = electroconvulsive therapy.
↑ = increased responsiveness. ↓ = decreased responsiveness. 0 = no change. — = not tested. Multiple symbols indicate mixed results.
[a]Demonstrated after long-term antidepressant treatment in patients with panic disorder.
[b]Mixed reuptake inhibitors include antidepressants that exhibit both norepinephrine and 5-HT reuptake inhibition, such as amitriptyline and imipramine.

is a blunted response of growth hormone to clonidine in depressed patients compared with healthy control subjects.[186] Antidepressant treatment with MAOIs, desipramine, and amitriptyline may decrease presynaptic α_2-adrenergic sensitivity as assessed by plasma MHPG response to clonidine challenges.[187,188] Other antidepressants, such as mianserin and trazodone, do not seem to affect α_2-adrenergic sensitivity.[189,190] Chronic antidepressant treatment in endogenously depressed patients did not affect the blunted response of growth hormone to clonidine, a response that is thought to be mediated by the postsynaptic α_2-adrenergic receptor.[187,189–192] This consistent finding may suggest a trait marker for, or perhaps a predisposition to, depression. Also suggestive of diminished postsynaptic α_2-adrenergic sensitivity was the finding that yohimbine, when administered to depressed patients and control subjects, resulted in a blunted cortisol but an unchanged plasma MHPG response in the depressed patients.[193] Chronic antidepressant treatment does not consistently alter platelet tritiated yohimbine and tritiated dihydroergotamine binding;[194] however, chronic treatment with imipramine, amitriptyline, or lithium has been shown to decrease platelet tritiated clonidine binding.[195,196]

α_1-Adrenergic–mediated responsiveness in depressed patients has been studied by measuring the pressor and iris-dilating response to phenylephrine.[197,198] Amphetamine-induced NE release increases plasma cortisol levels via α_1-adrenergic receptors. Evidence with these paradigms demonstrates variable effects of α_1-adrenergic–mediated responsiveness secondary to antidepressant treatment.[199,200]

Clinical studies of β-adrenergic receptor function are limited. β-Adrenergic receptor–mediated melatonin secretion in many but not all studies of depressed patients is blunted when compared with control subjects. However, contrasting preclinical findings suggesting that antidepressants decrease β-adrenergic receptor sensitivity, chronic desipramine treatment enhances β-adrenergic receptor–mediated melatonin secretion.[201,202] The reason for this disparity remains unclear. Studies of β-adrenergic receptor–mediated cardiovascular function in depressed patients demonstrate a hyposensitivity to β-adrenergic agonists as compared with healthy control subjects.[203] Tricyclic antidepressant treatment in patients with panic disorder resulted in decreased β_1-adrenergic responsiveness as measured by attenuation of isoproterenol-induced increases in systolic blood pressure.[204]

A limitation of these clinical studies is that they assess NE function in regions and systems that may not be relevant to mood regulation. A clinical paradigm to deplete brain catecholamines involves administration of α-methyl-*p*-tyrosine (AMPT) via inhibition of the rate-limiting step in catecholamine synthesis,[205] thereby reducing plasma homovanillic acid and MHPG by 71% and 44%, respectively. AMPT has been administered to healthy control subjects, drug-free depressed patients, and patients whose depression remitted with antidepressant medication. The first two groups of subjects demonstrated no significant change in mood, whereas successfully medicated patients commonly demonstrated a transient depressive relapse. Patients medicated with potent NE or dopamine reuptake inhibitors had a markedly greater propensity for depressive relapse than did those medicated with SSRIs. All patients receiving mazindol ($n = 2$) and desipramine ($n = 3$) relapsed, in contrast to only 1 of 9 patients treated with SSRIs.

In summary, the results of clinical studies, mostly neuroendocrine challenge tests, suggest that chronic antidepressant treatment commonly, but not universally, results in decreased responsiveness of presynaptic α_2-adrenergic function. Clinical studies of β-adrenergic function are limited and contradict preclinical findings. One paradigm for measuring β_1-adrenergic function clinically suggests a decreased sensitivity after antidepressant treatment, findings that are in accord with preclinical data. Preclinical and clinical investigations have demonstrated the ability of antidepressants to modify presynaptic α_2-adrenergic sensitivity, a finding more strongly and consistently associated with NE reuptake inhibitors and MAOIs. Nevertheless, no clear association exists between an antidepressant's potency in altering NE receptor regulation and clinical efficacy. In other words, some patients demonstrating antidepressant-mediated receptor regulation may not show clinical improvement, and conversely, some patients who demonstrate little or no antidepressant-mediated receptor regulation show great clinical improvement. Nevertheless, NE transmission is relevant to the mechanism of action of antidepressants. Catecholamine depletion, via use of AMPT, in medicated, remitted depressed patients can produce a depressive relapse. This relapse occurs more commonly in patients treated with antidepressants that directly affect the catecholamine systems (i.e., desipramine and mazindol). Therefore, intact catecholamine neurotransmission may be required for the action of some antidepressants.

Therapeutic Studies

Therapeutic studies and observations contradict the role of β-adrenergic receptor regulation in the clinical action of antidepressant treatment. Preclinical studies demonstrated that coadministration of yohimbine and desipramine resulted in a rapid reduction in β-adrenergic receptor function within 4 days, as compared to the 2 or more weeks required with desipramine administration alone.[206,207] In a therapeutic trial with 20 patients, however, coadministration of desipramine and yohimbine did not result in rapid clinical improvement.[208]

In addition, agents that block β-adrenergic receptor function may be expected to be associated with the same clinical effect of β-adrenergic receptor downregulation that is seen with chronic antidepressant treatment. Nevertheless, β-adrenergic receptor antagonists, such as propranolol, are associated with an increased incidence of depression.[209]

Furthermore, agents that attenuate the antidepressant-induced downregulation of β-adrenergic receptors might be additionally expected to attenuate clinical effects. Nevertheless, triiodothyronine, which upregulates β-adrenergic receptors and blocks tricyclic antidepressant-induced downregulation of β-adrenergic receptors, has demonstrated clinical efficacy in augmenting tricyclic antidepressants.[210,211]

Summary

Overall, chronic antidepressant treatment results in β- and α_2-adrenergic desensitization, as well as α_1-adrenergic hypersensitization. These findings are commonly but not consistently found. Further studies are needed to reconcile the discrepancy of findings for β-adrenergic function among preclinical, clinical, and therapeutic studies. Studies on α_2-adrenergic function are needed to sort out the specific effects of antidepressants on presynaptic and postsynaptic function, as well as the functional distinctions of the various α_2-adrenergic receptor subtypes. Clinical studies of central α_1-adrenergic function are needed, because most studies to date have assessed peripheral function.

Dopamine Function and the Mechanism of Action of Antidepressants

Randrup et al.[212] first hypothesized that deficits in dopamine function contribute to the neurobiology of affective disorders. Several lines of evidence associate dopamine function with depression.[213–216] Reserpine and α-methlydopa, antihypertensive agents that deplete dopamine from synaptic vesicles, are associated with depressive symptoms. Also, Parkinson's disease, which is characterized by a degeneration of dopaminergic neurons, confers a 10-fold increased risk of major depression.[217] Many findings support the hypothesis of deficient dopamine transmission in depression.

Preclinical Studies

Antidepressant administration does not consistently alter dopamine, subtype 2 (D_2), receptor density[218–220] but may decrease D_1 receptor binding in limbic areas.[219,221] Antidepressant effects on the limbic and cortical D_3, D_4, and D_5 receptors have not yet been studied. Mesolimbic dopamine function, as assessed by apomorphine-induced spontaneous locomotor activity, is enhanced by electroconvulsive therapy, tricyclic antidepressants, and mianserin, possibly via increased postsynaptic responsiveness.[222] Nigrostriatal dopamine function, as assessed by dopamine agonist-stimulated stereotypy, shows less consistent results.[223]

Clinical Studies

Clinical studies of dopamine-mediated neuroendocrine function do not consistently demonstrate altered function in either drug-free or medicated patients as compared with healthy control subjects. The paradigm employed in these studies is the apomorphine-induced growth hormone increase or PRL decrease. The lack of consistent findings may reflect a differential regulation of the dopaminergic neurons arising from the hypothalamus versus those arising from the ventral tegmental area.

Therapeutic Studies

Administration of dopamine precursors (levodopa and tyrosine) and agonists (amphetamine, bromocriptine, and piribedil) may improve mood in some patients, but not robustly.[223] Depressed bipolar patients may be more sensitive than depressed unipolar patients to amphetamine-, bromocriptine-, or levodopa-induced mood enhancement.[224–226] The NE and dopamine reuptake inhibitor nomifensine, in over 20 double-blind and controlled studies, demonstrated antidepressant efficacy comparable to that of standard treatments.[223,227] Patients demonstrating lower HVA levels in CSF and greater psychomotor retardation may be more responsive to nomifensine.[228] Although nomifensine has been removed from the market due to its causing hemolytic anemia, other dopamine reuptake inhibitors, such as α-amineptine, bupropion, and mazindol, have been shown to be effective antidepressants.[229–231] Deprenyl, an MAOI of the B subtype, has been shown to have antidepressant efficacy in some but not all studies.[232]

Summary

Further studies are needed to determine the differential role of dopamine in the treatment of various subtypes of depression, as well as to characterize the differential role of various dopamine receptor subtypes.

Other Neurotransmitter Systems and the Mechanism of Action of Antidepressants

$GABA_B$ Receptor Upregulation

Initial studies showed that chronic administration of many antidepressants were associated with increased $GABA_B$ receptor density in the rodent frontal cortex;[233–237] however, subsequent studies failed to confirm these observations.[238–240] Functional biochemical assays show that chronic antidepressant administration generally increases[236,241] or leaves unchanged[164,237,242] $GABA_B$ function as measured by the effects of baclofen challenge in vitro and in vivo. Baclofen, a $GABA_B$ agonist, potentiates NE-stimulated cAMP production. This potentiation is further enhanced by long-term administration of imipramine. When baclofen and imipramine are coadministered, β-adrenergic receptor density and NE-stimulated cAMP accumulation is decreased. Administered separately, baclofen and imipramine do not induce these effects.[243]

Behavioral and clinical studies do not support the hypothesis of $GABA_B$ upregulation. Chronic antidepressant dosing did not alter $GABA_B$ agonist–induced motor suppressant effects as compared with unmedicated rats.[164] In humans, chronic antidepressant treatment did not alter baclofen-induced growth hormone responses as compared with healthy control subjects.[244] In one therapeutic study making use of the $GABA_B$ hypothesis of depression,[245] five patients were administered L-baclofen in a double-blind manner. Two patients demonstrated no change, whereas three demonstrated slightly increased and more variable scores on the Hamilton Rating Scale for Depression.[245a] This study suggests that, because a $GABA_B$ agonist may worsen depression, $GABA_B$ antagonists such as D-baclofen[246] may potentially possess antidepressant efficacy. Further studies are needed to reassess both the preclinical and clinical effects of antidepressant treatment on the $GABA_B$ system.

Cholinergic Function

It has been hypothesized that cholinergic activity or sensitivity is increased in patients with depression.[247] Cholinomimetic agents, such as specific organophosphate insecticides,[248] arecoline,[249] and physostigmine,[250] are associated with depressive symptoms in healthy and depressed subjects. In clinical studies, cholinomimetic agents induce the release of adrenocorticotropin hormone and β-endorphin.[251] This response is enhanced in depressed patients.[252] In behavioral studies, cholinomimetics lead to shortened induction of rapid-eye-movement (REM) sleep, an effect that is further shortened in depressed patients.[253,254] Further studies are needed to assess the effect of antidepressant treatment on cholinergic function, to characterize the function of specific receptor subtypes, and to better define antidepressant effects on the cholinergic system.

Excitatory Amino Acid Systems: NMDA Receptors

Little direct evidence suggests that excitatory amino acids, such as glutamate and aspartate, are involved in the pathophysiology of major depression. Nevertheless, a growing body of literature suggests that antidepressants modulate the function of the *N*-methyl-D-aspartate (NMDA) subtype of glutamate receptors. Plasma glutamate levels have been shown to be higher in drug-free patients with mood disorders than in control subjects.[255] However, glutamate and aspartate levels in CSF do not differ in medicated and unmedicated depressed patients.[256] Furthermore, no change in NMDA receptor density was found in postmortem studies of depressed suicide victims versus matched control subjects.[257]

Results of preclinical studies[258,259] suggest that some antidepressants are noncompetitive NMDA receptor antagonists. This activity is demonstrated only at antidepressant blood levels that exceed commonly achieved clinical levels. The 50% inhibiting concentrations (IC_{50}s) of antidepressants range from approximately 10–100 μM, roughly 1–2 orders of magnitude weaker than the NMDA antagonist ketamine. Neuroleptics also inhibit NMDA receptor binding; their IC_{50}s range from approximately 50–200 μM.[258,259] Conversely, NMDA antagonists and partial antagonists to the glycine modulatory site demonstrate acute but not chronic antidepressant activity in preclinical animal models, such as the forced-swim and tail-suspension tests.[260–262]

NMDA is highly important in the modulation of monoamine transmission.[263] Conversely, glutamate systems are profoundly modulated by monoamine function.[264] Therefore, it may be difficult to differentiate the direct effects of chronic antidepressant treatment on indices of glutamate function from indirect effects that may be mediated via primary alterations in monoamine function. Chronic but not acute administration of noncompetitive NMDA antagonists are associated with a decreased density of β-adrenergic receptors in mouse cortex.[265] In one study,[266] chronic imipramine administration reduced binding to the strychnine-insensitive glycine modulatory site of the NMDA receptor in cerebral cortex; in another study,[258] however, chronic desipramine, conversely, resulted in increased total NMDA receptor binding. In a behavioral study,[267] acute and chronic administration of desipramine desensitized NMDA-induced biting and scratching behavior. This effect was inhibited by the administration of 5-HT_{1A} antagonist,[267] suggesting that it may be secondary to 5-HT–related mechanisms. In clinical investigations, the administration of NMDA antagonists phencyclidine and ketamine to humans may result in mild euphoria, as well as heightened anxiety.[268]

It is unlikely that NMDA antagonism is a primary mechanism of antidepressant action. Antidepressants that block NMDA receptor function do so at blood levels that are much higher than therapeutic levels. Nevertheless, NMDA antagonism may contribute to the range of behavioral effects produced by antidepressants. For example, at blood levels associated with desipramine-induced psychosis and delirium, desipramine would be expected to occupy roughly 30% of NMDA receptors in the brain, an amount of binding predicted to be comparable to subanesthetic doses of ketamine.[259,268] NMDA antagonism may also contribute to the anticonvulsant properties of the antidepressants. Given the high level of interaction between glutamatergic and monoamine systems, coupled with evidence of direct modulation of NMDA receptors by antidepressants, further studies will be needed to define the role of glutamate receptor systems in the actions of antidepressants.

Neuropeptides: CRH and the Hypothalamic-Pituitary-Adrenal Axis

Recent studies of neuropeptides have implicated their function in multiple pathological processes. Elevated secretion of corticotropin-releasing hormone (CRH) may contribute to major depression,[269] and conversely, antidepressant treatment may work via reducing CRH secretion. Most[270–274] but not all[275] studies of depressed patients demonstrate higher CSF CRH levels than in control groups. However, this finding has been reported in patients with obsessive-compulsive disorder[276] and anorexia nervosa.[277] Postmortem studies in suicide victims demonstrate lower frontal cortical CRH receptor density than in control subjects.[278] The adrenocorticotropic hormone response to CRH has consistently been found to be blunted in patients with major depression, a response also found in patients with posttraumatic stress disorder,[279] panic disorder,[280] and a history of alcohol abuse.[281,282]

Preclinical Studies

In animal behavioral studies,[283] exogenous CRH promoted stress-associated phenomena such as hypercortisolism, anorexia, decreased sexual behaviors, and hyperarousal. Acute and chronic stress result in elevated CRH concentrations in the locus ceruleus. In an electrophysiologic study,[284] chronic desipramine treatment attenuated the stress-induced activation of locus ceruleus neurons mediated by CRH neurotransmission, and chronic sertraline treatment altered locus ceruleus discharge in a manner functionally opposing the actions of CRH on the locus ceruleus (i.e., sertraline enhances the evoked-to-tonic locus ceruleus discharge rate).

Chronic imipramine and desipramine administration did not alter CRH binding in most regions of rat brain except in the brain stem, where chronic imipramine dosing reduced binding.[285] In a behavioral study, chronic administration of desipramine enhanced the locomotor-activating effect of CRH.[286] In laboratory animals, chronic administration of fluoxetine,[145] phenelzine,[145] and imipramine[287] resulted in decreased hypothalamic CRH mRNA expression. For the most part, these studies suggest that antidepressant treatment decreases CRH transmission and responses.

Clinical Studies

A reduction in CRH concentration in CSF has been associated with long-term antidepressant treatment with electroconvulsive therapy,[288] fluoxetine,[289] and 2 days of desipramine (Table 12–6).[290] In another study,[291] a decrease in CRH levels in CSF after antidepressant treatment was significant only in the group of depressed patients who sustained a remission for 6 months or longer.

Perhaps the most studied clinical neuroendocrine assay is the dexamethasone suppression test. In patients with major depression, as well as in those with other psychiatric disorders, dexamethasone administration may be associated with failure of negative feedback regulation and, consequently, persistent cortisol secretion. No study has demonstrated differential effects of antidepressant treatments on this test. In addition, the test itself has limited potential in predicting outcome. A recent metaanalysis[292] of over 140 articles on the dexamethasone suppression test concluded that a baseline dexamethasone suppression test does not correlate with outcome, that baseline nonsuppression is associated with a poorer response to placebo, and that nonsuppression of dexamethasone after antidepressant treatment is associated with early relapse as well as poor outcome.

It remains to be determined whether CRH function is more closely associated with specific symptoms of depression, such as anxiety and neurovegetative changes, or whether it plays a more pervasive role in the pathophysiology of depression and the mecha-

Table 12–6. Effects of chronic antidepressant treatment on neuropeptide systems

Antidepressant category	CRH: Rat CRH mRNA	CRH: Human CSF CRH	Neuropeptide Y: Rat brain levels: Cortex	Neuropeptide Y: Rat brain levels: Hippocampus	Neuropeptide Y: Rat brain levels: Hypothalamus	Neuropeptide Y: mRNA levels: Cortex	Neuropeptide Y: mRNA levels: Hippocampus	Neuropeptide Y: mRNA levels: Locus ceruleus	Somatostatin: Brain content	Somatostatin: Receptor density
NE reuptake inhibitors	↓	↓	0	0	—	↓	0	—	—	↑[a]
Mixed reuptake inhibitors[b]	↓	↓	↑↓	0	↑0	0	0	—	0	—
5-HT reuptake inhibitors	↓	↓	0↑	0	↑	0	0	—	↓	—
MAOIs	↓	—	—	—	—	—	—	—	—	—
ECT	—	↓	↑	↑	—	—	—	↑	—	—
Other antidepressants										
Trazodone	—	—	—	—	—	—	—	—	—	—
Bupropion	—	—	—	—	—	—	—	—	—	—
Mianserin	—	—	—	—	—	—	—	—	0	—

Note. CRH = corticotropin-releasing hormone. CSF = cerebrospinal fluid. NE = norepinephrine. 5-HT = 5-hydroxytryptamine (serotonin). MAOIs = monoamine oxidase inhibitors. ECT = electroconvulsive therapy.
↑ = increased responsiveness. ↓ = decreased responsiveness. 0 = no change. — = not tested. Multiple symbols indicate mixed results.
[a]In nucleus accumbens only.
[b]Mixed reuptake inhibitors include antidepressants that exhibit both norepinephrine and 5-HT reuptake inhibition, such as amitriptyline and imipramine.

nism of antidepressant action. In support of the former notion, the CRH antagonist α-helical CRH blocks the anxiogenic-like response of rats withdrawing from alcohol.[293] This finding in an animal paradigm not resembling depression suggests that CRH may be a mediator of "stress" and anxiety that is not specific to depression. In addition, although the behavioral effects of intracerebroventricular administration of CRH are rapid and antidepressant treatment is associated with a rapid decrease of CRH levels in CSF,[290] the effects of antidepressant treatment are delayed by several weeks.

Therapeutic Studies

Several therapeutic studies indirectly support the role of modification of the hypothalamic-pituitary-adrenal axis in the mechanism of action of antidepressants. Given that major depression is a hypercortisolemic and hyper-CRH state, agents that lower these parameters might effectively treat depression.[294]

In two recent open-trial studies,[295,296] patients with refractory depression consistently demonstrated clinical improvement on a regimen of steroid suppressant therapy via the administration of aminoglutethimide, metyrapone, and/or ketoconazole. In the first study,[296] 6 subjects who completed the study, of an initial 10 subjects, demonstrated either full ($n = 4$) or partial ($n = 2$) remission. In the second study,[295] the 7 subjects who completed the study, of an initial 10 subjects, demonstrated an average 30% decrease in Hamilton rating scores. These robust results in patients with refractory depression further support the role of the hypothalamic-pituitary-adrenal axis in mood regulation.

Recent work from groups led by Nemeroff and Gold has identified CRH as an important focus of study that is relevant in the pathophysiology of depression and the mechanism of antidepressant action. Further clinical and therapeutic studies in humans are needed to elucidate and distinguish the role of CRH in depression and anxiety. This avenue of study may provide innovative treatments for these disorders.

Neuropeptides

Neuropeptide Y

Another studied neuropeptide implicated in depression is neuropeptide Y (NPY). This peptide is colocalized with NE, somatostatin, GABA, and galanin. The known functions of NPY include mediation of pituitary hormone release, autonomic function, and a variety of behaviors in animals.[297] In postmortem studies of suicide victims with likely diagnoses of depression, concentrations of NPY immunoreactivity were significantly reduced in the frontal cortex and caudate nucleus.[298] NPY levels in CSF have been found to be reduced in depressed patients.[299]

In preclinical studies in rats, chronic administration of zimelidine,[300] imipramine,[300] and electroconvulsive therapy[301–303] increased NPY immunoreactivity in inconsistent brain regions. Expression of NPY mRNA after chronic antidepressant dosing also showed variable results.[303,304] Recent evidence suggests that chronic desipramine treatment results in decreased NPY-Y2, but not NPY-Y1, receptor density in rat hippocampus and frontal cortex.[305] Further studies are needed to demonstrate the effects of antidepressant treatment on the NPY system.

Somatostatin

Somatostatin, a tetradecapeptide, is rich in the hypothalamus, amygdala, and nucleus accumbens. Somatostatin receptors are located in the cortex, cingulate cortex, claustrum, locus ceruleus, and limbic system.[306] Somatostatin is involved in the modulation of slow-wave and REM sleep, food consumption, locomotor activity, analgesia, learning, and regulation of other neurotransmitter systems, including dopamine, NE, 5-HT, and acetylcholine.[307]

Depressed patients have consistently been shown to have decreased concentrations of somatostatin in CSF.[308,309] This is a nonspecific finding that is also noted in patients with Parkinson's disease, multiple sclerosis, and dementia.[306,307] Chronic antidepressant dosing with clomipramine[310,311] and zimelidine,[310,311] but not with imipramine,[311] maprotiline,[311] or mianserin,[312] resulted in a widespread reduction in somatostatin levels in rat brain. Chronic desipramine dosing in rats resulted in increased binding to somatostatin receptors in the nucleus accumbens but not the hippocampus, cortex, or striatum.[313] In a preliminary clinical study, successful antidepressant treatment was not associated with altered somatostatin levels in CSF.[291] Further studies are necessary to confirm and elaborate these preliminary results.

Concluding Comments

The preceding sections provide an overview of the neurobiological changes associated with antidepressant administration. It is clear from this review that no simple neurotransmitter or neuropeptide system can account for the mechanism of action of all antidepressant treatments. Nevertheless, there is evidence suggesting the critical involvement of monoamine neurotransmitters.

The results of both preclinical and clinical investigations support an important role of 5-HT in the therapeutic effects of many antidepressant treatments. Through adaptive alteration in 5-HT receptor subtype function, most antidepressants increase 5-HT neurotransmission. SSRIs are effective antidepressants, and antidepressants of several different classes have been demonstrated to enhance 5-HT function in clinical studies. Further, the reversal of the therapeutic effects of SSRIs and MAOIs by TRP depletion emphasizes the importance of 5-HT in antidepressant action.

Results of preclinical studies have shown that the administration of antidepressants has consistent effects on specific aspects of NE system activity, most notably a reduction in β-adrenergic receptor function. Some, but not all, antidepressants decrease α_2-adrenergic receptor function, and a few preclinical studies indicate that the sensitivity of α_1-adrenergic receptors is increased. Selective NE reuptake inhibitors are effective antidepressants. Clinical investigations have been limited by an inability to adequately assess brain β-adrenergic receptor function.

Insufficient attention has been directed to the role of dopamine in affective disorders, particularly in the light of the identification of at least five different dopamine receptor subtypes. Preclinical studies generally suggest that dopamine neuronal activity is increased by antidepressant administration, but effects on the recently discovered dopamine receptor subtypes have not been examined. Dopamine reuptake inhibitors are effective antidepressants. Unfortunately, clinical research has been hampered by the lack of methods to assess dopamine function in the brain regions that are relevant to antidepressant action. The depressive relapse induced by AMPT in patients maintained on dopamine or NE reuptake inhibitors supports the involvement of these monoamines in antidepressant efficacy.

The role of neuropeptides in antidepressant action is just beginning to be explored. Preclinical and clinical studies highlight the potential importance of neuropeptides, especially CRH, in the pathophysiology and treatment of depression. A major limitation of current efforts is that, aside from CSF measurements, it has been difficult to develop methods capable of assessing brain neuropeptide function in human subjects.

Beyond the Monoamine Hypothesis of Antidepressant Action

In this review, we suggest that no single monoaminergic mechanism exists that underlies the therapeutic effects of antidepressant treatment. This failure creates a scientific dilemma for the research endeavors that have spanned several decades and have sought to identify the final common pathway for antidepressant action. Clinical studies have not been consistently successful in correlating any measure of monoamine or neuropeptide function to therapeutic response. Also, the brain structures that mediate antidepressant action have not been identified. Thus, there is the need to critically reexamine the role of brain monoamine function in the pathophysiology of depression and the mechanism of action of antidepressant drugs. The findings of several recent clinical research investigations may be most salient partly because they begin to distinguish clinical response and aspects of the biochemical response that may be unrelated to the clinical efficacy of antidepressants.

In both drug-free depressed patients and healthy subjects, TRP depletion and AMPT did not produce marked changes in mood.[79,314] These results suggest that alterations in 5-HT, dopamine, and NE systems may not reflect the primary pathology causing depressive illness. An alternative explanation is that in depressed patients these systems are sufficiently dysfunctional that further manipulations do not worsen depressive systems.

To date, there are no convincing data to suggest that the SSRIs and NE reuptake inhibitors have differential efficacy in treating depression. Most depressed patients respond to the first trial of either antidepressant class. Yet patients who do not respond to maximal trials with one class of antidepressant generally do not respond to the second class.[315] These data argue against the propositions that specific subtypes of depressive illness exist on the basis of alterations in function of a single monoaminergic system and that these drugs work solely by distinct monoamine-related mechanisms. The findings may be viewed as consistent with the idea that both the primary pathology of depression and the mechanisms of action of antidepressant treatments may be due to an abnormality in a yet-to-be-discovered neuronal system that is highly regulated by the brain's monoamine systems.

Tryptophan depletion, which reduces brain 5-HT function, reverses the therapeutic effects of SSRIs but not of NE reuptake inhibitors. In contrast, depletion of NE and dopamine as a consequence of AMPT administration reverses the remission induced by NE (desipramine) and dopamine (mazindol) reuptake inhibitors, but not SSRIs. These data further call into question the mediation of antidepressant action through a common monoaminergic mechanism. SSRIs and NE reuptake inhibitors may work via primary actions on 5-HT and NE function, respectively. Alternatively, these two classes of antidepressant drugs may exert their therapeutic properties by affecting the function of an as-yet-unspecified neuronal system modulated by these monoamine systems or by common effects on postreceptor signal transduction.

Postreceptor Signal Transduction

Recently, the search for a common mechanism of antidepressant action has led to investigations of the effects of antidepressants on intracellular function.[316,317] These studies suggest that antidepressants may have effects on the production of coupling factors, regulatory phosphoproteins, second messengers, and gene expression. Multiple transmitters may act on similar target neurons to effect the cascade of events that are eventually responsible for clinical improvement. It is known, for example, that many transmitters converge on particular neurons in rat hippocampal tissue.[318] Released neurotransmitters stimulate multiple receptor subtypes that subsequently activate second- and third-messenger systems. Via this mechanism, cell functioning may immediately change in response to neurotransmission; however, some changes require longer to emerge. Among these latter changes are altered gene expression, which may be regulated by gene transcription, RNA translation, RNA turnover, and/or protein turnover. These latter biochemical changes that require longer to emerge are of particular interest because the timing of their emergence parallels the timing of clinical improvement. Current research strategies focusing on characterization of the antidepressant-induced changes in second and third messengers, as well as identification of potential target genes of antidepressant treatment, may lead to important breakthroughs in our understanding of antidepressant mechanisms.

Alterations in receptor function produced by chronic antidepressant treatment could depend upon the direct effects of second- and third-messenger systems. As reviewed earlier, receptor desensitization produced by chronic antidepressant treatment arises in part by uncoupling of primary- to second-messenger systems.[319] This result may be achieved by decreasing intraneuronal levels of G protein in many regions. Supporting this hypothesis are results showing that multiple antidepressant treatments decrease the levels of mRNA and inhibitory and/or stimulatory G proteins in rat cerebral cortex.[312] Other studies, however, do not confirm this finding.[320] Findings of downregulation of G_s is in accord with preclinical evidence that chronic antidepressant treatment commonly leads to decreased isoproterenol-stimulated cAMP accumulation in rat brain. Also, some[321,322] but not all[153,319] studies have shown that chronic antidepressant treatment increases guanosine triphosphate (GTP) stimulation of adenylate cyclase in rat cortex.

More recent studies have elucidated antidepressant effects beyond second messengers. Chronic antidepressant treatment promotes a nuclear translocation of cAMP-dependent protein kinases,[323] as well as altered enzymatic activity.[324] Alterations in protein kinase activity and protein phosphorylation suggest subsequent alterations beyond this level of intracellular functioning.

Ultimately, chronic antidepressant treatment affects gene expression. Antidepressant-induced changes in gene expression have been demonstrated for G proteins (see above), neurotrophin,[325] the β-adrenergic receptor,[326] and the 5-HT_2 receptor.[327] The relationship between mRNA and protein expression is complex, affected by mRNA and protein turnover and/or processing. The exact mechanism by which antidepressant treatment regulates the expression of receptor mRNA has not been identified, but studies suggest that activation of the cAMP system is important in regulation of β-adrenergic receptor mRNA.[328–330]

Antidepressant regulation of gene expression must involve drug-induced changes in transcription factors, cellular proteins that bind to DNA and subsequently alter the expression of specific genes.[331] Acute and chronic antidepressant treatment have been demonstrated to influence, in complex ways, *Fos* and immediate-early gene transcription factors in multiple brain regions.[332–336] These transcription factors would be expected to target multiple genes, such as those coding for monoamine receptors, neurotrophins, G proteins, and many others yet to be identified.

The complexity of and interdependency among neurotransmitter, receptor, and intracellular messenger systems in the brain suggest that antidepressant action may lie not in the modification of a single protein but in the up- or downregulation of the expression of multiple proteins in multiple neuronal cell types. The target protein(s) that may be crucial in the therapeutic action of antidepressants remains to be determined. Through the study of intracellular messenger systems and neuronal gene expression, it may be possible to unravel the complex actions of antidepressants on brain function that together result in their therapeutic effects.

Neuroanatomy of Antidepressant Action

A daunting research dilemma is how to identify brain neuronal systems that are functionally related to monoamine systems and that may be involved in antidepressant action. Preclinical studies documenting the effects of antidepressants on the functional interactions between monoamines and neuropeptides are needed, and this area is the focus of several prominent research laboratories. Work with CRH should be emphasized, because it has been shown to have regulatory relationships with NE and 5-HT neuronal systems.[289,337]

Another potentially useful approach could be the use of animal models of depression to help identify relevant neuronal systems and brain structures. However, animal models of depression have proven to be of limited predictive, face, and construct validity.[338]

Functional brain imaging in depressed patients may prove to be critical in discovering the brain structures that mediate antidepressant efficacy. Relatively few functional brain imaging investigations have been designed to study the mechanism of action of antidepressant drugs. In addition, interpretation of most of these studies are limited by insufficient drug washout periods, lack of uniform antidepressant treatments, and imprecise brain structure localization. In drug-free depressed patients, the most consistent findings with positron-emission tomography (PET) and single photon emission computerized tomography (SPECT) is a reduction in frontal cortex metabolism and blood flow, specifically, the left anterolateral prefrontal cortex.[339–347] A notable exception is the observation of Drevets et al.[348] that depressed patients had increased blood flow in an area extending from the left ventrolateral prefrontal cortex onto the medial prefrontal cortical surface and no evidence of alteration in the left anterolateral prefrontal cortex. Unfortunately, careful analysis does not reveal obvious reasons for the discrepancy.

Consistent changes in cerebral metabolism and blood flow after effective antidepressant treatments have not been identified. Baxter et al.[340] reported that a decrease in anterolateral prefrontal cortex metabolism was normalized when remission was induced by antidepressant treatment. In contrast, Drevets et al.[348] found that the increase in frontal blood flow was reduced with effective antidepressant drug treatment.

Despite the somewhat confusing results obtained thus far, functional brain imaging has great potential to increase our knowledge of the brain sites and neurochemicals that mediate antidepressant action. Major advances in camera resolution and image coregistration and the development of neuroreceptor ligands for functional brain imaging provide a basis for this optimism.

Implications for Novel Treatment Approaches to Depressive Illness

It is likely that the future development of antidepressant treatment will move beyond drugs whose therapeutic properties relate to monoamine reuptake or metabolism inhibition. As more monoamine receptor subtypes and neuropeptides are implicated in the mechanism of antidepressant action, more novel treatment strategies will be unveiled (Table 12–7).

Antidepressants that are safer and more effective in terms of therapeutic onset and magnitude may be discovered by developing drugs with selective and potent effects on specific 5-HT receptor subtypes. Preliminary data suggest that 5-HT_2 receptor antagonists such as ritanserin may have antidepressant properties.[349] However, this has not been fully explored in terms of dose-response and placebo-controlled investigations. 5-HT_{1A} agonists appear to have antianxiety and antidepressant efficacy, but most of the drugs tested are partial agonists with insufficient selectivity for pre- and postsynaptic 5-HT_{1A} receptors. Identification of the therapeutic profiles

Table 12–7. Novel treatment strategies for depression

5-HT	▌ *Full 5-HT$_{1A}$ receptor presynaptic antagonists:* To enhance 5-HT neuronal firing and turnover. Would provide useful test of 5-HT hypothesis of mechanism of antidepressant action. Such drugs are not clinically available.
	▌ *Full 5-HT$_{1A}$ receptor postsynaptic agonists:* Preclinical neurophysiological and behavioral investigations suggest potential for antidepressant action. Preliminary findings with partial agonist gepirone suggest antidepressant efficacy.
	▌ *5-HT$_{2/1C}$ receptor antagonists:* Would allow evaluation of relevance of downregulation of 5-HT$_{2/1C}$ receptors by antidepressants. Ritanserin is available for antidepressant testing.
Norepinephrine	▌ *α_2 Receptor antagonists:* To enhance neuronal firing and turnover. Would provide useful test of role of NE transmission in antidepressant action. Idazoxan, an α_2 receptor antagonist, is currently being tested in antidepressant trials.
	▌ *α_1 Receptor agonists:* Evaluation of clinical relevance of the potentiation of α_1 receptor function produced by antidepressants. Centrally active α_1 receptor agonists are not available.
Dopamine	▌ *DA reuptake inhibitors:* To enhance DA function. Nomifensine, a DA reuptake inhibitor, was shown to have robust antidepressant activity but is no longer available because of side effects. Agents in development include amineptine.
Peptides	▌ *CRH partial antagonists:* In animals, antagonists reverse or block stress-associated behaviors. For peptide agents
	▌ *Corticosteroid synthesis inhibitors or corticosteroid partial antagonists:* Preliminary studies with ketoconazole and metyrapone suggest efficacy.

Note. CRH = corticotropin-releasing hormone.

of drugs with full agonist effects on postsynaptic 5-HT$_{1A}$ receptors, as well as full antagonist effects on presynaptic 5-HT$_{1A}$ receptors, will be important. Of interest, a recent open-label study has suggested that SSRI augmentation with the 5-HT$_{1A}$ antagonist pindolol robustly enhances and hastens clinical response.[350] As the functional properties of other 5-HT receptor subtypes, such as the 5-HT_{2C} and 5-HT_{1D} receptors, become ascertained, drugs with actions on those receptors may prove to have antidepressant properties.

Further clinical evaluation of the efficacy of potent dopamine reuptake inhibitors is warranted. The role of recently identified dopamine receptor subtypes in depression should be investigated and may lead to new ideas for antidepressant drug discovery.

The hypothesized involvement of neuropeptides in the pathophysiology of depression has not yet been clinically exploited. Improved drug delivery systems to the brain need to be developed so that the efficacy of neuropeptide agents such as CRH antagonists can be tested in depressed patients. Finally, further understanding of the effects of antidepressant drug action at sites distal to receptor recognition sites may provide new approaches for developing new classes of antidepressant drugs.[351,352]

References

1. Schildkraut JJ: The catecholamine hypothesis of affective disorders: a review of supporting evidence. Am J Psychiatry 122:509–522, 1965
2. Bunney WE Jr, Davis JM: Norepinephrine in depressive reactions. Arch Gen Psychiatry 13:483–494, 1965
3. Coppen A: The biochemistry of affective disorders. Br J Psychiatry 113:1237–1264, 1967
4. Lapin IP, Oxenkrug GF: Intensification of the central serotonergic processes as a possible determinant of the thymoleptic effect. Lancet 1:132–136, 1969
5. Price LH, Charney DS, Heninger GR: Effects of tranylcypromine treatment on neuroendocrine, behavioral, and autonomic responses to tryptophan in depressed patients. Life Sci 37:809–818, 1985
6. Charney DS, Menkes DB, Heninger GR: Receptor sensitivity and the mechanism of action of antidepressant treatment. Arch Gen

Psychiatry 38:1160–1180, 1981
7. Heninger GR, Charney DS: Mechanism of action of antidepressant treatments: implications for the etiology and treatment of depressive disorders, in Psychopharmacology: The Third Generation of Progress. Edited by Meltzer HY. New York, Raven, 1986, pp 535–544
8. deMontigny C, Aghajanian GK: Tricyclic antidepressants: long-term treatment increases responsivity of rat forebrain neurons to serotonin. Science 202:1303–1306, 1978
9. Peroutka SJ: 5-Hydroxytryptamine receptors. J Neurochem 60:408–416, 1993
10. Pazos A, Hoyer D, Dieti MM, et al: Autoradiography of serotonin receptors, in Neuronal Serotonin. Edited by Osborne NN, Hamon M. Chichester, England, Wiley, 1988, pp 507–543
11. Welner SA, deMontigny C, Desroches J, et al: Autoradiographic quantification of serotonin$_{1A}$ receptors in rat brain following antidepressant drug treatment. Synapse 4:347–352, 1989
12. Wieland S, Fischette CT, Lucki I: Effect of chronic treatments with tandospirone and imipramine on serotonin-mediated behavioral responses and monoamine receptors. Neuropharmacology 32:561–573, 1993
13. Hensler JG, Kovachich GB, Frazer A: A quantitative autoradiographic study of serotonin$_{1A}$ receptor regulation: effect of 5,7-dihydroxytryptamine and antidepressant treatments. Neuropsychopharmacology 4:131–144, 1991
14. Lund A, Mjellem-Jolly N, Hole K: Desipramine, administered chronically, influences 5-hydroxytryptamine$_{1A}$ receptors, as measured by behavioral tests and receptor binding in rats. Neuropharmacology 31:25–32, 1992
15. Pandey SC, Isaac L, Davis JM, et al: Similar effects of treatment with desipramine and electroconvulsive shock on 5-hydroxytryptamine$_{1A}$ receptors in rat brain. Eur J Pharmacol 202:221–225, 1991
16. Mizuta T, Segawo T: Chronic effects of imipramine and lithium on postsynaptic 5-HT$_{1A}$ and 5-HT$_{1B}$ sites and on presynaptic 5-HT$_3$ sites in rat brain. Jpn J Pharmacol 47:107–113, 1988
17. Hamon M, Emerit MB, El Mestikawy S, et al: Pharmacological,

biochemical and functional properties of 5-HT_{1A} receptor binding sites labelled by [^{3}H]8-hydroxy-2-(di-*N*-propylamino)tetralin in the rat brain, in Brain 5-HT_{1A} Receptor. Edited by Dourish CT, Ahlenius S, Hutson PH. London, England, Ellis Hartwood, 1987, pp 34–51

18. Akiyoshi J, Tsuchiyama K, Yamada K, et al: Effect of IAP and chronic antidepressant administration on the 5HT_{1A} receptor in rat cortical membranes. Prog Neuropsychopharmacol Biol Psychiatry 16:339–349, 1992
19. Pazos A, Palacios JM: Quantitative autoradiographic mapping of serotonin receptors in the rat brain, I: serotonin-1 receptors. Brain Res 346:205–230, 1985
20. Palacios JM, Hoyer WD, Mengod G: Distribution of serotonin receptors. Ann N Y Acad Sci 600:36–52, 1990
21. Waeber CP, Schoeffter JM, Palacios JM, et al: Molecular pharmacology of 5-HT_{1D} recognition sites: radioligand binding studies in human, pig, and calf membranes. Naunyn Schmiedebergs Arch Pharmacol 337:595–601, 1988
22. Montero D, DeFelipe MC, DelRio J: Acute or chronic antidepressants do not modify [^{125}I]cyanopindolol binding to 5-HT_{1B} receptors in rat brain. Eur J Pharmacol 196:327–329, 1991
23. Frankfurt M, McKittrick CR, McEwen BS: Changes in serotonin receptor subtypes induced by short- and long-term antidepressant treatment. Society for Neuroscience Abstracts 564:2, 1993
24. Waeber C, Dietl MM, Hoyer D, et al: Visualization of a novel serotonin recognition site (5-HT_{1D}) in the human brain by autoradiography. Neurosci Lett 88:11–16, 1988
25. Schilicker E, Fink K, Gothert M: The pharmacologic properties of the presynaptic autoreceptor in the pig brain cortex conform to the 5-HT_{1D} receptor subtype. Naunyn Schmiedebergs Arch Pharmacol 340:135–138, 1989
26. Galzin AM, Poirier MF, Lista A, et al: Characterization of the 5-HT autoreceptor modulating the release of 3H-5-HT in slices of the human cortex. J Neurochem 59:1293–1301, 1992
27. Hartig PR: Molecular biology of 5-HT receptors. Trends Pharmacol Sci 10:64–69, 1989
28. Hoyer D: Molecular pharmacology and biology of 5-HT_{1C} recep-

tors. Trends Pharmacol Sci 9:89–94, 1988
29. Pazos A, Probst A, Palacios JM: Serotonin receptors in the human brain, IV: autoradiographic mapping of serotonin-2 receptors. Neuroscience 21:123–139, 1987
30. Green AR, Heal OJ, Goodman GM: The effects of electroconvulsive therapy and antidepressant drugs on monoamine receptors in rodent brain, in Antidepressant and Receptor Function. Edited by Porter R, Bock G, Clark S. New York, Wiley, 1986, pp 246–259
31. Butler MO, Morinobu S, Duman RS: Chronic electroconvulsive seizures increase the expression of serotonin$_2$ receptor mRNA in rat frontal cortex. J Neurochem 61:1270–1276, 1993
32. Whiteford HA, Jarvis MR, Stedman TJ, et al: Mianserin-induced up-regulation of serotonin receptors on normal human platelets in vivo. Life Sci 53:371–376, 1993
33. Scott JA, Crews FT: Down-regulation of serotonin$_2$, but not of beta-adrenergic receptors during chronic treatment with amitriptyline is independent of stimulation of serotonin$_2$ and beta-adrenergic receptors. Neuropharmacology 25:1301–1306, 1986
34. Quik M, Azmita E: Selective destruction of the serotonergic fibers of the fornix fimbria and cingulum bundle increases 5-HT$_1$ but not 5-HT$_2$ receptors in rat midbrain. Eur J Pharmacol 90:377–384, 1983
35. Richelson E: Synaptic pharmacology of antidepressants: an update. Paper presented at the annual meeting of the American Psychiatric Association, Washington, DC, May 1986
36. Wander TJ, Nelson A, Okazaki H, et al: Antagonism by antidepressants of serotonin S_1 and S_2 receptors of normal brain in vitro. Eur J Pharmacol 132:115–121, 1986
37. Blackshear MA, Friedman RL, Sanders-Bush E: Acute and chronic effects of serotonin antagonists on serotonin binding sites. Naunyn Schmiedebergs Arch Pharmacol 324:125–129, 1983
38. Leysen JE, Van Gompel P, Gommeren W, et al: Down regulation of serotonin-S_2 receptor sites in rat brain by chronic treatment with the serotonin-S_2 antagonists: ritanserin and setoperone. Psychopharmacology 88:434–444, 1986

39. Pazos A, Hoyer D, Dietl MM: Autoradiography of serotonin receptors, in Neural Serotonin. Edited by Osborne NN, Hamon M. Chichester, England, Wiley, 1988, pp 507–543
40. Jenck F, Moreau J-L, Mutel V, et al: Evidence for a role of 5-HT_{1C} receptors in the antiserotonergic properties of some antidepressant drugs. Eur J Pharmacol 231:223–229, 1993
41. Pranzatelli MR, Murthy JN, Tailor PT: Novel regulation of 5-HT_{1C} receptors: down-regulation induced both by 5-$HT_{1C/2}$ receptor agonists and antagonists. Eur J Pharmacol 244:1–5, 1993
42. Andrade R, Nicoll RA: Pharmacologically distinct action of serotonin on single pyramidal neurons of the rat hippocampus recorded in vitro. J Physiol (Lond) 394:99–124, 1987
43. Granoff MI, Lee C, Jackson A, et al: The interaction of 5-HT_{1A} and 5-HT_2 receptors in the rat medial prefrontal cortex: behavioral studies. Society for Neuroscience Abstracts 18:1330 1992
44. Ashby CR Jr, Wang RY: The interaction of 5-HT_{1A} and 5-HT_2 receptors in the rat medial prefrontal cortex: iontophoretic studies. Society for Neuroscience Abstracts 18:1330, 1992
45. Pratt GD, Bowery NG, Kilpatric GJ, et al: Consensus meeting agrees distribution of 5-HT_3 receptors in mammalian hindbrain. Trends Pharmacol Sci 11:135–136, 1990
46. Kilpatric GJ, Jones BJ, Tyers MB: Identification and distribution of 5-HT_3 receptors in rat brain using radioligand binding. Nature 330:746–747, 1987
47. Waeber C, Hoyer D, Palacios JM: 5-Hydroxytryptamine-3 receptors in human brain: autoradiographic visualization using 3HICSS205-930. Neuroscience 31:393–400, 1989
48. Bockaert J, Fozard JR, Dumuis A, et al: The 5-HT_4 receptor: a place in the sun. Trends Pharmacol Sci 13:141–145, 1992
49. Costall B, Naylor RJ: The pharmacology of the 5-HT_4 receptor. Int Clin Psychopharmacol 2 (suppl 8):11–18, 1993
50. Plassat JL, Bosohert U, Amlaiky N, et al: The mouse 5-HT_5 receptor reveals a remarkable heterogeneity within the 5-HT_{1D} receptor family. EMBO J 11:4779–4786, 1992
51. Monsma FJ Jr, Shen Y, Ward RP, et al: Cloning and expression of a novel serotonin receptor with high affinity for tricyclic psychotropic drugs. Mol Pharmacol 43:320–327, 1993

52. Ruat M, Traiffort E, Arrang JM, et al: A novel rat serotonin (5-HT_6) receptor: molecular cloning, localization, and stimulation of cAMP accumulation. Biochem Biophys Res Commun 193: 268–276, 1993
53. Ruat M, Traiffort E, Arrang JM, et al: Pharmacologic properties and localization of a novel cloned rat serotonin receptor (5-HT_7). Society for Neuroscience Abstracts 480:4, 1993
54. Lovenberg TW, Baron BM, deLecea L, et al: A novel adenyl cyclase-activating serotonin receptor (5-HT_7) implicated in the regulation of mammalian circadian rhythms. Neuron 11:449–458, 1993
55. Dewar KM, Grondin L, Nenonene EK, et al: [^{3}H]Paroxetine binding and serotonin content of rat brain: absence of changes following antidepressant treatments. Eur J Pharmacol 235:137–142, 1993
56. Graham D, Tahraoui L, Langer SZ: Effect of chronic treatment with selective monoamine oxidase inhibitors and specific 5-hydroxytryptamine uptake inhibitors on [^{3}H]paroxetine binding to cerebral cortical membranes of the rat. Neuropharmacology 26:1087–1092, 1987
57. Gleiter CH, Nutt DJ: Repeated electroconvulsive shock does not change [^{3}H]paroxetine binding to the 5-HT uptake site in rat cortical membranes. Psychopharmacology 95:68–70, 1988
58. Lesch KP, Aulakh CS, Wolozin BL, et al: Regional brain expression of serotonin transporter mRNA and its regulation by reuptake inhibiting antidepressants. Mol Brain Res 17:31–35, 1993
59. Martensson B, Wagner A, Beck O, et al: Effects of clomipramine treatment on cerebrospinal fluid monoamine metabolites and platelet ^{3}H-imipramine binding and serotonin uptake and concentration in major depressive disorder. Acta Psychiatr Scand 83:125–133, 1991
60. Wgner A, Montero D, Martensson B, et al: Effects of fluoxetine treatment on platelet ^{3}H-imipramine binding, 5-HT uptake, and 5-HT content in major depressive disorder. J Affective Disord 20:101–113, 1990
61. Arora RC, Meltzer HY: Effect of desipramine treatment on ^{3}H-imipramine binding in the blood platelets of depressed patients.

Biol Psychiatry 23:397–404, 1988

62. Cowen PJ, Geaney DP, Schachter M, et al: Desipramine treatment in normal subjects: effects on neuroendocrine responses to tryptophan and on platelet serotonin (5-HT)-related receptors. Arch Gen Psychiatry 43:61–67, 1986
63. Langer SZ, Sechter D, Loo H, et al: Electroconvulsive shock therapy and maximum binding of platelet tritiated imipramine binding in depression. Arch Gen Psychiatry 43:949–952, 1986
64. Maj M, Mastronardi P, Cerreta A, et al: Changes in platelet ^{3}H-imipramine binding in depressed patients receiving electroconvulsive therapy. Biol Psychiatry 24:469–472, 1988
65. Suranyi-Cadotte BE, Quirion R, Nair NPV, et al: Imipramine treatment differentially affects platelet ^{3}H-imipramine binding and serotonin uptake in depressed patients. Life Sci 36:795–799, 1985
66. DeMet EM, Gerner RH, Bell KM, et al: Changes in platelet ^{3}H-imipramine binding with chronic imipramine treatment are not state-dependent. Biol Psychiatry 26:478–488, 1989
67. Suranyi-Cadotte BE, LaFaille F, Schwartz G, et al: Unchanged platelet ^{3}H-imipramine binding in normal subjects after imipramine administration. Biol Psychiatry 20:1237–1240, 1985
68. Asarch KB, Shih JC, Kulcsar A: Decreased ^{3}H-imipramine binding in depressed males and females. Communications in Psychopharmacology 4:425–432, 1980
69. Newman ME, Shapira B, Lerer B: Regulation of 5-hydroxytryptamine$_{1A}$ receptor function in rat hippocampus by short- and long-term administration of 5-hydroxytryptamine$_{1A}$ agonists and antidepressants. J Pharmacol Exp Ther 260:16–20, 1992
70. Newman ME, Lerer B: Chronic electroconvulsive shock and desipramine reduce the degree of inhibition by 5-HT and carbochol of forskolin-stimulated adenylate cyclase in rat hippocampal membranes. Eur J Pharmacol 148:257–560, 1988
71. Newman ME, Drummer D, Lerer B: Single and combined effects of desipramine and lithium on serotonergic receptor number and second messenger function in rat brain. J Pharmacol Exp Ther 252:826–831, 1990
72. Sleight AJ, Marsden CA, Palfreyman MG, et al: Chronic MAO A

and MAO B inhibition decreases the 5-HT-1a receptor-mediated inhibition of forskolin stimulated adenylate cyclase. Eur J Pharmacol 154:255–261, 1988
73. Varrault A, Leviel V, Bockaert J: 5-HT_{1A}-sensitive adenylyl cyclase of rodent hippocampal neurons: effects of antidepressant treatments and chronic stimulation with agonists. J Pharmacol Exp Ther 257:433–438, 1991
74. Kusumi I, Mikuni M, Takahashi K: Effect of subchronic antidepressant administration on serotonin-stimulated phosphoinositide hydrolysis in para-chlorophenylalanine-treated rat hippocampal slices. Prog Neuropsychopharmacol Biol Psychiatry 15:393–403, 1991
75. Godfrey PP, McClue SJ, Young MM, et al: 5-Hydroxytryptamine-stimulated inositol phospholipid hydrolysis in the mouse cortex has pharmacological characteristics compatible with mediation via 5-HT_2 receptors but this response does not reflect altered 5-HT_2 function after 5,7-dihydroxytryptamine lesioning or repeated antidepressant treatments. J Neurochem 50:730–738, 1988
76. Kendall DA, Nahorski SR: 5-Hydroxytryptamine-stimulated inositol phospholipid hydrolysis in rat cerebral cortex slices: pharmacological characterization and effects of antidepressants. J Pharmacol Exp Ther 233:473–479, 1985
77. Briley M, Moret C: Neurobiological mechanisms involved in antidepressant therapies. Clin Neuropharmacol 16:387–400, 1993
78. Blier P, deMontigny C, Chaput Y: Modifications of the serotonin system by antidepressant treatments: implications for the therapeutic response in major depression. J Clin Psychopharmacol 7:24S–35S, 1987
79. Chaput Y, deMontigny C, Blier P: Presynaptic and postsynaptic modifications of the serotonin system by long-term administration of antidepressant treatments: an in vivo electrophysiologic study in the rat. Neuropsychopharmacology 5:219–229, 1991
80. Blier P, deMontigny C, Chaput Y: A role for the serotonin system in the mechanism of action of antidepressant treatments: preclinical evidence. J Clin Psychiatry 51 (suppl 4):14–20, 1990
81. Blier P, Lista A, deMontigny C: Differential properties of pre- and

postsynaptic 5-hydroxytryptamine$_{1A}$ receptors in the dorsal raphe and hippocampus, II: effect of pertussis and cholera toxins. J Pharmacol Exp Ther 265:16–23, 1993
82. Blier P, Lista A, deMontigny C: Differential properties of pre- and postsynaptic 5-hydroxytryptamine$_{1A}$ receptors in the dorsal raphe and hippocampus, I: effect of spiperone. J Pharmacol Exp Ther 265:7–15, 1993
83. Blier P, Bouchard C: Effect of repeated electroconvulsive shocks on serotonergic neurons. Eur J Pharmacol 211:365–373, 1992
84. Blier P, deMontigny C, Tardif D: Short-term lithium treatment enhances responsiveness of postsynaptic 5-HT$_{1A}$ receptors without altering 5-HT autoreceptor sensitivity: an electrophysiological study in the rat brain. Synapse 1:225–232, 1987
85. Willner P: Antidepressants and serotonergic neurotransmission: an integrative review. Psychopharmacology 85:387–404, 1985
86. Green AR: Evolving concepts on the interactions between antidepressant treatments and monoamine neurotransmitters. Neuropharmacology 26(7B):815–822, 1987
87. Eison AS, Yocca FD, Gianutsos G: Effect of chronic administration of antidepressant drugs on 5-HT$_2$-mediated behavior in the rat following noradrenergic or serotonergic denervation. J Neural Transm Gen Sect 84:19–32, 1991
88. Lucki I: Behavioral studies of serotonin receptor agonists as antidepressant drugs. J Clin Psychiatry 52 (suppl 12):24–31, 1991
89. Goodwin GM: The effects of antidepressant treatments and lithium upon 5-HT$_{1A}$ receptor function. Prog Neuropsychopharmacol Biol Psychiatry 13:445–451, 1989
90. Hutson PH, Donohue TP, Curzon G: Hypothermia induced by the putative 5-HT$_{1A}$ agonists LY165163 and 8-OH-DPAT is not prevented by 5-HT depletion. Eur J Pharmacol 143:221–228, 1987
91. Maj J, Moryl E: Effects of fluoxetine given chronically on the responsiveness of 5-HT receptor subpopulations to their agonists. Eur Neuropsychopharmacol 3:85–94, 1993
92. Maj J, Moryl E: Effects of sertraline and citalopram given repeatedly on the responsiveness of 5-HT receptor subpopulations. J Neural Transm Gen Sect 88:143–156, 1992
93. Frances H, Khidichian F: Chronic but not acute antidepressants

interfere with serotonin (5-HT$_{1B}$) receptors. Eur J Pharmacol 179:173–176, 1990

94. Frances H, Lienard C, Fermanian J: Improvement of the isolation-induced social behavioural deficit involves activation of the 5-HT$_{1B}$ receptors. Prog Neuropsychopharmacol Biol Psychiatry 14:91–102, 1990
95. Lucki I, Minugh-Purvis N: Serotonin-induced head shaking behavior in rats does not involve receptors located in the frontal cortex. Brain Res 420:403–406, 1987
96. Cadogan AK, Marsden CA, Tulloch I, et al: Evidence that chronic administration of paroxetine or fluoxetine enhances 5-HT$_2$ receptor function in the brain of the guinea pig. Neuropharmacology 32:249–256, 1993
97. Charney DS, Heninger GR, Sternberg DE: Serotonin function and the mechanism of action of antidepressant treatment: effects of amitriptyline and desipramine. Arch Gen Psychiatry 41:359–364, 1984
98. Price LH, Charney DS, Delgado PL, et al: Lithium treatment and serotonergic function. Arch Gen Psychiatry 46:13–19, 1989
99. Price LH, Charney DS, Delgado PL, et al: Effects of desipramine and fluvoxamine treatment on the prolactin response to tryptophan. Arch Gen Psychiatry 46:625–631, 1989
100. Price LH, Charney DS, Heninger GR: Effects of trazodone treatment on serotonergic function in depressed patients. Psychiatry Res 24:165–175, 1988
101. Shapira B, Reiss A, Kaiser N, et al: Effect of imipramine treatment on the prolactin response to fenfluramine and placebo challenge in depressed patients. J Affective Disord 16:1–4, 1989
102. Palazidou E, Stephenson J, McGregor A, et al: Evidence for 5-HT$_{1A}$ receptor involvement in the control of prolactin secretion in man. Neuropsychopharmacology 9 (suppl 2):157S, 1993
103. O'Keane V, McLoughlin D, Dinan TG: D-Fenfluramine-induced prolactin and cortisol release in major depression: response to treatment. J Affective Disord 26:143–150, 1992
104. Shapira B, Yagmur MJ, Gropp C, et al: Effect of clomipramine and lithium on fenfluramine-induced hormone release in major depression. Biol Psychiatry 31:975–983, 1992

105. Shapira B, Cohen J, Newman ME, et al: Prolactin response to fenfluramine and placebo challenge following maintenance pharmacotherapy withdrawal in remitted depressed patients. Biol Psychiatry 33:531–535, 1993
106. Shapira B, Lerer B, Kindler S, et al: Enhanced serotonergic responsivity following electroconvulsive therapy in patients with major depression. Br J Psychiatry 160:223–229, 1992
107. Kasper S, Vieira A, Schmidt R, et al: Multiple hormone responses to stimulation with dl-fenfluramine in patients with major depression before and after antidepressive treatment. Pharmacopsychiatry 23:76–84, 1990
108. Shapira B, Newman M, Lerer B: Serotonergic mechanisms of ECT: neuroendocrine evidence. Clin Neuropharm 15 (suppl 1):673A–674A, 1992
109. Moreno AG, Ansseau M, Pitchot W, et al: Effect of ritanserin on the neuroendocrine and temperature responses to flesinoxan. Neuropsychopharmacology 9 (suppl 2):99S, 1993
110. Moreno AG, Ansseu M, Pitchot W, et al: Effect of pindolol on the neuroendocrine and temperature responses to flesinoxan. Neuropsychopharmacology 9:2S, 1993
111. Lesch KP, Lerer B: The 5-HT receptor–G-protein–effector system complex in depression, I: effect of glucocorticoids. J Neural Transm Gen Sect 84:3–18, 1991
112. Lesch KP, Disselkamp-Tietze J, Schmidtke A: 5-HT_{1A} receptor function in depression: effect of chronic amitriptyline treatment. J Neural Transm Gen Sect 80:157–161, 1990
113. Lesch KP, Hoh A, Schulte HM, et al: Long-term fluoxetine treatment decreases 5-HT_{1A} receptor responsivity in obsessive-compulsive disorder. Psychopharmacology 105:415–420, 1991
114. Delgado PL, Charney DS, Price LH, et al: Serotonin function and the mechanism of antidepressant action. Arch Gen Psychiatry 47:411–418, 1990
115. Miller HL, Delgado PL, Salomon RM, et al: Acute tryptophan depletion: a method of studying antidepressant action. J Clin Psychiatry 53 (suppl 10):28–35, 1992
116. Delgado PL, Miller HL, Salomon RM, et al: Tryptophan depletion challenge in depressed patients treated with desipramine or flu-

oxetine: implications for the role of serotonin in the mechanism of antidepressant action. Arch Gen Psychiatry, in press
117. Salomon RM, Delgado PL, Miller HL, et al: Serotonin function in depression. Psyche 1:7–16, 1993
118. deMontigny C, Grunberg F, Mayer A, et al: Lithium induces rapid relief of depression in tricyclic antidepressant drug nonresponders. Br J Psychiatry 138:252–256, 1981
119. Heninger GR, Charney DS, Sternberg DE: Lithium carbonate augmentation of antidepressant treatment: an effective prescription for treatment-refractory depression. Arch Gen Psychiatry 40:1335–1342, 1983
120. deMontigny C, Cournoyer G, Morrissette R, et al: Lithium carbonate addition in tricyclic antidepressant-resistant depression: correlations with the neurobiologic actions of tricyclic antidepressant drugs and lithium ion on the serotonin system. Arch Gen Psychiatry 40:1327–1334, 1983
121. Nelson JC, Byck R: Rapid response to lithium in phenelzine nonresponders. Am J Psychiatry 141:85–86, 1982
122. Price LH, Conwell Y, Nelson JC: Lithium augmentation of combined neuroleptic-tricyclic treatment in delusional depression. Am J Psychiatry 140:318–322, 1983
123. Birkhimer LJ, Alderman AA, Schmitt CE, et al: Combined trazodone-lithium therapy for refractory depression. Am J Psychiatry 140:1382–1383, 1983
124. Joyce PR, Hewland HR, Jones AV: Rapid response to lithium in treatment-resistant depression. Br J Psychiatry 142:204–205, 1983
125. Louie AK, Meltzer HY: Lithium potentiation of antidepressant treatment. J Clin Psychopharmacol 4:316–321, 1984
126. deMontigny C, Elie R, Caille C: Rapid response to the addition of lithium in iprindole-resistant unipolar depression: a pilot study. Am J Psychiatry 142:220–223, 1984
127. Schrader GD, Levien HEM: Response to sequential administration of clomipramine and lithium carbonate in treatment-resistant depression. Br J Psychiatry 147:573–575, 1985
128. Roy A, Pickar D: Lithium potentiation of imipramine in treatment-resistant depression. Br J Psychiatry 147:582–583, 1985

129. Nelson JC, Mazure CM: Lithium augmentation in psychotic depression refractory to combined drug treatment. Am J Psychiatry 143:363–366, 1986
130. Kushnir SL: Lithium-antidepressant combinations in the treatment of depressed, physically ill geriatric patients. Am J Psychiatry 143:378–379, 1986
131. Price LH, Charney DS, Heninger GR: Variability of response to lithium augmentation in refractory depression. Am J Psychiatry 143:1387–1392, 1986
132. Cowen PJ, McCance SL, Ware CJ, et al: Lithium in tricyclic-resistant depression correlation of increased brain 5-HT function with clinical outcome. Br J Psychiatry 159:341–346, 1991
133. McCance-Katz E, Price LH, Charney DS, et al: Serotonergic function during lithium augmentation of refractory depression. Psychopharmacology 108:93–97, 1992
134. Pope HG Jr, McElroy SL, Nixon FA: Possible synergism between fluoxetine and lithium in refractory depression. Am J Psychiatry 145:1292–1294, 1988
135. Fontaine R, Ontiveros A, Elie R, et al: Lithium carbonate augmentation of desipramine and fluoxetine in refractory depression. Biol Psychiatry 29:946–948, 1991
136. Dinan TG: Lithium augmentation in sertraline-resistant depression: a preliminary dose-response study. Acta Psychiatr Scand 88:300–301, 1993
137. Kramlinger KG, Post RM: The addition of lithium to carbamazepine: antidepressant efficacy in treatment resistant depression. Arch Gen Psychiatry 46:794–800, 1989
138. Price LH, Charney DS, Delgado PL, et al: Lithium and serotonin function: implications for the serotonin hypothesis of depression. Psychopharmacology 100:3–12, 1990
139. Price LH, Charney DS, Delgado PL, et al: Fenfluramine augmentation in tricyclic-refractory depression. J Clin Psychopharmacol 10:312–317, 1990
140. Melia KR, Nestler EJ, Duman RS: Chronic imipramine treatment normalizes levels of tyrosine hydroxylase in the locus coeruleus of chronically stressed rats. Psychopharmacology 108: 23–26, 1992

141. Nestler EJ, McMahon A, Sabban EL, et al: Chronic antidepressant administration decreases the expression of tyrosine hydroxylase in the rat locus coeruleus. Proc Natl Acad Sci U S A 87:7522–7526, 1990
142. Moret C, Briley M: Effect of antidepressant drugs on monoamine synthesis in brain in vivo. Neuropharmacology 31:679–684, 1992
143. Melia KR, Rasmussen K, Terwilliger RZ, et al: Coordinate regulation of the cyclic AMP system with firing rate and expression of tyrosine hydroxylase in the rat locus coeruleus: effects of chronic stress and drug treatments. J Neurochem 58:494–502, 1992
144. Brady LS, Gold PW, Herkenham M, et al: The antidepressants fluoxetine, idazoxan and phenelzine alter corticotropin-releasing hormone and tyrosine hydroxylase mRNA levels in rat brain: therapeutic implications. Brain Res 55:121–133, 1992
145. Racagni G, Mocchetti I, Calderini G, et al: Temporal sequence of changes in central noradrenergic system of rat after prolonged antidepressant treatment: receptor desensitization and neurotransmitter interactions. Neuropharmacology 22:415–424, 1983
146. Biegon A: Effect of chronic desipramine treatment on dihydroalprenolol, imipramine, and desipramine binding sites: a quantitative autoradiographic study in the rat brain. J Neurochem 47:77–80, 1986
147. Modigh K: Long term effects of electroconvulsive shock therapy on synthesis, turnover and uptake of brain monoamines. Psychopharmacology 49:170–185, 1976
148. Minchin MCW, Williams J, Bowdler JM, et al: Effect of electroconvulsive shock on the uptake and release of noradrenaline and 5-hydroxytryptamine in rat brain slices. J Neurochem 40:765–768, 1983
149. Gleiter CH, Nutt DJ: Repeated electroconvulsive shock increases the number of [^{3}H]desipramine binding sites in rat cerebral cortex. Psychopharmacology 96:426–427, 1988
150. Bauer ME, Tejani-Butt SM: Effects of repeated administration of desipramine or electroconvulsive shock on norepinephrine up-

take sites measured by [^{3}H]nisoxetine autoradiography. Brain Res 582:208–214, 1992

151. Sugrue MF: Chronic antidepressant therapy and associated changes in central monoaminergic receptor functioning. Pharmacol Ther 21:1–33, 1983
152. Costa E, Ravizza ML, Barbaccia ML: Evaluation of current theories on the mode of action of antidepressants, in Mode of Action of Antidepressants. Edited by Bartholini G, Lloyd KG, Morselli PL. New York, Raven, 1986, pp 9–21
153. Duman RS, Strada SJ, Enna SJ: Effect of imipramine and adrenocorticotropin administration on the rat brain norepinephrine-coupled cyclic nucleotide generating system: alterations in alpha and beta adrenergic components. J Pharmacol Exp Ther 234:409–414, 1985
154. Garcha G, Smokcum RW, Stephenson JD, et al: Effect of some atypical antidepressants on beta adrenoceptor binding and adenylate cyclase activity in the rat forebrain. Eur J Pharmacol 108:1–7, 1985
155. Hyttel J, Overo KF, Arnt J: Biochemical effects and drug levels in rats after long-term treatment with the specific 5-HT uptake inhibitor, citalopram. Psychopharmacology 83:20–27, 1984
156. Nalepa I, Vetulani J: Enhancement of the responsiveness of cortical adrenergic receptors by chronic administration of the 5-hydroxytryptamine uptake inhibitor citalopram. J Neurochem 60:2029–2035, 1993
157. Areso P, Gambarana C, Tejani-Bu HS, et al: Antidepressant-induced downregulation of central b_1 adrenoceptors: regional selective effects. Neurosci Abstr 15:1318, 1989
158. Sugrue MF: Current concepts on the mechanisms of action of antidepressant drugs. Pharmacol Ther 13:219–247, 1981
159. Sulser F: New perspectives on the molecular pharmacology of affective disorders. European Archives of Psychiatry and Neurological Sciences 238:231–239, 1989
160. Gillespie DD, Manier DH, Sanders-Bush E, et al: The serotonin norepinephrine link in brain, II: the role of serotonin in the regulation of beta adrenoceptors in the low agonist affinity conformation. J Pharmacol Exp Ther 244:154–159, 1988

161. Lacroix D, Blier P, Curet O, et al: Effects of long-term desipramine administration on noradrenergic neurotransmission: electrophysiological studies in the rat brain. J Pharmacol Exp Ther 257:1081–1090, 1991
162. Olpe HR, Schellenberg A: Reduced sensitivity of neurons to noradrenaline after chronic treatment with antidepressant drugs. Eur J Pharmacol 63:7–13, 1980
163. Schultz JE, Siggins GR, Schocker FW: Effects of prolonged treatment with lithium and tricyclic antidepressants on discharge frequency, norepinephrine responses and beta receptor binding in rat cerebellum: electrophysiological and biochemical comparison. J Pharmacol Exp Ther 216:28–38, 1981
164. McManus DJ, Greenshaw AJ: Differential effects of chronic antidepressants in behavioural tests of B-adrenergic and $GABA_B$ receptor function. Psychopharmacology 103:204–208, 1991
165. Przegalinski E, Baran L, Siwanowicz J, et al: Repeated treatment with antidepressant drugs prevents salbutamol-induced hypoactivity in rats. Pharmacol Biochem Behav 21:695–698, 1984
166. Cohen RM, Aulakh CS, Campbell IC, et al: Functional subsensitivity of $alpha_2$ adrenoceptors accompanies reductions in yohimbine binding after clorgyline treatment. Eur J Pharmacol 81:145–148, 1982
167. Sugrue MF: A study of the sensitivity of rat brain $alpha_2$-adrenoceptors during chronic antidepressant treatments. Naunyn Schmiedebergs Arch Pharmacol 320:90–96, 1982
168. Pilc A, Enna SJ: Synergistic interaction between α- and β-adrenergic receptors in rat brain cortical slices: possible site for antidepressant drug action. Life Sci 37:1183–1193, 1985
169. Wang RY, Aghajanian GK: Enhanced sensitivity of amygdaloid neurons to serotonin and norepinephrine by antidepressant treatments. Commun Psychopharmacol 4:83–90, 1980
170. Scuvee-Moreau JJ, Svensson TH: Sensitivity in vivo of central a_2- and opiate receptors after chronic treatment with various antidepressants. Journal of Neural Transmission 54:51–63, 1982
171. Spyraki C, Fibiger HC: Functional evidence for subsensitivity of noradrenergic $alpha_2$ receptors after chronic desipramine treatment. Life Sci 27:1863–1876, 1980

172. Heal DJ, Lister S, Smith SL, et al: The effects of acute and repeated administration of various antidepressant drugs on clonidine-induced hypoactivity in rats and mice. Neuropharmacology 22:983–992, 1983
173. Heal DJ, Akagi A, Bowdler JM, et al: Repeated electroconvulsive shock attenuates clonidine-induced hypoactivity in rodents. Eur J Pharmacol 75:231–237, 1981
174. Kostowski W, Obersztyn M: Chronic administration of desipramine and imipramine but not zimelidine attenuates clonidine induced depression of avoidance behavior in rats. Polish Journal of Pharmacology and Pharmacy 40:341–349, 1988
175. McKenna KF, Baker GB, Coutts RT, et al: Chronic administration of the antidepressant-antipanic drug phenelzine and its N-acetylated analogue: effects on monoamine oxidase, biogenic amines, and α_2-adrenoreceptor. J Pharm Sci 81:832–835, 1992
176. Davis M, Menkes DB: Tricyclic antidepressants vary in decreasing alpha$_2$-adrenoceptor sensitivity with chronic treatment: assessment with clonidine inhibition of acoustic startle. Br J Pharmacol 77:217–222, 1982
177. Gorka Z, Zacny E: The effect of single and chronic administration of imipramine on clonidine-induced hypothermia in the rat. Life Sci 28:2847–2854, 1981
178. Menkes DB, Kehne JH, Gallager DW, et al: Functional supersensitivity of CNS alpha$_1$ adrenoceptors following chronic antidepressant treatment. Life Sci 33:181–188, 1983
179. Hong KW, Rhim BY, Lee WS: Enhancement of central and peripheral alpha$_1$ adrenoceptor sensitivity and reduction of alpha$_2$ adrenoceptor sensitivity following chronic imipramine treatment in rats. Eur J Pharmacol 120:275–283, 1986
180. Maj J, Rogoz Z, Skuza G, et al: Repeated treatment with antidepressant drugs potentiates the locomotor response to (+)-amphetamine. J Pharm Pharmacol 36:127–130, 1984
181. Maj J, Klimek V, Nowak G: Antidepressant drugs given repeatedly increase binding to alpha$_1$ adrenoceptors in the rat cortex. Eur J Pharmacol 119:113-116, 1985
182. Menkes DB, Aghajanian GK: α_2-adrenoceptor-mediated responses in the lateral geniculate nucleus are enhanced by

chronic antidepressant treatment. Eur J Pharmacol 74:27–35, 1981

183. Menkes DB, Aghajanian GK, McCall RB: Chronic antidepressant treatment enhances α-adrenergic and serotonergic responses in the facial nucleus. Life Sci 27:45–55, 1980
184. Sapena R, Morin D, Zini R, et al: Evaluation of central adrenergic receptor signal transmissions after an antidepressant administration to the rat. Biochem Pharmacol 44:1067–1072, 1992
185. Richelson E: Antidepressants: pharmacology and clinical use, in Treatments of Psychiatric Disorders, Vol 3. Edited by Karasu T. Washington, DC, American Psychiatric Association, 1989, pp 1773–1787
186. Siever LJ, Uhde TW, Silberman EK, et al: The growth hormone response to clonidine as a probe of noradrenergic receptor responsiveness in affective disorder patients and controls. Psychiatry Res 6:171–183, 1982
187. Charney DS, Heninger GR, Sternberg DE, et al: Presynaptic adrenergic receptor sensitivity in depression: the effect of long-term desipramine treatment. Arch Gen Psychiatry 38:1334–1340, 1981
188. Charney DS, Heninger GR, Sternberg DE: Alpha$_2$ adrenergic receptor sensitivity and the mechanism of action of antidepressant therapy: the effect of long-term amitriptyline treatment. Br J Psychiatry 142:265–275, 1983
189. Charney DS, Heninger GR, Sternberg DE: The effect of mianserin on alpha-2 adrenergic receptor function in depressed patients. Br J Psychiatry 144:407–416, 1984
190. Price LH, Charney DS, Heninger GR: Effects of trazodone treatment on alpha-2 adrenoreceptor function in depressed patients. Psychopharmacology 89:38–44, 1986
191. Siever LJ, Uhde TW, Insel TR, et al: Growth hormone response to clonidine unchanged by chronic clorgyline treatment. Psychiatry Res 7:139–144, 1982
192. Charney DS, Heninger GR, Sternberg DE: Failure of chronic antidepressant treatment to alter growth hormone response to clonidine. Psychiatry Res 7:135–138, 1982
193. Heninger GR, Charney DS, Price LH: α_2-Adrenergic receptor

sensitivity in depression: the plasma MHPG, behavioral and cardiovascular responses to yohimbine. Arch Gen Psychiatry 45: 165–175, 1988
194. Piletz JE, Schubert DSP, Halaris A: Evaluation of studies on platelet alpha$_2$ adrenoreceptors in depressive illness. Life Sci 39:1589–1616, 1986
195. Garcia-Sevilla JA, Zis AP, Hollingsworth PJ, et al: Platelet α_2-adrenergic receptors in major depressive disorder: binding of tritiated clonidine before and after tricyclic antidepressant drug treatment. Arch Gen Psychiatry 38:1327–1333, 1981
196. Garcia-Sevilla JA, Guimon J, Garcia-Vallejo P, et al: Biochemical and functional evidence of supersensitive platelet α_2-adrenoceptors in major affective disorder: effect of long-term lithium carbonate treatment. Arch Gen Psychiatry 43:51–57, 1986
197. Shur E, Checkley SA: Pupil studies in depressed patients: an investigation of the mechanism of action of desipramine. Br J Psychiatry 140:181–184, 1982
198. Shur E, Checkley S, Delgado I: Failure of mianserin to affect autonomic function in the pupils of depressed patients. Acta Psychiatr Scand 67:50–55, 1983
199. Checkley SA: Corticosteroid and growth hormone responses to methylamphetamine in depressive illness. Psychol Med 9:107–115, 1979
200. Sachar EJ, Asnis G, Nathan S: Dextro amphetamine and cortisol in depression: morning plasma cortisol levels suppressed. Arch Gen Psychiatry 37:755–757, 1980
201. Murphy DL, Tamarkin L, Sunderland T, et al: Human plasma melatonin is elevated during treatment with the monoamine oxidase inhibitors clorgyline and tranylcypromine but not deprenyl. Psychiatry Res 17:119–127, 1986
202. Palazidou E, Papadopoulos A, Ratcliff H, et al: Noradrenaline uptake inhibition increases melatonin secretion, a measure of noradrenergic neurotransmission, in depressed patients. Psychol Med 22:309–315, 1992
203. Bertschy G, Vandel S, Puech A, et al: Cardiac beta-adrenergic sensitivity in depression: relation with endogenous subtype and desipramine response. Neuropsychobiology 21:177–181, 1989

204. Pohl R, Yeragani VK, Balon R: Effects of isoproterenol in panic disorder patients after antidepressant treatment. Biol Psychiatry 28:203–214, 1990
205. Delgado PL, Miller HL, Salomon RM, et al: Monoamines and the mechanism of antidepressant action: effects of catecholamine depletion on mood of patients treated with antidepressants. Psychopharmacol Bull 29:389–396, 1994
206. Paul SM, Crews FT: Rapid desensitization of cerebral cortical β-adrenergic receptors induced by desmethylimipramine and phenoxybenzamine. Eur J Pharmacol 62:349–350, 1980
207. Johnson RW, Reisine T, Spotnitz S, et al: Effects of desipramine and yohimbine on α_2- and β-adrenoreceptor sensitivity. Eur J Pharmacol 67:123–127, 1980
208. Charney DS, Price LH, Heninger GR: Desipramine-yohimbine combination treatment of refractory depression: implications for the β-adrenergic receptor hypothesis of antidepressant action. Arch Gen Psychiatry 43:1155–1161, 1986
209. Avorn J, Everitt DE, Weiss S: Increased antidepressant use in patients prescribed β-blockers. JAMA 255:357–360, 1986
210. Mason GA, Bondy SC, Nemeroff CB, et al: The effects of thyroid state on beta-adrenergic and serotonergic receptors in rat brain. Psychoneuroendocrinology 12:261–270, 1987
211. Goodwin FK, Prange AJ, Post RM, et al: Potentiation of antidepressant effect of triiodothyronine in tricyclic nonresponders. Am J Psychiatry 139:34–38, 1982
212. Randrup A, Munkvad I, Fog R, et al: Mania, depression, and brain dopamine, in Current Developments of Psychopharmacology, Vol 2. Edited by Essman WB, Valzelli L. New York, Spectrum Publications, 1975, pp 206–248
213. Durlach-Misteli C, VanRee JM: Dopamine and melatonin in the nucleus accumbens may be implicated in the mode of action of antidepressant drugs. Eur J Pharmacol 217:15–21, 1992
214. Guitart X, Nestler EJ: Chronic administration of lithium or other antidepressants increases levels of DARPP-32 in rat frontal cortex. J Neurochem 59:1164–1167, 1992
215. Diehl DJ, Gershon S: The role of dopamine in mood disorders. Compr Psychiatry 33:115–120, 1992

216. Brown AS, Gershon S: Dopamine and depression. J Neural Transm Gen Sect 91:75–109, 1993
217. Mayeux R: Parkinson's Disease. J Clin Psychiatry 51 (suppl 7):20–23, 1990
218. Antkiewicz-Michaluk L, Rokosz-Pelc A, Vetulani J: Increased low-affinity ^{3}H-spiroperidol binding to rat cortical membranes after chronic antidepressant treatments. Polish Journal of Pharmacology and Pharmacy 37:317–323, 1985
219. Martin KF, Needham PL, Atkinson J, et al: Rat striatal and mesolimbic D-1 receptor binding is not altered by antidepressant treatments including ECS and sibutramine HCl. Br J Pharmacol 95:896–899, 1988
220. Willner P: Dopamine and depression: a review of recent evidence, III: the effects of antidepressant treatments. Brain Research Reviews 6:237–246, 1983
221. Klimek V, Nielsen M: Chronic treatment with antidepressants decreases the number of [^{3}H]SCH 23390 binding sites in the rat striatum and limbic system. Eur J Pharmacol 139:163–169, 1987
222. Serra G, Cully M, D'Augulia PS, et al: On the mechanisms involved in the behavioral supersensitivity to DA-agonists induced by chronic antidepressants, in Dopamine in Mental Depression. Edited by Gessa GL, Serra G. Oxford, England, Pergamon, 1990, pp 121–138
223. Kapur S, Mann JJ: Role of the dopaminergic system in depression. Biol Psychiatry 32:1–17, 1992
224. Silberman EK, Reus VI, Jimerson DC, et al: Heterogeneity of amphetamine response in depressed patients. Am J Psychiatry 138:1302–1307, 1981
225. Silverstone T: Response to bromocriptine distinguishes bipolar from unipolar. Lancet 1:903–904, 1984
226. Murphy DL, Brodie HKH, Goodwin FK, et al: Regular induction of hypomania by L-dopa in "bipolar" manic-depressive patients. Nature 229:135–136, 1971
227. Kinney JL: Nomifensine maleate: a new second-generation antidepressant. Clinical Pharmacy 4:625–636, 1985
228. van Scheyen JD, van Praag HM, Koft J: Controlled study compar-

ing nomifensine and clomipramine in unipolar depression, using the probenecid technique. Br J Clin Pharmacol 4:179S–184S, 1977
229. Kemali D: A multicenter Italian study of amineptine (Survector 100). Clin Neuropharmacol 12 (suppl 2):41–50, 1989
230. Mendis N, Hanwella DR, Weerasinghe C, et al: A double-blind comparative study: amineptine (Survector 100) versus imipramine. Clin Neuropharmacol 12 (suppl 2):58-65, 1989
231. Paes de Sousa M, Tropa J: Evaluation of the efficacy of amineptine in a population of 1,229 depressed patients: results of a multicenter study carried out by 135 general practitioners. Clin Neuropharmacol 12 (suppl 2):77–86, 1989
232. Mann JJ, Aarons SF, Wilner PJ, et al: A controlled study of the antidepressant efficacy and side effects of (–)-deprenyl: a selective monoamine oxidase inhibitor. Arch Gen Psychiatry 46:45–50, 1989
233. Lloyd KG, Zukovic B, Scatton B, et al: The GABAergic hypothesis of depression. Prog Neuropsychopharmacol Biol Psychiatry 13:341–351, 1989
234. Suzdak PD, Gianstsos G: Parallel changes in the sensitivity of gamma-aminobutyric acid and noradrenergic receptors following chronic administration of antidepressant and GABAergic drugs: a possible role in affective disorders. Neuropharmacology 24:217–222, 1985
235. Lloyd KG, Thuret F, Pilc A: Upregulation of g-aminobutyric acid $(GABA)_B$ binding sites in rat frontal cortex: a common action of repeated administration of different classes of antidepressants and electroshock. J Pharmacol Exp Ther 235:191–199, 1985
236. Suzdak PD, Gianutsos G: Effect of chronic imipramine or baclofen on $GABA_B$ binding and cyclic AMP production in cerebral cortex. Eur J Pharmacol 131:129–133, 1986
237. Szekely AM, Barbaccia ML, Costa E: Effect of a protracted antidepressant treatment on signal transduction and $[^3H](-)$-baclofen binding at $GABA_B$ receptors. J Pharmacol Exp Ther 243:155–159, 1987
238. McManus DJ, Greenshaw AJ: Differential effects of antidepressants on $GABA_B$ and β-adrenergic receptors in rat cerebral cor-

tex. Biochem Pharmacol 42:1525–1528, 1991

239. Cross JA, Horton RW: Are increases in $GABA_B$ receptors consistent findings following chronic antidepressant administration? Eur J Pharmacol 141:159–162, 1987
240. Cross JA, Horton RW: Effects of chronic oral administration of the antidepressants, desmethyl imipramine and zimelidine on rat cortical $GABA_B$ binding sites: a comparison with 5-HT_2 binding site changes. Br J Pharmacol 93:331–336, 1988
241. Gray JA, Green AR: Increased $GABA_B$ receptor function in mouse frontal cortex after repeated administration of antidepressant drugs or electroconvulsive shocks. Br J Pharmacol 92: 357–361, 1987
242. Bowery NG, Hill DR, Hudson AL, et al: (–)-Baclofen decreases neurotransmitter release in the mammalian CNS by an action at a novel GABA receptor. Nature 283:92–94, 1980
243. Enna SJ, Karbon EW, Duman RS: $GABA_B$ agonists and imipramine-induced modifications in rat brain β-adrenergic receptor binding and function, in GABA and Mood Disorders. Edited by Bartholini G, Lloyd G, Morselli PL. New York, Raven, 1986, pp 23–31
244. Monteleone P, Maj M, Iovino M, et al: GABA, depression and the mechanism of action of antidepressant drugs: a neuroendocrine approach. J Affective Disord 20:1–5, 1990
245. Post RM, Ketter TA, Joffe RT, et al: Lack of beneficial effects of L-Baclofen in affective disorder. Int Clin Psychopharmacol 6:197–207, 1991

245a. Hamilton M: A rating scale for depression. J Neurol Neurosurg Psychiatry 23:56–62,1960

246. Sawynok J, Dickson C: D-Baclofen is an antagonist at baclofen receptors mediating antinociception in the spinal cord. Pharmacology 31:248–259, 1985
247. Dilsaver SC, Coffman JA: Cholinergic hypothesis of depression: a reappraisal. J Clin Psychopharmacol 9:173–179, 1989
248. Gershon S, Shaw FH: Psychiatric sequelae of chronic organophosphorus insecticides. Lancet 1:1371–1374, 1961
249. Risch SC, Janowsky DS, Seiver LJ, et al: Correlated cholinomimetic-stimulated beta-endorphin and prolactin release in

humans. Peptides 3:319–322, 1982

250. Janowski DS, Risch SC, Judd LL, et al: Behavioural and neuroendocrine effects of physostigmine in affect disorder patients, in Treatment of Depression. Edited by Clayton PJ, Barrett JR. New York, Raven, 1983, pp 61–74
251. Janowski DS, Risch SC: Role of acetylcholine mechanisms in the affective disorders, in Psychopharmacology: The Third Generation of Progress. Edited by Meltzer HY. New York, Raven, 1987, pp 527–533
252. Risch SC: Beta-endorphin hypersecretion in depression: possible cholinergic mechanism. Biol Psychiatry 17:1071–1079, 1982
253. Numberger JI Jr, Berrettini W, Mendelson W, et al: Measuring cholinergic sensitivity, I: arecoline effects in bipolar patients. Biol Psychiatry 25:610–617, 1989
254. Sitaram N, Nurnberger JI, Gershon ES, et al: Faster cholinergic REM sleep induction in euthymic patients with primary affective illness. Science 20S:200–203, 1980
255. Altamura CA, Mauri MC, Ferrara A, et al: Plasma and platelet excitatory amino acids in psychiatric disorders. Am J Psychiatry 150:1731–1733, 1993
256. Pangalos MN, Malizia AL, Francis PT, et al: Effect of psychotropic drugs on excitatory amino acids in patients undergoing psychosurgery for depression. Br J Psychiatry 160:638–642, 1992
257. Holemans S, Paermentier F, Horton RW, et al: NMDA glutamatergic receptors, labelled with [^{3}H]MK-801, in brain samples from drug-free depressed suicides. Brain Res 616:138–143, 1993
258. Kitamura Y, Zhao X-H, Takei M, et al: Effects of antidepressants on the glutamatergic system in mouse brain. Neurochem Int 19:247–253, 1991
259. Reynolds IJ, Miller RJ: Tricyclic antidepressants block *N*-methyl-D-aspartate receptors: similarities to the action of zinc. Br J Pharmacol 95:95–102, 1988
260. Trullas R, Skolnick P: Functional antagonists at the NMDA receptor complex exhibit antidepressant actions. Eur J Pharmacol 185:1–10, 1990
261. Skolnick P, Miller R, Young A, et al: Chronic treatment with 1-

aminocyclopropanecarboxylic acid desensitizes behavioral responses to compounds acting at the *N*-methyl-D-aspartate receptor complex. Psychopharmacology 107:489–496, 1992
262. Trullas R, Folio T, Young A, et al: 1-Aminocyclopropanecarboxylates exhibit antidepressant and anxiolytic actions in animal models. Eur J Pharmacology 203:379–385, 1991
263. Javitt DC, Zukin SR: Recent advances in the phencyclidine model of schizophrenia. Am J Psychiatry 148:1301–1308, 1991
264. Lewis DA, Hayes TL, Lund JS, et al: Dopamine and the neural circuitry of primate prefrontal cortex: implications for schizophrenia research. Neuropsychopharmacology 6:127–134, 1992
265. Paul IA, Trullas R, Skolnick P, et al: Down-regulation of cortical β-adrenoceptors by chronic treatment with functional NMDA antagonists. Psychopharmacology 106:285–287, 1992
266. Nowak G, Trullas R, Layer RT, et al: Adaptive changes in the N-methyl-D-aspartate receptor complex after chronic treatment with imipramine and 1-aminocyclopropanecarboxylic acid. J Pharmacol Exp Ther 265:1380–1386, 1993
267. Mjellem N, Lund A, Hole K: Reduction of NMDA-induced behaviour after acute and chronic administration of desipramine in mice. Neuropharmacology 32:591–595, 1993
268. Krystal JH, Karper LP, Seibyl JP, et al: Subanesthetic effects of the NMDA antagonist, ketamine, in humans: psychomimetic, perceptual, cognitive, and neuroendocrine effects. Arch Gen Psychiatry 51:199–214, 1994
269. Owens MJ, Nemeroff CB: The role of corticotropin-releasing factor in the pathophysiology of affective and anxiety disorders: laboratory and clinical studies, in Corticotropin-Releasing Factor. CIBA Foundation Symposium 172. Chichester, England, Wiley, 1993, pp 296–316
270. Banki CM, Karmacsi L, Bissette G, et al: Cerebrospinal-fluid neuropeptides: a biochemical subgrouping approach. Neuropsychobiology 26:37–42, 1992
271. Banki CM, Karmacs L, Bissette G, et al: Cerebrospinal fluid neuropeptides in mood disorder and dementia. J Affective Disord 25:39–46, 1992
272. Banki CM, Bissette G, Arato M, et al: CSF corticotropin-releasing

factor-like immunoreactivity in depression and schizophrenia. Am J Psychiatry 144:873–877, 1987

273. Bissette G, Spielman F, Stanley M, et al: Further studies of corticotropin-releasing factor-like immunoreactivity in CSF of patients with affective disorders. Society for Neuroscience Abstracts 11:133, 1985
274. Nemeroff CB, Widerlov E, Bissette G, et al: Elevated concentrations of CSF corticotropin-releasing factor-like immunoreactivity in depressed patients. Science 226:1342–1344, 1984
275. Roy A, Pickar D, Paul S, et al: CSF corticotropin-releasing hormone in depressed patients and normal control subjects. Am J Psychiatry 144:641–645, 1987
276. Altemus M, Pigott T, Kalogeras KT, et al: Abnormalities in the regulation of vasopressin and CSF corticotropin-releasing factor secretion in obsessive-compulsive disorder. Arch Gen Psychiatry 49:9–20, 1992
277. Gwirtsman HE, Guze BH, Yager J, et al: Fluoxetine treatment of anorexia nervosa: an open clinical trial. J Clin Psychiatry 51: 378–382, 1990
278. Nemeroff CB, Owens MJ, Bissette G, et al: Reduced corticotropin-releasing factor (CRF) binding sites in the frontal cortex of suicides. Arch Gen Psychiatry 45:577–579, 1988
279. Smith MA, Davidson J, Ritchie JC, et al: The corticotropin-releasing hormone test in patients with post-traumatic stress disorder. Biol Psychiatry 26:349–355, 1989
280. Roy-Byrne PP, Uhde T, Post R, et al: The corticotropin-releasing hormone stimulation test in patients with panic disorder. Am J Psychiatry 143:896–899, 1986
281. Heuser I, Von Bardeleben U, Boll E, et al: Response of ACTH and cortisol to human corticotropin-releasing hormone after short-term abstention from alcohol abuse. Biol Psychiatry 24:316–321, 1988
282. Adinoff B, Martin PR, Bone GHA, et al: Hypothalamic-pituitary-adrenal axis functioning and cerebrospinal fluid corticotropin releasing hormone and corticotropin levels in alcoholics after recent and long-term abstinence. Arch Gen Psychiatry 47:325–330, 1990

283. Dunn AJ, Berridge CW: Physiological and behavioral responses to corticotropin-releasing factor administration: is CRF a mediator of anxiety or stress responses? Brain Research Reviews 15:71–100, 1990
284. Valentino RJ, Curtis AL: Antidepressant interactions with corticotropin-releasing factor in the noradrenergic nucleus locus coeruleus. Psychopharmacol Bull 27:263–269, 1991
285. Grigoriadis DE, Pearsall D, DeSouza EB: Effects of chronic antidepressant and benzodiazepine treatment on corticotropin-releasing-factor receptors in rat brain and pituitary. Neuropsychopharmacology 2:53–60, 1989
286. Ehlers CL, Chaplin RI, Koob GF: Antidepressants modulate the CNS effects of corticotropin-releasing factor in rats. Medical Science Research 15:719–720, 1987
287. Brady LS, Whitfield HJ Jr, Fox RJ, et al: Long-term antidepressant administration alters corticotropin-releasing hormone, tyrosine hydroxylase, and mineralocorticoid receptor gene expression in rat brain: therapeutic implications. J Clin Invest 87:831–837, 1991
288. Nemeroff CB, Bissette G, Akil H, et al: Neuropeptide concentrations in the CSF of depressed patients treated with electroconvulsive therapy. Br J Psychiatry 158:59–63, 1991
289. DeBellis MD, Gold PW, Geracioti TD Jr, et al: Association of fluoxetine treatment with reductions in CSF concentrations of corticotropin-releasing hormone and arginine vasopressin in patients with major depression. Am J Psychiatry 150:656–657, 1993
290. Veith RC, Lewis N, Langohr JI, et al: Effect of desipramine on cerebrospinal fluid concentrations of corticotropin-releasing factor in human subjects. Psychiatry Res 46:1–8, 1993
291. Banki CM, Karmacsi L, Bissette G, et al: CSF corticotropin-releasing hormone and somatostatin in major depression: response to antidepressant treatment and relapse. Eur Neuropsychopharmacol 2:107–113, 1992
292. Ribeiro SCM, Tandon R, Grunhaus L, et al: The DST as a predictor of outcome in depression: a meta-analysis. Am J Psychiatry 150:1618–1629, 1993

293. Baldwin HA, Rassnick S, Rivier J, et al: CRF antagonist reverses the "anxiogenic" response to ethanol withdrawal in the rat. Psychopharmacology 103:227–232, 1991
294. Murphy BEP, Wolkowitz OM: The pathophysiologic significance of hyperadrenocorticism: antiglucocorticoid strategies. Psychiatry Annals 23:682–690, 1993
295. Wolkowitz OM, Reus VI, Manfredi F, et al: Ketoconazole administration in hypercortisolemic depression. Am J Psychiatry 150: 810–812, 1993
296. Murphy BEP, Dhar V, Ghadirian AM, et al: Response to steroid suppression in major depression resistant to antidepressant therapy. J Clin Psychopharmacol 11:121–126, 1991
297. Heilig M, Widerlov E: Neuropeptide Y: an overview of central distribution, functional aspects, and possible involvement in neuropsychiatric illnesses. Acta Psychiatr Scand 82:95–114, 1990
298. Widdowson PS, Ordway GA, Halaris AE: Reduced neuropeptide Y concentrations in suicide brain. J Neurochem 59:73–80, 1992
299. Stenfors C, Theordorsson E, Mathe AA: Effect of repeated electroconvulsive treatment on regional concentrations of tachykinins, neurotensin, vasoactive intestinal polypeptide, neuropeptide Y, and galanin in rat brain. J Neurosci Res 24:445–450, 1989
300. Heilig M, Wahlestedt C, Ekman R, et al: Antidepressant drugs increase the concentration of neuropeptide Y (NYP)-like immunoreactivity in the rat brain. Eur J Pharmacol 147:465–467, 1988
301. Wahlestedt C, Blendy JA, Kellar KJ, et al: Electroconvulsive shocks increase the concentration of neocortical and hippocampal neuropeptide Y (NPY)-like immunoreactivity in the rat. Brain Res 507:65–68, 1990
302. Widerlov E, Heilig M, Ekman R, et al: Neuropeptide Y: possible involvement in depression and anxiety, in Nobel Conference on Neuropeptide Y. Edited by Mutt V, Fuxe K, Hokefelt T. New York, Raven, 1989, pp 331–342
303. Kapal S, Austin MC, Underwood MD, et al: Electroconvulsive shock increases tyrosine hydroxylase and neuropeptide Y messenger RNA in the locus coeruleus. Society for Neuroscience

Abstracts 18:578.7, 1992
304. Bellman R, Gunther S: Effects of antidepressant drug treatment on levels of NPY or prepro-NPY-mRNA in the rat brain. Neurochem Int 22:183–187, 1993
305. Widdowson PS, Halaris AE: Chronic desipramine treatment reduces regional neuropeptide Y binding to Y2-type receptors in rat brain. Brain Res 539:196–202, 1991
306. Vecsei L, Widerlov E: Brain and CSF somatostatin concentrations in patients with psychiatric or neurological illness: an overview. Acta Psychiatr Scand 78:657–667, 1988
307. Rubinow DR, Davis CL, Post RM: Somatostatin in neuropsychiatric disorders. Prog Neuropsychopharmacol Biol Psychiatry 12:S137–S155, 1988
308. Gerner RH, Yamada T: Altered neuropeptide concentrations in cerebrospinal fluid of psychiatric patients. Brain Res 1238:298–302, 1982
309. Rubinow DR, Gold PW, Post RM, et al: CSF somatostatin in affective illness. Arch Gen Psychiatry 40:409–412, 1983
310. Kakigi T, Maeda K: Effect of serotonergic agents on regional concentrations of somatostatin- and neuropeptide Y–like immunoreactivities in rat brain. Brain Res 599:45–50, 1992
311. Kakigi T, Maeda K, Kaneda H, et al: Repeated administration of antidepressant drugs reduces regional somatostatin concentrations in rat brain. J Affective Disord 25:215–220, 1992
312. Duman RS, Terwilliger RZ, Nestler EJ: Chronic antidepressant regulation of G_sa and cyclic AMP-dependent protein kinase. American Society for Pharmacology and Experimental Therapeutics Abstracts 59, 1989
313. Gheorvassaki EG, Thermos K, Liapakis G, et al: Effects of acute and chronic desipramine treatment on somatostatin receptors in brain. Psychopharmacology 108:363–366, 1992
314. Engelman K, Horwitz D, Jequier E, et al: Biochemical and pharmacologic effects of α-methyltyrosine in man. J Clin Invest 47:577–594, 1968
315. Nolen WA, van de Putte JJ, Dijken WA, et al: Treatment strategy in depression, I: non-tricyclic and selective reuptake inhibitors in resistant depression: a double-blind partial crossover study on

the effects of oxaprotiline and fluvoxamine. Acta Psychiatr Scand 78:668–675, 1988

316. Hudson CJ, Young LT, Li PP, et al: CNS signal transduction in the pathophysiology and pharmacotherapy of affective disorders and schizophrenia. Synapse 13:278–293, 1993
317. Nestler EJ, Duman RS: Intracellular messenger pathways as mediators of neural plasticity, in Psychopharmacology: The Fourth Generation of Progress. Edited by Bloom F, Kupfer D. New York, Raven (in press)
318. Nicoll RA: The coupling of neurotransmitter receptors to ion channels in the brain. Science 241:545–551, 1988
319. Okada F, Tokumitsu Y, Ui M: Desensitization of β-adrenergic receptor-coupled adenylate cyclase in cerebral cortex after in vivo treatment of rats with desipramine. J Neurochem 47:454–459, 1986
320. Li PP, Emamghoreishi M, Sibony D, et al: Chronic antidepressant treatment does not alter the levels of Bs and Gi a-subunit transcript and immunoreactivity in rat cortex. Society for Neuroscience Abstracts 19:763.12, 1993
321. Newman ME, Soloman H, Lerer B: Electroconvulsive shock and cyclic AMP signal transduction: effects distal to the receptor. J Neurochem 46:1667–1669, 1986
322. Menkes DB, Resenick MM, Wheeler MA, et al: Guanosine triphosphate activation of brain adenylate cyclase: enhancement by long-term antidepressant treatment. Science 219:65–67, 1983
323. Nestler EJ, Terwilliger RZ, Duman RS: Chronic antidepressant administration alters subcellular distribution of cyclic AMP–dependent protein kinase in rat frontal cortex. J Neurochem 53:1644–1647, 1989
324. Perez J, Tinelli D, Brunello N, et al: cAMP-dependent phosphorylation of soluble and crude microtubule fractions of rat cerebral cortex after prolonged desmethylimipramine treatment. Eur J Pharmacol 172:305–316, 1989
325. Morinobu S, Duman RS: Induction of BDNF on RNA by electroconvulsive seizure (ECS) and antidepressants in rat frontal cortex. Society for Neuroscience Abstracts 19:499, 1993

326. Hosoda K, Duman RS: Regulation of β1-adrenergic receptor mRNA and ligand binding by antidepressant treatments and norepinephrine depletion in rat frontal cortex. J Neurochem 60:1335–1343, 1993
327. Butler MO, Morinobu S, Duman RS: Chronic electroconvulsive seizures increase the expression of serotonin$_2$ receptor mRNA in rat frontal cortex. J Neurochem 61:1–7, 1993
328. Collins S, Bouvier M, Bolanowski MA, et al: cAMP stimulates transcription of the β2-adrenergic receptor gene in response to short-term agonist exposure. Proc Natl Acad Sci U S A 86:4853–4857, 1989
329. Hadcock JR, Malbon CC: Agonist regulation of gene expression of adrenergic receptors and G proteins. J Neurochem 60:1–9, 1993
330. Hosoda K, Feussner G, Fishman PH, et al: β1-Adrenergic receptor down-regulation in C6 glioma cells: evidence for inhibition of b1AR gene transcription by a transient repressor. Society for Neuroscience Abstracts 18:816, 1992
331. Comb M, Hyman SE, Goodman HM: Mechanisms of trans-synaptic regulation of gene expression. Trends Neurosci 10:473–478, 1987
332. Winston SM, Hayward MD, Nestler EJ, et al: Chronic electroconvulsive seizures down regulate expression of the immediate-early genes c-fos and c-jun in rat cerebral cortex. J Neurochem 54:1920–1925, 1990
333. Duncan GE, Johnson KB, Breese GR: Imipramine antagonizes neuroanatomically selective alterations of 2-DG uptake and induction of Fos-like immunoreactivity induced by stress. Proceedings of the 1992 Annual Meeting of the American College of Neuropsychopharmacology, December 1992, p 85
334. Hope BT, Kelz M, Duman RS, et al: Chronic administration of ECS produces a long-lasting AP-1 complex in rat cerebral cortex of altered composition and characteristics. J Neurosci 14:4318–4328, 1994
335. Strausbaugh HJ, Morinobu S, Duman RS: Modulation of c-fos expression by electroconvulsive seizure (ECS) and antidepressants in rat frontal cortex. Society for Neuroscience Abstracts

19:449, 1993
336. Winston SM, Hayward MD, Nestler EJ, et al: Chronic electroconvulsive seizures down regulate expression of the c-fos protooncogene in rat cerebral cortex. J Neurochem 54:1920–1925, 1990
337. DeSouza EB, Insel TR, Perrin MH, et al: Corticotropin-releasing factor receptors are widely distributed within the rat central nervous system: an autoradiographic study. J Neurosci 5:3189–3203, 1985
338. Willner P: Animal models of depression, in Handbook of Depression and Anxiety: A Biological Approach. Edited by denBoer JA, Sitsen JA. New York, Marcel Dekker, 1994, pp 291–316
339. Baxter LR Jr, Phelps ME, Mazziotta JC, et al: Cerebral metabolic rates for glucose in mood disorders: studies with positron emission tomography and fluorodeoxyglucose F 18. Arch Gen Psychiatry 42:441–447, 1985
340. Baxter LR Jr, Schwartz JM, Phelps ME, et al: Reduction of prefrontal cortex glucose metabolism common to three types of depression. Arch Gen Psychiatry 46:243–250, 1989
341. Martinot JL, Hardy P, Feline A, et al: Left prefrontal glucose hypometabolism in the depressed state. Am J Psychiatry 147: 1313–1317, 1990
342. Mayberg HS, Starkstein SE, Sadzot B, et al: Selective hypometabolism in the inferior frontal lobe in depressed patients with Parkinson's Disease. Ann Neurol 28:57–64, 1990
343. Bench CJ, Friston KJ, Brown RG, et al: The anatomy of melancholia—focal abnormalities of cerebral blood flow in major depression. Psychol Med 22:6071615, 1992
344. Bromfield EB, Altshuler L, Leiderman DB, et al: Cerebral metabolism and depression in patients with complex partial seizures. Arch Neurol 49:617–623, 1992
345. Andreason PJ, Altemus M, Zametkin AJ, et al: Regional cerebral glucose metabolism in bulimia nervosa. Am J Psychiatry 149: 1506–1513, 1992
346. Dolan RJ, Bench CJ, Brown RG, et al: Regional cerebral blood flow abnormalities in depressed patients with cognitive impairment. J Neurol Neurosurg Psychiatry 55:768–773, 1992

347. George MS, Ketter TA, Post RM: SPECT and PET imaging in mood disorders. J Clin Psychiatry 54 (suppl 11):6–13, 1993
348. Drevets WC, Videen TO, Price JL, et al: A functional anatomical study of unipolar depression. J Neurosci 12:3628–3641, 1992
349. Bakish D, Lapierre YD, Weinstein R, et al: Ritanserin, imipramine, and placebo in the treatment of dysthymic disorder. J Clin Psychopharmacol 13:409–414, 1993
350. Artigas F, Perez V, Alvarez E: Pindolol induces a rapid improvement of depressed patients treated with serotonin reuptake inhibitors. Arch Gen Psychiatry 51:248–251, 1994
351. Wachtel H: The second-messenger dysbalance hypothesis of affective disorders. Pharmacopsychiatry 23:27–32, 1990
352. Wachtel H: Intraneuronal signalling systems as targets for the development of novel mood-stabilizing drugs. Clin Neuropharmacol 15:198–199, 1992

CHAPTER

13

Dopamine and Schizophrenia Revisited

René S. Kahn, M.D., Ph.D.
Michael Davidson, M.D.
Kenneth L. Davis, M.D.

The dopamine hypothesis of schizophrenia postulated that schizophrenia is related to increased dopamine function.[1] The foundations of this hypothesis rested mainly upon indirect evidence gained from the study of dopamine antagonists and agonists. Specifically, the ability of neuroleptics to displace dopamine antagonists in vitro robustly correlates with the clinical potency of these agents.[2,3] Conversely, drugs that increase dopamine activity generally worsen the symptoms of schizophrenia.[4–6]

Data have accumulated, however, that are inconsistent with the notion of hyperdopaminergia in all schizophrenic patients. For example, a substantial proportion of schizophrenic patients do not respond to treatment with neuroleptics. Furthermore, schizophrenic-like symptoms are rarely, if ever, induced in nonschizophrenic individuals exposed to drugs that augment dopaminergic activity. Moreover, neuroleptics are only partially effective in alleviating "negative," or deficit, symptoms of schizophrenic patients,[7] particularly after resolution of the acute phase of the illness. This in turn suggests that deficit state symptoms may be unrelated to increased dopamine activity.

Of interest is that data are accumulating that the negative symptoms of schizophrenia, as well as the cognitive deficits, may be related to decreased dopamine function in the prefrontal cortex. In contrast, the positive symptoms of schizophrenia appear to be related to increased dopamine turnover in the striatum. Schizophrenia may thus be characterized by increased and decreased dopamine activity, possibly present simultaneously in the same patient, albeit in different brain areas. That dopamine activity in the prefrontal cortex has been shown in animal studies to display an inhibitory regulatory control on dopamine activity in the striatum suggests an interrelationship between these two dopaminergic systems. It also indicates the possibility of a relationship between the negative and positive symptoms of schizophrenia. In this chapter, we review the available evidence for this proposition and examine its implications for the treatment of schizophrenia.

Anatomy of the Dopamine System

The dopamine system consists of a number of subsystems, whereas the dopamine receptor system consists of multiple subreceptors. The nigrostriatal system projects from the substantia nigra to the neostriatum (i.e., putamen and caudate nucleus). The mesolimbic system has its cell bodies in the ventral tegmental area of the midbrain and in the substantia nigra and projects to the nucleus accumbens, olfactory tubercle, and amygdala. The mesocortical system has its cell bodies mainly in the ventral tegmental area, its neurons projecting to the prefrontal cortex, the nucleus accumbens, septum, and the olfactory tubercles.[8,9]

The effects of neuroleptics on these different dopamine neuronal systems are not equivalent. In the nigrostriatal and mesolimbic dopamine systems, a single dose of a neuroleptic increases dopamine neuron firing.[10,11] This is probably due to blockade of presynaptic dopamine, subtype 2 (D_2), receptors and subsequent decreased inhibition of dopamine activity.[11,12] Chronic (3- to 4-week) neuroleptic administration decreases dopamine neuron firing in both A-9 and A-10 below pretreatment levels, an effect that can be reversed by apomorphine, a phenomenon called depolarization blockade.[12,13] Atypical neuroleptics, that is, antipsychotics that do not induce extrapyramidal side effects, such as clozapine, are anatomically more selective in their effect on dopamine neuronal firing than are typical neuroleptics in that they induce depolarization blockade in A-10 only.[11]

Dopamine receptors can be subdivided into several subclasses. D_1 receptors are coupled to adenylate cyclase, have a low binding affinity to [^{3}H]spiperone, and are found predominantly in the cortex of humans.[14,15] D_2 receptors are negatively coupled to adenylate cyclase, display high binding affinity to [^{3}H]spiperone,[16] and are most prominent in the striatal and limbic structures in humans. Their presence in the human cortex, if they are present at all, is limited.[15,17] The D_2 receptor has also been cloned, and two D_2 isoforms, labeled D_{2a} and D_{2b}, have been identified.[18,19]

The D_3 receptor has been cloned and is primarily present in the nucleus accumbens and in very low levels in the caudate and putamen.[20] In one study, no linkage was found in four Icelandic pedigrees between schizophrenia and the D_3 receptor gene.[21] The D_3 receptor resembles neither D_1 nor D_2 systems.[22] D_4 receptors displaying a higher affinity for the atypical neuroleptic clozapine have been identified.[23]

D_5 receptors have a pharmacology similar to D_1 receptors but have a higher affinity for dopamine than do D_1 receptors.[24] Whereas the D_1 receptor is widely distributed in the brain, however, the D_5 receptor appears to be limited to the hippocampus and thalamus.[25]

The identification of these various dopamine receptors has important implications. The high affinity of clozapine to the D_4 receptor, for instance, raises the issue of whether atypical neuroleptics are effective by blocking D_4 receptors more effectively than they do D_2 receptors. Indeed, it has been argued that blockade of D_4 receptors is related to the efficacy of neuroleptics, whereas blockade of D_2 receptors is related to their extrapyramidal side effect profile.[26]

The anatomical localization of D_3 receptors to limbic regions has intriguing possibilities for the development of antipsychotic compounds.

Increased Dopamine Function in Patients With Schizophrenia

Postmortem studies

Studies of homovanillic acid (HVA) and dopamine concentrations in postmortem brains of schizophrenic patients consistently show differences between patients and control subjects (Table 13–1). The differences in the anatomical areas where the abnormalities are found, however, are not consistent (Table 13–1). For example, HVA concentrations in the caudate and nucleus accumbens[27] and the cortex[28] of schizophrenic patients were found to be higher than those in normal brains. The difference in the concentrations found in the caudate was attributable to prior medication history, whereas the finding in the nucleus accumbens applied only in the medication-free patients.

Similarly, although dopamine concentrations in the nucleus accumbens were found to be higher in schizophrenic patients than in control subjects,[29] another study[30] found increased dopamine concentrations in the caudate but not in the nucleus accumbens of schizophrenic patients. Finally, Reynolds[31] reported increased dopamine concentrations in the amygdala of schizophrenic patients, with the most pronounced increase in the left hemisphere. These inconsistencies may be due to differences in the medication statuses of the patients studied, differences in the analytical and statistical methods used, or to genuine anatomical specificity of dopamine abnormalities in patients with schizophrenia.

Receptor studies have also been fairly consistent. D_2, but not D_1, receptors have been found to be increased in the striatum of schizophrenic patients (Table 13–2).[27,32–36] Although this could be the result of prior exposure to neuroleptics, most studies show that

Table 13–1. Postmortem studies of dopamine and HVA concentrations in brains of schizophrenic patients

				Results		
Study	**SCZ on**	**SCZ off**	**Controls**	**Site**	**Dopamine/ HVA**	**Comparison**
Reynolds 1983[31]	22		19	Amygdala	Dopamine	SCZ > Controls
Bacopoulos et al. 1979[28]	18–25	3	20–28	Temporal cortex	HVA	On > off = Controls
				Cingulate cortex	HVA	On > off = Controls
				Frontal cortex	HVA	On > off = Controls
				Putamen	HVA	SCZ = Controls
Toru et al. 1988[27]	5	5	10	Caudate	Dopamine	On = off = Controls
					HVA	On > off = Controls
				Accumbens	Dopamine	On = off = Controls
					HVA	Off > on = Controls
Mackay et al. 1982[29]	34		37	Accumbens	Dopamine	SCZ > Controls
				Caudate	Dopamine	SCZ = Controls
Owen et al. 1978[30]	15		15	Caudate	Dopamine	SCZ > Controls
				Accumbens	Dopamine	SCZ = Controls

Note. HVA = homovanillic acid. SCZ = schizophrenia. On = on neuroleptic prior to autopsy. Off = off neuroleptic prior to autopsy.

Table 13–2. Postmortem studies of dopamine receptor densities in brains of schizophrenic patients

Study	SCZ on	SCZ off	Controls	Results Site	Receptor	Comparison
Toru et al. 1988[27]	5	5	10	Putamen	D_2	On > Controls Off > Controls
Mackay et al. 1982[29]	9	3	17	Caudate	D_2	On > Controls Off = Controls
Seeman et al. 1987[33]	92		242	Striatum	D_2 D_1	On > Controls On = Controls
Crow et al. 1978[32]	14	5	19	Caudate	D_2	On > Controls Off > Controls
Cross et al. 1981[34]	8	7	8	Caudate	D_2 D_1	On = off > Controls SCZ = Controls
Hess et al. 1987[36]	8		8	Caudate	D_2 D_1	SCZ > Controls SCZ < Controls

Note. SCZ = schizophrenia. D_1 and D_2 = dopamine, subtype 1 and 2, receptors. On = on neuroleptic prior to autopsy. Off = off neuroleptic prior to autopsy.

striatal D_2 receptors were also increased in patients who had been drug naive or neuroleptic free for at least 1 year before the study. Of interest is that, when D_2 receptors were examined in patients who were not schizophrenic (i.e., those with Alzheimer's or Huntington's disease) but who had previously been treated with neuroleptics, striatal dopamine receptors were found to be increased by only 25%, in contrast to the increases of greater than 100% that were found in schizophrenic patients.[33] This finding suggests that neuroleptics account for only some of the increase in D_2 receptor numbers seen in patients with schizophrenia. The available data thus strongly suggest that D_2 (but not D_1) receptor density is increased in patients with schizophrenia.

Positron-Emission Tomography Studies

In contrast to the findings of postmortem studies, in vivo measurement of D_2 receptor affinity in humans with positron-emission tomography (PET) has provided conflicting results. An increase in D_2 receptor numbers in the striatum of 10 neuroleptic-naive schizophrenic patients, using [^{11}C]methylspiperone as a D_2 ligand, has been reported.[37] In contrast, no differences in D_2 receptor density were observed in 15[38] and 18[39] similarly drug-naive schizophrenic patients and in control subjects when studied with [^{11}C]raclopride. Similarly, when [^{76}Br]bromospiperone was used to compare D_2 receptor density in 12 schizophrenic patients (who were either drug naive or drug free for at least 1 year) with that in 12 control subjects, no differences in D_2 receptor density were found between the groups.[40] Interestingly, the more acutely ill patients had higher D_2 receptor density in the striatum than did the more chronically ill patients or the control subjects, suggesting that D_2 receptor density may be state dependent.

Part of these conflicting data may be due to the ligand used. For instance, methylspiperone, but not raclopride, binds potently to 5-HT_2 receptors. Moreover, the methods with which PET data were analyzed varied among studies. Finally, as suggested by the study in which [^{76}Br]bromospiperone was used, differences in patient population may partly explain the different D_2 receptor densities found in schizophrenic patients.

Peripheral Measures of Dopamine Function

Studies in cerebrospinal fluid. Generally, studies in which HVA concentrations in cerebrospinal fluid (CSF) of schizophrenic patients and healthy control subjects are compared have failed to yield differences between patients and control subjects.[41] However, decreased HVA concentrations in CSF have been found in subgroups of schizophrenic patients, such as those who respond poorly to neuroleptics[41] and those with predominantly negative symptoms. A negative correlation between HVA concentrations in CSF and the ventricle-to-brain ratio[42,43] and, more specifically, a negative correlation between prefrontal brain atrophy and HVA concentrations in CSF have been found.[44] Finally, the ability to activate the prefrontal cortex during cognitive tasks that depend on activity of that area is negatively related to HVA concentrations in CSF.[45] Thus, the cortical hypofunctionality[45–47] and atrophy[48] found in patients with schizophrenia may be associated with diminished cortical dopamine activity.

Studies in plasma. The finding that depolarization blockade in A-10 is a characteristic of all neuroleptics suggests that decreasing dopamine firing (in A-10) may be an important mechanism of action of antipsychotics. Because obtaining direct evidence linking the antipsychotic effect of neuroleptics to their effect on dopamine cell firing in humans has been impossible, however, indirect measurements of dopamine activity must be obtained. Measurement of levels of the dopamine metabolite HVA in plasma (pHVA) may be such a measure.

The HVA found in plasma is produced primarily by brain dopamine neurons and peripheral noradrenergic neurons. Secondary sources of HVA are peripheral dopamine and brain noradrenergic neurons. Studies in animals and humans suggest that brain dopamine turnover can be reflected by pHVA concentrations.[49,50] Although the precise proportion of pHVA deriving from brain HVA has not been fully elucidated,[51,52] measurement of this dopamine metabolite in the plasma of schizophrenic patients appears to be a valid method to investigate dopamine in this disorder, provided that certain conditions are met.[51]

Results of measurements of pHVA in humans are consistent with animal data; that is, neuroleptics initially increase and subsequently decrease dopamine firing. When neuroleptics are suddenly discontinued, pHVA levels increase,[53–55] a result mostly confined to those patients who clinically decompensate (Table 13–3).[54] Thus, pHVA concentrations rise dramatically during the first few days of neuroleptic treatment.[56,57] This rise in pHVA coincides with the increase in striatal dopamine firing observed in animals after acute administration of neuroleptics. After chronic (1 week or more) administration of neuroleptics, pHVA levels decrease to below baseline,[58,59] an observation that is consistent with the depolarization blockade observed in animals after chronic administration of neuroleptics (Table 13–4).

Table 13–3. Studies of HVA concentrations in plasma of schizophrenic patients after discontinuation of neuroleptic treatment

Study	Subjects	Weeks since drug discontinuation	Effect
Pickar et al. 1986[53]	SCZ (*N* = 11)	5	Increase
Davidson et al. 1991[54]	SCZ (*N* = 24)	6	Increase
Glazer et al. 1989[55]	SCZ (*N* = 13)	3	Increase
Kirch et al. 1988[64]	SCZ (*N* = 22)	6	No change

Note. HVA = homovanillic acid. SCZ = schizophrenia.

Table 13–4. Studies of HVA concentrations in plasma of schizophrenic patients during neuroleptic treatment

Study	Subjects	Duration of treatment	Effect
Davidson et al. 1987[6]	SCZ (*N* = 30)	6 weeks	Increase day 1
Pickar et al. 1986[53]	SCZ (*N* = 16)	5 weeks	Decrease week 3.5
Sharma et al. 1989[58]	SCZ (*N* = 11)	4 weeks	No change
	PSY (*N* = 6)		
Davila et al. 1988[52]	SCZ (*N* = 14)	4 weeks	Increase day 4
Bowers et al. 1989[57]	PSY (*N* = 37)[a]	9 days	Decrease day 7
Bowers et al. 1984[59]	PSY (*N* = 29)[b]	10 days	Decrease day 21
Wolkowitz et al. 1988[90]	SCZ (*N* = 12)	10 weeks	Decrease R
Chang et al. 1990[91]	SCZ (*N* = 33)	6 weeks	No change
Davidson et al. 1991[54]	SCZ (*N* = 20)	5 weeks	Decrease R

Note. HVA = homovanillic acid. SCZ = schizophrenic patients. PSY = psychotic patients. R = patients who responded to treatment.
[a]Only four patients were schizophrenic.
[b]Only two patients were schizophrenic.

When HVA is examined during the steady state in schizophrenic patients, however, inconsistent results have been obtained (Table 13–5). pHVA measured at drug-free baseline differentiates patients from control subjects in only some studies, and results of studies trying to link pHVA concentrations to specific schizophrenic symptoms, or even to severity of illness, have also been contradictory.

Table 13–5. Studies of HVA concentrations in plasma of schizophrenic patients before neuroleptic treatment

Study	Subjects	Mean weeks without drug	Correlation[a]
Maas et al. 1988[50]	SCZ (N = 23)	2	+
Pickar et al. 1986[53]	SCZ (N = 11)	5	+
Sharma et al. 1989[58]	SCZ (N = 11) PSY (N = 6)	2, 5	–
Davis et al. 1985[60]	SCZ (N = 18)	4	+
Davidson and Davis 1988[61]	SCZ (N = 14) controls (N = 14)	3	+
Pickar et al. 1984[62]	SCZ (N = 8)	2	+
Van Putten et al. 1989[63]	SCZ (N = 22)	4	–
Kirch et al. 1988[64]	SCZ (N = 22)	6	–

Note. HVA = homovanillic acid. SCZ = schizophrenic patients. PSY = psychotic patients.

[a]Correlation = whether a positive correlation was found between severity of symptoms and HVA concentrations in plasma. + = significant correlations were found; – = significant correlations were not found.

Five such studies found a positive correlation between pHVA levels and clinical severity,[50,53,60–62] whereas three studies did not.[58,63,64]

Thus, although the use of HVA as an indication of baseline dopamine function yields conflicting results, the use of HVA as an index of change in dopamine function yields results that are remarkably uniform. The latter consistency may hinge on the relatively large changes in HVA production when dopamine activity is manipulated. For instance, administration to rats of 1 mg of apomorphine per kg reduces striatal HVA by about one-third and pHVA by about one-fourth.[65] Haloperidol (1 mg/kg) almost quadruples HVA levels in striatum and nearly doubles them in plasma of rats.[66] A single administration of haloperidol roughly doubles pHVA concentrations in human subjects.[67] Thus, the changes induced by perturbation of dopamine function lead to large changes in both central and peripheral HVA concentrations. It is possible that when dopamine function is manipulated the changes that occur are profound enough to be detected in metabolite concentrations in CSF or plasma.

In contrast, when steady-state dopamine function is assessed, dopamine metabolite concentrations may be much more prone to multiple confounding factors. These are indeed legion. Metabolite concentrations in CSF are affected by age, height, and weight,[68] as well as by circadian and seasonal variations.[69] As explained by Maas et al.[70,71] only 15%–35% of pHVA may be derived from central sources, and consequently pHVA may reflect central dopamine turnover only when central dopamine metabolism is drastically altered.

Decreased Dopamine Function in Patients With Schizophrenia

Decreased Cortical Function

The negative or deficit symptoms of schizophrenia, for example, decreased social interaction, apathy, and avolition, are considered to be the core symptoms of the disorder.[7] It was Bleuler[71a] who proposed that these symptoms are characteristic for schizophrenia and are at the root of the poor social and work functions that almost define chronic schizophrenia. The importance of the frontal cortex for initiating and maintaining social interactions has been suggested by studies in primates: monkeys with frontal lobe ablations display social deficits that resemble the negative symptoms of schizophrenia.[72]

In only a handful studies have attempts been made to directly link decreased activity of the frontal cortex in patients with schizophrenia with negative symptoms. Decreased function of the frontal lobes has been repeatedly demonstrated with both measurements of cerebral blood flow, as measured by single photon emission computed tomography (SPECT), and PET.[47] In a cognitive task linked to frontal lobe function, the Wisconsin Card Sorting Test,[73] schizophrenic patients failed to show an increase in cerebral blood flow to the same degree as that seen in control subjects.[46] Facility at this task has been associated with the dorsolateral prefrontal lobe.[74] Similarly, schizophrenic patients showed decreased blood flow and activation of the left mesial frontal cortex on performing the "tower of London" task, another test thought to depend on activation of the prefrontal cortex.[47] This lack of activation and decreased blood flow was similar in drug-naive and medicated patients but occurred only in patients with high negative symptom scores.[47] Indeed, negative symptomatology has been associated with prefrontal hypometabolism on PET,[75] a finding that appears to be unrelated to medication effects.[76] Frontal hypofunction, then, seems to be a key feature of schizophrenia, particularly in patients with prominent negative or deficit symptoms. Of interest is preliminary evidence indicating that the decreased function of the prefrontal cortex may be associated with decreased activity in the mesocortical dopamine system.

Decreased Dopamine Function

Results of animal studies suggest that some of the cognitive deficits, as well as the negative symptoms, found in patients with schizophrenia may be due to decreased mesocortical dopamine activity. Surgical ablation of the prefrontal cortex or selective destruction of mesocortical dopamine neurons in monkeys impaired performance of the spatial delayed-response task, a test thought to depend on activation of the frontal cortical areas in monkeys.[77] Iontophoretically applied dopamine in area 46 (corresponding to the dorsolateral aspects of the prefrontal cortex in humans) improved performance in the delayed-response task in monkeys.[78] Administration of D_1 antagonists produced dose-dependent deficits in performance during the delayed-response task, whereas the selective D_2 antagonist raclopride did not.[78]

Because the terminals of the mesocortical dopamine system consists of the D_1 receptor subtype,[8] these findings suggest that the mesocortical dopamine system is important for memory and retrieval functions in high-order primates and, by inference, in humans as well. These data are consistent with the notion that the decreased cognitive performance on frontally mediated tasks in patients with schizophrenia may be the result of decreased activity of the mesocortical (D_1/D_5) system. Indirect evidence has suggested that cortical hypofunctionality is associated with diminished cortical dopamine activity in patients with schizophrenia. For example, a strong positive correlation was found between the ability to activate the prefrontal cortex (on the Wisconsin Card Sorting Test) and HVA concentrations in CSF.[45] Indeed, cognitive deficits attributed to activity of the frontal cortex, such as performance on the Wisconsin Card Sorting Test, were associated with lowered HVA concentrations in CSF, suggesting a relationship between decreased dopamine function and impaired frontally mediated cognitive function.[79] Moreover, blood flow in the prefrontal cortex increases in schizophrenic patients after administration of the dopamine agonists amphetamine[79a] and apomorphine,[80] suggesting that the hypofrontality found in schizophrenic patients can be redressed by increasing dopamine activity in the prefrontal cortex. The increase in prefrontal blood flow after amphetamine administration also correlated significantly with improved performance on the Wisconsin Card Sorting Test,[79a] indicating that increasing dopamine activity improves a cognitive deficit linked to diminished prefrontal cortical activity.

That negative symptoms are associated with decreased dopamine function (in the mesocortical dopamine system) is also suggested by findings of treatment studies in schizophrenic patients. Various studies have attempted to improve schizophrenic symptoms by increasing dopamine activity. Most have failed to find clinically meaningful effects.[81] Recently, however, the dopamine reuptake inhibitor mazindole (2 mg per day) improved negative symptoms as compared with placebo.[82] In that study, mazindole or placebo were added to neuroleptic treatment after patients had been stabilized on neuroleptic medication for 4 weeks. Large, well-controlled studies are needed, however, to explore the efficacy of increasing dopamine activity in the negative symptoms of schizophrenia, although the data reviewed here certainly encourage such an approach.

Linking Increased With Decreased Dopamine Function

The central finding enabling the linkage of decreased with increased dopamine function has been the elucidation of an interaction between cortical and striatal dopamine systems, that is, an inhibitory regulation of cortical dopamine systems on striatal dopamine neurons. When dopamine-receptive neurons are lesioned in the prefrontal cortex in rats, increased levels of dopamine and its metabolites, as well as increased D_2 receptor binding sites and D_2 receptor responsivity, are found in striatum.[83–87] Conversely, injection of the dopamine agonist apomorphine in the prefrontal cortex of rats reduces the dopamine metabolites HVA and dihydroxyphenylacetic acid by about 20% in the striatum.[88] This finding suggests that decreased activity of the mesocortical dopamine system may lead to overactivity of the mesolimbic (striatal) dopamine system.

In a modification of the model proposed by Pycock et al.[83] Deutch[89] proposed that the effect of dopamine depletion in the prefrontal cortex on striatal dopamine activity is particularly revealed after the animal has been stressed. Specifically, when animals were stressed, larger increases in striatal dopamine activity in those whose mesocortical dopamine neurons had been lesioned were found than in those with intact prefrontal cortex dopamine systems.[89] This finding suggests that the sensitivity of striatal (mesolimbic) dopamine neurons to physiological (i.e., stress) challenge is enhanced when dopamine function in the prefrontal cortex is decreased.

The results of these studies indicate that decreasing prefrontal cortical dopamine activity increases striatal dopamine turnover, D_2 receptor sensitivity, and D_2 receptor function, whereas increased dopamine function in the prefrontal cortex decreases striatal dopamine activity. Decreased activity in the prefrontal cortex may render the subject particularly sensitive to stress-induced increases in subcortical dopamine activity.

Conclusions

The finding that decreased mesocortical dopamine activity may be related to the cognitive deficits and negative symptoms of schizophrenia has important therapeutic implications. As indicated, the mesocortical dopamine neurons are of the D_1 and D_5 type, whereas the dopamine receptors in the subcortical areas (mesolimbic system) are of the D_2 type. This difference has important implications for possible treatment: negative symptoms and cognitive deficits appear to be related to decreased activity of the mesocortical dopamine neurons, not the mesolimbic neurons. Thus, one would expect increasing dopamine activity at D_1/D_5 neurons to have beneficial effects on negative symptoms and cognitive deficits in patients with schizophrenia. However, increasing dopamine activity at D_2 receptors (in the subcortical areas) may be deleterious because it is expected to increase psychotic symptoms in patients with schizophrenia. Consistent with the findings reported above that increasing prefrontal cortical dopamine activity reduces striatal dopamine activity, treatment with D_1 agonists could decrease the hypothesized increased dopamine activity in subcortical dopamine neurons and thus be useful (in combination with traditional D_2 antagonists) in the treatment of acute psychoses as well.

In summary, the possibility of simultaneously increased and decreased dopamine activity in various brain areas involving different dopamine receptor systems has broadened the perception of the role of dopamine in schizophrenia. It provides an interesting and heuristically useful model to examine the role of dopamine in schizophrenia and offers new avenues for drug development. Indeed, the findings may have far-reaching and important implications for the role of dopamine in schizophrenia: they suggest the usefulness of increasing dopamine activity (in the prefrontal cortex at D_1 or D_5 receptors) as treatment for negative symptoms. Even more important, via increasing dopamine function in the prefrontal cortex, dopamine agonists may be used to prevent (stress-induced) increases in subcortical dopamine activity. This may eventually lead to using dopamine agonists as maintenance treatment in patients with schizophrenia.

References

1. Matthysse S: Antipsychotic drug actions: a clue to the neuropathology of schizophrenia? Federal Proceedings 32:200–205,

1973
2. Creese I, Burt DR, Snyder SH: DA receptor binding predicts clinical and pharmacological potencies of antischizophrenic drugs. Science 192:481–483, 1976
3. Seeman P, Lee T, Chau-Wong M, et al: Antipsychotic drug doses and neuroleptic/DA receptors. Nature 261:717–719, 1976
4. Angrist B, Peselow E, Rubinstein M, et al: Amphetamine response and relapse risk after depot neuroleptic discontinuation. Psychopharmacology 85:277–283, 1975
5. Lieberman JA, Kane JM, Gadaletta D, et al: Methylphenidate challenge as a predictor of relapse in schizophrenia. Am J Psychiatry 141:633–638, 1984
6. Davidson M, Losonczy, MF, Mohs RC, et al: Effects of debrisoquin and haloperidol on plasma homovanillic acid concentration in schizophrenic patients. Neuropsychopharmacology 1:17–23, 1987
7. Andreasen NC, Olsen SA: Negative vs positive schizophrenia: definition and validation. Arch Gen Psychiatry 39:789–794, 1982
8. Bannon ML, Roth RH: Pharmacology of mesocortical dopamine neurons. Pharmacol Rev 35:53–68, 1983
9. Swanson LW: The projections of the ventral tegmental area and adjacent regions: a combined fluorescent retrograde tracer and immunofluorescence study in the rat. Brain Res Bull 9:321–353, 1982
10. Bunney BS, Grace AA: Acute and chronic haloperidol treatment: comparison effects on nigral dopaminergic cell activity. Life Sci 23:1715–1728, 1978
11. Chiodo LA, Bunney BS: Typical and atypical neuroleptics: differential effects of chronic administration on the activity of A9 and A10 midbrain dopaminergic neurons. J Neurosci 3:1607–1619, 1983
12. Huff RM, Adams RN: Dopamine release in n. accumbens and striatum by clozapine: simultaneous monitoring by in vivo electrochemistry. Neuropharmacology 19:587–590, 1980
13. White FJ, Wang RY: A10 dopamine neurons: role of autoreceptors determining firing rate and sensitivity to dopamine agonists.

Life Sci 34:1161–1170, 1984
14. Bunzow JR, Van Tol HHM, Grandy DK, et al: Cloning and expression of a rat D2 DA receptor cDNA. Nature 336:783–787, 1988
15. Selbie LA, Hayes G, Shine J: The major dopamine D2 receptor: molecular analysis of the human DA2a subtype. DNA 8:683–689, 1989
16. Robakis NK, Mohamadi M, Fu DY, et al: Human retina D2 receptor cDNA's have multiple polyadenylation sites and differ from a pituitary clone at the 5' non-coding region. Nucleic Acids Res 18:1299, 1990
17. Grandy DK, Marchionni MA, Makam H, et al: Cloning of the cDNA gene for a human D2 dopamine receptor. Proc Natl Acad Sci U S A 86:9762–9766, 1989
18. Todd RD, Khurana TS, Sajovic P: Cloning of ligand-specific cell lines via gene transfer: identification of a D2 dopamine receptor subtype. Proc Natl Acad Sci U S A 86:10134–10138, 1989
19. Dal Toso R, Sommer B, Ewert M, et al: The dopamine D2 receptor: two molecular forms generated by alternative splicing. EMBO J 8:4025–4034, 1989
20. Landwehrmeyer-B, Mengod G, Palacios JM: Dopamine D_3 receptor mRNA and binding sites in human brain. Brain Res Mol Brain Res 18:187–192, 1993
21. Wiese C, Lannfelt L, Kristbjarnarson H, et al: No evidence of linkage between schizophrenia and D_3 dopamine receptor gene locus in Icelandic pedigrees. Psychiatry Res 46:69–78, 1993
22. Sokoloff P, Giros B, Martres MP, et al: Molecular cloning and characterization of a novel dopamine receptor (D3) as a target for neuroleptics. Nature 347:146–151, 1990
23. Van Tol HHM, Bunzow IJ, Hong-Chang E: Cloning of the gene for a human dopamine D_4 receptor with high affinity for the antipsychotic clozapine. Nature 350:610–614, 1991
24. Sunahara RK, Hong Chang G, O'Dowd BF, et al: Cloning of the gene for a human dopamine D_5 receptor with higher affinity for dopamine than D_1. Nature 350:614–619, 1991
25. Meader-Woodruff JH, Mansour A, Grandy D, et al: Distribution of D5 dopamine receptor mRNA in rat brain. Neurosci Lett 145: 209–212, 1992

26. Seeman PH: Dopamine receptor sequences: therapeutic levels of neuroleptics occupy D_2 receptors, clozapine occupies D_4. Neuropsychopharmacology 7:261–284, 1992
27. Toru M, Watanabe S, Shibuya H, et al: Neurotransmitters, receptors and neuropeptides in post-mortem brains of chronic schizophrenic patients. Acta Psychiatr Scand 78:121–137, 1988
28. Bacopoulos NC, Spokes EG, Bird ED, et al: Antipsychotic drug action in schizophrenic patients: effect on cortical DA metabolism after long-term treatment. Science 205:1405–1407, 1979
29. Mackay AVP, Iversen LL, Rossor M, et al: Increased brain DA and DA receptors in schizophrenia. Arch Gen Psychiatry 39:991–997, 1982
30. Owen F, Crow TJ, Poulter M, et al: Increased DA-receptor sensitivity in schizophrenia. Lancet 29:223–225, 1978
31. Reynolds GP: Increased concentrations and lateral asymmetry of amygdala DA in schizophrenia. Nature 305:527–529, 1983
32. Crow TJ, Johnstone EC, Longden AJ, et al: Dopaminergic mechanisms in schizophrenia: the antipsychotic effect and the disease process. Life Sci 23:563–568, 1978
33. Seeman P, Bzowej NH, Guan HC, et al: Human brain D1 and D2 DA dopamine receptors in schizophrenia, Alzheimer's, Parkinson's, and Huntington's diseases. Neuropsychopharmacology 1:5–15, 1987
34. Cross AJ, Crow TJ, Owen F: 3H-flupenthixol binding in post-mortem brains of schizophrenics: evidence for a selective increase in dopamine D2 receptors. Psychopharmacology 74: 122–124, 1981
35. Mita T, Hanada S, Nishino N: Decreased serotonin S_2 and increased dopamine D_2 receptors in chronic schizophrenics. Biol Psychiatry 21:1407–1414, 1986
36. Hess EJ, Bracha S, Kleinman JE, et al: Dopamine receptor subtype imbalance in schizophrenia. Life Sci 40:1487–1497, 1987
37. Wong DF, Wagner HN, Tune LE, et al: Positron emission tomography reveals elevated D2 DA receptors in drug-naive schizophrenics. Science 234:1558–1563, 1986
38. Farde L, Weisel F, Hall H, et al: No D2 receptor increase in PET study of schizophrenia. Arch Gen Psychiatry 44:671–672, 1987

39. Farde L, Wiesel FA, Stone-Elander S, et al: D2 dopamine receptors in neuroleptic-naive schizophrenic patients: a positron emission tomography study with [11C]raclopride. Arch Gen Psychiatry 47:213–219, 1990
40. Martinot JL, Peron-Magnan P, Huret JD, et al: Striatal D2 dopaminergic receptors assessed with positron emission tomography and 76Br-bromospiperone in untreated schizophrenic patients. Am J Psychiatry 147:44–50, 1989
41. Widerlov E: A critical appraisal of CSF monoamine metabolite studies in schizophrenia. Ann N Y Acad Sci 537:309–323, 1988
42. Losonczy MF, Song IS, Mohs RC, et al: Correlates of lateral ventricular size in chronic schizophrenia, II: biological measures. Am J Psychiatry 143:1113–1118, 1986
43. Nyback H, Berggren B, Hindmarsh T, et al: Cerebroventricular size and cerebrospinal fluid monoamine metabolites in schizophrenic patients and healthy volunteers. Psychiatry Res 9:301–308, 1983
44. Doran AR, Rubinow DR, Wolkowitz OM, et al: Fluphenazine treatment reduces CSF somatostatin in patients with schizophrenia: correlations with CSF HVA. Biol Psychiatry 25:431–439, 1989
45. Weinberger DR, Berman KF, Illowsky BP: Physiological dysfunction of dorsolateral prefrontal cortex in schizophrenia, III: a new cohort and evidence for a monoaminergic mechanism. Arch Gen Psychiatry 45:609–615, 1988
46. Weinberger DR, Berman KF, Chase TN: Prefrontal cortex physiological activation in Parkinson disease: effect of L-dopa. Neurology 36 (suppl):170, 1986
47. Andreasen NC, Rezai K, Alliger R, et al: Hypofrontality in neuroleptic-naive patients and in patients with chronic schizophrenia: assessment with Xenon 133 single-photon emission computed tomography and the tower of London. Arch Gen Psychiatry 12:943–958, 1992
48. Andreasen N, Nasrallah HA, Dunn V, et al: Structural abnormalities in the frontal system in schizophrenia. Arch Gen Psychiatry 43:136–144, 1986
49. Bacopoulos NG, Hattox SE, Roth RH: 3,4-Dihydroxyphenylacetic

acid and homovanillic acid in rat plasma: possible indicators of dopaminergic activity. Eur J Pharmacol 56:225–236, 1979

50. Maas JW, Contreras SA, Seleshi E, et al: Dopamine metabolism and disposition in schizophrenic patients. Arch Gen Psychiatry 45:553–560, 1988
51. Davidson M, Giordani A, Mohs, RC, et al: Control of extraneous factors affecting plasma homovanillic acid concentrations. Psychiatry Res 20:307–312, 1987
52. Davila R, Manero E, Zumarraga-Andia I, et al: Plasma homovanillic acid as a predictor of response to neuroleptics. Arch Gen Psychiatry 45:564–567, 1988
53. Pickar D, Labarca R, Doran A, et al: Longitudinal measurement of plasma homovanillic acid levels in schizophrenic patients. Arch Gen Psychiatry 43:669–676, 1986
54. Davidson M, Kahn RS, Knott P, et al: The effect of neuroleptic treatment on plasma homovanillic acid concentrations and schizophrenic symptoms. Arch Gen Psychiatry 48:910–913, 1991
55. Glazer WM, Bowers MBJ, Charney DS, Heninger GR: The effect of neuroleptic discontinuation on psychopathology, involuntary movements, and biochemical measures in patients with persistent tardive dyskinesia. Biol Psychiatry 46:224–233, 1989
56. Kopin I, Bankiewicz KS, Harvey-White J: Assessment of brain dopamine metabolism from plasma HVA and MHPG during debrisoquin treatment: validation in monkeys treated with MPTP. Neuropsychopharmacology 1:119–126, 1988
57. Bowers MB, Swigar ME, Jatlow PI, et al: Plasma catecholamine metabolites and treatment response at neuroleptic state. Biol Psychiatry 25:734–738, 1989
58. Sharma R, Javaid JI, Janicak PH, et al: Plasma and CSF HVA before and after pharmacological treatment. Psychiatry Res 28:97–104, 1989
59. Bowers MB, Swigar ME, Jatlow PI, et al: Plasma catecholamine metabolism and early response to haloperidol. J Clin Psychiatry 45:284–251, 1984
60. Davis KL, Davidson M, Mohs RC, et al: Plasma homovanillic acid concentration and the severity of schizophrenic illness. Science

227:1601–1602, 1985

61. Davidson M, Davis KL: A comparison of plasma homovanillic acid concentrations in schizophrenics and normal controls. Arch Gen Psychiatry 45:561–563, 1988
62. Pickar D, Labarca R, Linnoila M, et al: Neuroleptic induced decrease in plasma homovanillic acid and antipsychotic activity in schizophrenic patients. Science 225:954–956, 1984
63. Van Putten T, Marder S, Aravagiri M, et al: Plasma homovanillic acid as a predictor of response to fluphenazine treatment. Psychopharm Bull 1:89–91, 1989
64. Kirch DG, Jaskiw G, Linnoila M, et al: Plasma amine metabolites before and after withdrawal from neuroleptic treatment in chronic schizophrenic inpatients. Psychiatry Res 25:233–242, 1988
65. Kendler KS, Heninger GR, Roth RH: Influence of dopamine agonists on plasma and brain levels of homovanillic acid. Life Sci 30:2063–2069, 1982
66. Kendler KS, Heninger GR, Roth RH: Brain contribution to the haloperidol-induced increase in plasma homovanillic acid. Eur J Pharmacol 71:321–326, 1981
67. Davila R, Zumarraga M, Perea K, et al: Elevation of plasma homovanillic acid level can be detected within four hours after initiation of haloperidol treatment. Arch Gen Psychiatry 44:837–838, 1987
68. Hartikainen P, Soininen H, Reinikainen KJ, et al: Neurotransmitter markers in the cerebrospinal fluid of normal subjects: effects of aging and other confounding factors. J Neural Transm Gen Sect 84:103–117, 1991
69. Losonczy MF, Mohs RC, Davis KL: Seasonal variations of human lumbar CSF neurotransmitter metabolite concentrations. Psychiatr Res 12:79–87, 1984
70. Maas JW, Contreras SA, Miller AI, et al: Studies of catecholamine metabolism in schizophrenic/psychosis, I. Neuropsychopharmacology 8:97–110, 1993
71. Maas JW, Contreras SA, Miller AI, et al: Studies of catecholamine metabolism in schizophrenic/psychosis, II. Neuropsychopharmacology 8:111–116, 1993

71a. Bleuler E: Dementia Praecox or the Group of Schizophrenia. Madison, CT, International Universities Press, 1950
72. Myers RE, Swett C, Miller M: Loss of social group affinity following prefrontal lesions in free-ranging macaques. Brain Res 64:257–269, 1973
73. Heaton R: Wisconsin Card Sorting Test. Odessa, TX, Psychological Assessment Resources, 1985
74. Milner B: Effects of different brain lesions on card sorting. Arch Neurol 9:90–100, 1963
75. Wolkin A, Sanfilipo M, Wolf AP, et al: Negative symptoms and hypofrontality in chronic schizophrenia. Arch Gen Psychiatry 49:959–965, 1992
76. Buchsbaum MS, Haier RJ, Potkin SG, et al: Frontostriatal disorder of cerebral metabolism in never-medicated schizophrenics. Arch Gen Psychiatry 49:935–942, 1992
77. Brozoski TJ, Brown RM, Rosvold HE, et al: Cognitive deficit caused by regional depletion of dopamine in prefrontal cortex of rhesus monkey. Science 205:929–931, 1979
78. Sawaguchi T, Goldman-Rakic PS: D_1 dopamine receptors in prefrontal cortex: involvement in working memory. Science 251: 947–950, 1991
79. Kahn RS, Harvey PD, Davidson M, et al: Neuropsychological correlates of central monoamine function in chronic schizophrenia: relationship between CSF metabolites and cognitive performance. Schizophr Res 11:217–224, 1994
79a. Daniel DG, Weinberger DR, Jones DW, et al: The effect of amphetamine on regional cerebral blood flow during cognitive activation in schizophrenia. J Neuroscience 11:1907–1917, 1991
80. Daniel DG, Berman KF, Weinberger DR, et al: The effect of apomorphine on regional cerebral blood flow in schizophrenia. J Neuropsychiatry 1:377–384, 1989
81. Gerlach J, Luhdorf K: The effect of L-dopa on young patients with simple schizophrenia, treated with neuroleptic drugs. Psychopharmacology 44:105–110, 1975
82. Krystal JH, Seibyl JP, Erdos J, et al: Neuroleptic augmentation with medications enhancing dopaminergic function: focus on mazindol. Proceedings of the American College of Neuropsycho-

pharmacology, San Juan, PR, December 1992, p 17

83. Pycock CJ, Kerwin RW, Carter CJ: Effect of lesion of cortical DA terminals on subcortical DA receptors in rats. Nature 286:74–77, 1980
84. Haroutunian V, Knott P, Davis KL: Effects of mesocortical DAergic lesions upon subcortical DAergic function. Psychopharmacol Bull 24:341–344, 1989
85. Roskin DL, Deutch AY, Roth RH: Alterations in subcortical dopaminergic function following dopamine depletion in the medial prefrontal cortex. Society of Neurosciences Abstracts 13:560, 1987
86. Leccesse AP, Lyness WH: Lesions of dopamine neurons in the medial prefrontal cortex: effects on self-administration of amphetamine and dopamine synthesis in the brain of the rat. Neuropharmacology 26:1303–1308, 1987
87. Glowinski J, Tassin JP, Thierru AM: The mesocortical- prefrontal DAergic neurons. Trends Neurosci 7:415–418, 1984
88. Jaskiw GE, Karoum F, Freed WJ, et al: Effect of medial prefrontal cortex lesions on dopamine turnover and dopamine agonism. Society of Neurosciences Abstracts 13:599, 1987
89. Deutch AY: The regulation of subcortical dopamine systems by the prefrontal cortex: interactions of central dopamine systems and the pathogenesis of schizophrenia. Journal of Neural Transmission 36 (suppl):61–89, 1982
90. Wolkowitz OM, Breier A, Doran A, et al: Alprazolam augmentation of the antipsychotic effect of fluphenazine in schizophrenic patients. Arch Gen Psychiatry 45:664–672, 1988
91. Chang WH, Chen TY, Lin SK, et al: Plasma catecholamine metabolites in schizophrenics: evidence for the two-subtype concept. Biol Psychiatry 27:510–518, 1990

CHAPTER

14

Pathophysiology of Schizophrenia: Insights From Neuroimaging

John Darrell Van Horn, Ph.D.
Karen Faith Berman, M.D.
Daniel R. Weinberger, M.D.

For the better part of this century, inquiries into the details of human brain anatomy and function were conducted by examining patients with known cortical lesions or by postmortem examination of brain tissues. With methods for imaging the brain developed in the past few decades, it is now possible to systematically and repeatedly examine the brains of living, conscious subjects.

Imaging the brain using computerized tomography (CT) or, more recently, magnetic resonance imaging (MRI) allows for the detailed representation of anatomical structures in vivo. The radionuclide-based technologies of single photon emission tomography (SPECT) and positron-emission tomography (PET) have aided researchers in visualizing and measuring brain blood flow and glucose consumption rates while also allowing assessment of neurotransmitter uptake or blocking sites. Physiological imaging during the performance of neuropsychological tasks using ^{15}O PET allows for visualization of the brain in action, indicating the location of changes in regional cerebral blood flow (rCBF). These techniques have opened new vistas for the development of models of human brain function and, in particular, of brain dysfunction in psychoses such as schizophrenia.

Early schizophrenia researchers, such as Wigan,[1,2] Alzheimer,[3] Kraepelin,[4] and Bleuler,[5] all believed that the fundamental source of clinical symptoms seen in patients with the illness resided in the brain. In recent years, schizophrenia researchers have been quick to recognize the potential of brain imaging techniques in understanding the brain deficits that may underlie schizophrenia. Indeed, a brief perusal through the imaging literature of the past two decades makes it clear that the brains of patients with schizophrenia have subtle morphological and functional abnormalities. Such findings have driven the bulk of research in this field back toward conceptualizing schizophrenia as a disorder of the brain and away from viewing it as a purely "functional psychosis" (DSM-III-R).[6]

From this growing body of literature have arisen several intriguing notions that have attempted to shed light on the mechanisms of schizophrenic symptomatology. In this chapter, we present a selective overview of several research areas that have gained much of their support from, or have been borne out of, evidence from studies using neuroimaging. Finally, we discuss the findings from neuroimaging studies within the context of the recent concept of schizophrenia as a neurodevelopmental disorder.

Evidence for Structural Abnormalities in Schizophrenia

Lateral Cerebral Ventricular Enlargement

Early studies in which pneumoencephalography was used[7,8] found mixed evidence for increased ventricular size relative to other psychiatric groups and nonpsychiatric control subjects. The inconsistent results were most likely due to inappropriate selection of control subjects, the potential for artifacts, and few scientific guidelines in psychiatric research during that time.[9] Although ventricular enlargement was identified in many patients, it was not until the availability of CT that this was clearly established. The first CT investigation of ventricular size in schizophrenic patients was conducted by Johnstone et al.,[10] who found ventricular size in patients to be significantly larger than that in control subjects. This finding was later confirmed by Weinberger et al.[11] and replicated often throughout the 1980s. Ventricular enlargement in patients with schizophrenia as observed from CT scans was reported so frequently in early studies that it was said to be "the most common structural abnormality in schizophrenic patients"[12] (p. 11). These studies demonstrated, for the first time, a measurable and replicable structural anomaly in the brains of schizophrenic patients in vivo and were instrumental in sparking a resurgence of interest in conceptualizing schizophrenia as a brain disease.

This neurobiological observation prompted a number of potential explanations. Perhaps the most influential was put forward by Crow,[13,14] who proposed the type I/type II conceptualization of schizophrenia. Patients with type I schizophrenia were characterized as having so-called "positive symptoms" (hallucinations, delusions, etc.), normal ventricular size, and possibly increased dopamine but with a promising prognosis. Those subjects with type II schizophrenia had "negative symptoms" (flattening of affect, poverty of speech, etc.), ventricular enlargement, and a poorer clinical outlook. This theory was the first to integrate the findings of ventricular size with symptomatology, chronicity of illness, and the long-suspected role of dopamine. It soon became apparent, however, that this conceptualization was too simplistic, because the type I/type II dichotomization found mixed support in further imaging studies. The hypothesis that schizophrenic ventricular size is a bimodal distribution reflecting two subtypes also was not confirmed.[15] As first-episode patients have been found to show ventricular enlargement, the finding is not an artifact of chronicity and is probably not an effect of treatment.[16–19]

Methodological problems characterize many of the early CT imaging studies of ventriculomegaly and complicate their interpretation. Variation among studies in indexing ventricular size and the selection of control groups may influence the statistical effect in size between schizophrenic and control subjects.[20–22] To date, two large metaanalytic assessments of ventricular size studies have been conducted.[23,24] In both of these studies, the existence of general ventricular enlargement in schizophrenic patients has been confirmed, but it was observed that the difference between schizophrenic patients and control subjects has decreased over time, reflecting increased experimental control. Despite these issues, it does seem that, as a group, schizophrenic patients have a certain degree of ventricular enlargement, though probably not as great as has been previously implied.

Some of the best evidence for ventricular changes has come from studies of monozygotic twins who are discordant for schizophrenia[25,26] and in which the affected twins consistently show greater ventricular size than their nonaffected co-twin. Such evidence, in which genetic factors are controlled, suggests that the increases in ventricular size are by and large not genetically determined. It should be remembered that ventricular enlargement reflects a nonspecific finding, perhaps involving pathology anywhere in the brain. More recent studies in which MRI techniques and postmortem histology have been used have begun to pinpoint the location of some of the structural changes.

Abnormalities of the Medial Temporal Lobe

Abnormalities of temporal lobe structures in patients with schizophrenia have been reported at many levels of anatomical detail. Postmortem investigations have identified gross abnormalities in the macroscopic temporal lobe[27] and hippocampus[28] in some patients, as well as microscopic evidence of pyramidal cell disorganization,[29,30] although the latter has failed to stand up to replication.[31,32] Jakob and Beckmann[33] have reported reduced cell counts and cytoarchitectural anomalies in the entorhinal cortex, as well as reduced thickness of the parahippocampal gyrus. Evidence for temporal lobe abnormalities are of importance to schizophrenia research in that conventional models of the hippocampal cortex stress its involvement in memory and its role in the processing of emotive information.[34,35]

Imaging studies, too, have verified structural abnormalities in the medial limbic system and temporal lobe. Studies in which MRI was used have identified significant reductions in the anterior hippocampus, amygdala, parahippocampal gyrus, and the superior temporal gyrus of schizophrenic patients.[36,37] In first-episode schizophrenic patients, reductions in hippocampal tissue and anterior temporal horn ventricular volumes, particularly among male schizophrenic patients, have been noted.[38] These findings appear to be independent of duration of neuroleptic treatment, although patients with chronic schizophrenia have been reported to have greater reductions in temporal lobe size than those with acute illness.[39] Reductions in the volume of the left anterior superior temporal gyrus have been found to correlate with severity of hallucinations,[40,41] an intriguing finding in the light of the fact that these areas involve the auditory association cortex.

Abnormalities of the temporal lobe might predict that schizophrenic patients would exhibit more profound amnesic symptoms than is typically observed in this illness.[42,43] Memory problems in patients with schizophrenia tend to involve "working memory" and other cognitive deficits that are more typically seen in patients with frontal lobe damage.[44] It may be, therefore, that temporal lobe abnormalities reflect involvement of a larger, distributed neural system that is responsible for memory-based cognition.

Evidence for Functional Abnormalities

Early researchers believed that brain dysfunction in patients with schizophrenia affected brain centers that were putatively concerned with higher mental functioning,[45–47] such as the frontal and temporal lobes. Of particular importance is the prefrontal cortex (PFC). This area has been shown in studies of patients with frontal lobe injury to be crucial in higher cognition, attention, the processing of error information, planning, and other "executive" functions.[48–51] Neuropsychological studies of schizophrenic patients have shown that they have cognitive deficits similar to those seen in subjects known to have frontal lobe damage.[52–55] These considerations, along with evidence from neuroimaging studies, suggest that certain cognitive deficits in patients with schizophrenia may be related to PFC abnormality.

Frontal Lobe Hypofunction

The role of the frontal lobes in schizophrenia regained popularity after the innovative rCBF studies of Ingvar and Frazen.[56–59] They observed decreased blood flow in the frontal lobes relative to other brain areas of schizophrenic patients (hypofrontality), whereas nonpsychiatric control subjects showed a relatively general increase in blood flow in this area. More severely affected patients showed the greatest reduction in frontal lobe activity.

Subsequent investigations, however, have not always confirmed hypofrontality, because findings have been susceptible to variation in the characteristics of the groups of patients and in the conditions under which patients are studied. For instance, in many of the [^{18}F]fluorodeoxyglucose and H_2O^{15} blood flow PET studies in which hypofrontality has been reported, chronically ill patients have been employed, whereas studies failing to confirm findings of hypofrontality have tended to include patients with more acute disease.[60–62] One potential explanation for these inconsistent findings may be that hypofrontality is related to neuroleptic treatment. On the other hand, studies in which hypofrontality was not found were almost invariably performed during a "resting" condition. This suggests the possibility that hypofrontality might be present only when frontal brain regions are "challenged" during neuropsychological tasks.

Is Frontal Lobe Hypofunction a Medication Effect?

The effect of neuroleptic drugs has been a controversial issue, but findings of reduced prefrontal activity in PET and SPECT studies of drug-free and drug-naive patients does not support the notion that hypofrontality is primarily a drug-related phenomenon.[63–65] In discordant monozygotic twins, it has been shown that the schizophrenic twin invariably showed greater hypofrontality than the unaffected co-twin, and this is unrelated to lifetime neuroleptic treatment.[66] Moreover, in the few studies in which the same patients have been examined while off and on antipsychotic drugs, the medications have not consistently caused frontal activity to diminish.[67] In short, the bulk of studies in which functional imaging techniques have been used in schizophrenic patients provide no compelling evidence to suggest that hypofrontality is an artifact related to medication.

Under What Conditions Would One Expect to Find Hypofrontality?

Some PET studies in the literature have been conducted at rest[65] or have used a control task not suitably matched for all but the cognitive component of interest.[63] Studies comparing rCBF during rest may show more rCBF variability because idiosyncratic activations are especially likely to occur during a resting state.[68,69] Our own studies of rCBF in patients with schizophrenia have shown hypofunction to be a reliable and replicable phenomenon only during certain neuropsychological tasks that place a localized physiological load on the dorsolateral PFC.

Neuropsychological studies using the Wisconsin Card Sorting Test,[70] an abstract-reasoning, problem-solving test, have found it to be sensitive to PFC damage.[49,50] Patients with frontal lobe damage perseverate, failing to adjust their responses in the face of changing rules. Schizophrenic patients performing the Wisconsin Card Sorting Test show generally poorer performance than control subjects; in particular, these patients commit more perseverative errors.[71] Studies of rCBF in normal subjects have found that the Wisconsin Card Sorting Test is associated with bilateral increases in rCBF in the PFC.[72–75] Schizophrenic patients have been found to show decreased activation of the frontal lobe relative to control subjects.

In contrast, during other conditions, such as when performing number matching, Raven's Matrices, or during rest, no frontal lobe abnormalities were found.[73,76,77] These results are consistent with those of other studies reporting frontal hypofunction during frontal cognitive activation[67] and suggest that frontal hypofunction in patients with schizophrenia is related to deficits in frontal-lobe cognitive processing.

Abnormalities of Prefrontal Function and Brain Neurochemistry

Abnormalities of neurochemistry in patients with schizophrenia are suggested by the fact that drug treatment with dopamine antagonists have for several decades been found to stabilize symptoms. Concentrations of homovanillic acid (a dopamine metabolite) in the cerebrospinal fluid of schizophrenic patients have been reported to correlate positively with clinical response to neuroleptics,[78] although findings to the contrary also exist.[79,80] Postmortem studies suggesting abnormal concentrations of dopamine and other neurochemicals or of dopamine receptors in schizophrenic patients have found differences but lack consistent techniques and results.[81] One of the major advantages of using PET and SPECT is that brain neurochemistry may be examined in vivo, thereby avoiding the pitfalls (such as variations in tissue fixation, postmortem intervals, and storage time) of investigations of postmortem tissue. Using isotopes with short half-lives tagged to known neurotransmitter precursors or receptor ligands allows for the measurement of their metabolites or binding in the living human brain.

Several studies have been published addressing dopamine receptor density in basal ganglia. Studies using [^{77}Br]bromospiperone[82] and [^{11}C]*N*-methylspiperone[83] have noted generally greater densities of dopamine, subtype 2 (D_2), receptor in the caudate nucleus of drug-naive patients. [^{11}C]Raclopride binding to D_2 receptors in the basal ganglia of drug-naive patients has been found to be normal.[84–86] A study of striatal D_2 receptor activity assayed with [^{76}Br]bromospiperone showed no association between receptor density and positive or negative symptoms.[87] The inconsistency in the findings of radiotracer studies are most likely to be related to differences in patient selection, sample sizes, radioligands, and modeling methods.[62,86] It is unclear at this time whether any of these reports can be considered valid.

Although all D_2 radioligand studies have been conducted during resting conditions, one area needing investigation is the cognitive specificity of dopamine activity.[88] For example, it is conceivable that malfunctions of dopaminergic systems of certain regions such as the PFC would be evident only during cognitive challenge. We have previously reported a strong positive correlation between homovanillic acid concentrations in cerebrospinal fluid and PFC activation during performance on the Wisconsin Card Sorting Test.[89] There was, however, no correlation between homovanillic acid concentration and rCBF in the dorsolateral PFC during a number-matching task. Although speculative, this observation suggests that regional changes in dopamine functioning may be evident only during certain cognitive operations. Further research linking the parameters of dopamine functioning with measurements of task-specific cognitive function may be useful in elucidating regional pharmacological mechanisms.

Structural-Functional Interactions

Functional neural networks describe how separate anatomical areas that are specialized for certain functions communicate via neural pathways to process complex cognitive operations. This implies that distant regions that are not directly linked to one another nonetheless work together to sort and manage incoming stimuli in the process of higher cognition. Concepts involving neural connectivity have been very popular and have given rise to distinct research areas within cognitive and computational psychology.[90] Researchers using functional imaging also have taken an interest in network theory and have attempted to identify brain areas correlating with cognitive task performance or symptomatology.

Role of Functional Networks in Psychosis

Two important PET studies investigating the role of functional networks in patients with schizophrenia were conducted by Liddle et al.[91] and Friston et al.[92] Factor analytic studies by Liddle[93] and Liddle and Barnes[94] have demonstrated three principal factor axes derived from schizophrenic symptom scores: 1) psychomotor poverty (decreased spontaneous movement, poverty of speech, and flatness of affect), 2) disorganization (disorders of form of thought and inappropriate affect), and 3) reality distortion (delusions and hallucinations). Liddle et al.[91] performed pixel-wise analyses of PET data from schizophrenic patients and observed significant correlations between psychomotor poverty scores and rCBF in the bilateral caudate, left dorsolateral PFC, and left superior parietal association cortex. Disorganization correlated with the right anterior cingulate gyrus, mediodorsal thalamus, right ventromedial PFC, left Broca's area, and bilateral angular gyri. Reality distortion was correlated with rCBF in the left temporal and frontal regions; left parahippocampal gyrus; left ventral striatum; and right posterior cingulate, right caudate, right posterior superior temporal region, and supramarginal gyrus. These results are consistent with those of previous discussions in the literature regarding areas believed to be dysfunctional in patients with schizophrenia,[95] particularly associations between reality distortion and temporofrontal areas. This study highlights that neuronal dysfunction underlying schizophrenic symptoms may not be limited to specific brain areas per se but are more likely to involve independent, distributed neural systems.

Our own work, in which structural and functional imaging has been used, has also indicated that important neuronal connections between prefrontal cortical and limbic structures may play a central role in the phenomenology of schizophrenic symptoms.[96] The behavioral implications of such dysfunctional intracortical connectivity may make itself known only during the performance of cognitive tasks that depend on the functional integrity of the cortical regions involved.

Functional abnormalities in specific brain regions may result from several possible sources, including structural changes in the region itself or its afferent or efferent pathways or neurochemical imbalances. Because brain systems are large, distributed, and dynamic, even subtle structural changes that are spatially located far from the site of functional abnormality may manifest themselves only during certain cognitive operations.[97] These changes may not be outwardly noticeable during cognitive conditions or other behaviors not involving the affected areas.

Asymmetry of Pathology or Pathology of Asymmetry?

Cerebral asymmetry and hemispheric dominance have been important concepts throughout this century and have been particularly prominent in theories of language function and brain evolution.[98] Dysfunctions or abnormalities of cerebral dominance have been proposed to underlie a number of neurological conditions, such as autism,[99,100] dyslexia,[101,102] and hysteria.[103,104] It may not be surprising, then, that researchers have considered schizophrenia to be a potential disease of cerebral lateralization. This hypothesis, too, had early origins, being a topic of much philosophical discussion in the last century.[105] According to the theories of Wigan,[1,2] for instance, an imbalance between the hemispheres was responsible for insanity, and patients could potentially learn to use their stronger hemisphere to overcome inappropriate thoughts and behaviors resulting from the affected hemisphere.

Current views of cerebral lateralization and schizophrenia have evolved from the findings of Flor-Henry[106,107] that patients with left temporal lobe epilepsy tended to have a greater number of schizophrenia-like symptoms than did other groups of patients. An extreme variation on the theme of lateralized pathophysiology and schizophrenia is the proposal that schizophrenia results from a mutation of a gene that is putatively responsible for normal asymmetric brain development.[108-114] It is important, however, not to confuse the concepts of asymmetric pathology with disease of the development of normal cerebral asymmetries. Mesulam[115] has astutely noted that "asymmetric disease need not imply disease of asymmetry" (p. 548) and that evidence from imaging studies must be interpreted carefully in this regard.

In terms of brain structure, imaging studies have frequently reported morphometric asymmetries in anatomical structure between schizophrenic and control subjects. Early CT studies claimed that schizophrenic patients showed "reversals" in the anatomical asymmetries of the occipital and frontal lobes normally seen in the human brain[116–119] and in asymmetries in CT scan density.[120–123] More recent studies have reported asymmetric increases in left temporal horn ventricular size and reductions in left temporal lobe area.[124] In terms of brain function, several PET investigations have suggested that schizophrenic patients have overactivation of the left hemisphere.[125–129] Still other studies have suggested that overactivation[130–132] or underactivation[133–134] might be localized to the left frontal lobes.

In general, imaging studies have reported mixed findings on abnormalities of structural and functional lateralization in the schizophrenic brain, although the left hemisphere is most often implicated. The reasons for the discrepancies are complex, and it is difficult to determine which studies are in conflict and which ones simply do not measure what previous researchers have measured. Variations in definition of asymmetry, methodology, and significance of cerebral asymmetries in the early CT studies are most likely responsible for the inconsistency in findings of reversed asymmetry. Uncertainty in the physiological meaning of CT scan reversals or asymmetric brain density makes it difficult to attach importance to hemispheric differences, apart from indicating that additional neurological problems may exist. Some PET studies find specific locations in each hemisphere where metabolism differs from that in control subjects, whereas others claim changes in the entire hemisphere. Lateralized findings in PET appear to occur as a moderate effect, often secondary to regional hypofunction. Although the notion of schizophrenia as a disease of laterality is an intriguing and, we believe, important question, we must concur with the statement made by Robertson and Taylor,[135] following their review of the neuropsychological literature on evidence of disturbances of laterality in patients with schizophrenia, that a clear demonstration of abnormal laterality in patients with schizophrenia remains "not proven."

Implications of Abnormal Neurodevelopment in Patients With Schizophrenia

The topics chosen for discussion highlight an increasing level of complexity achieved in the literature over the years in models of brain dysfunction in patients with schizophrenia. Neuroimaging has made a strong impact on schizophrenia research, not simply by its role in determining differences between patients and control subjects, but also in its heuristic value for understanding the schizophrenic disease process. It is clear from this overview that notions of what is wrong in the schizophrenic brain have spanned many areas, and the story underlying schizophrenic symptomatology is unlikely to be as simple as being a subtle localized brain abnormality. Each of the phenomena described, in their own way, may characterize certain aspects of brain dysfunction underlying this illness and represent components of a broader scenario of brain abnormality. The etiology of the primary brain abnormality is increasingly being assumed to involve brain development.

Requirements of a Neurodevelopmental Model

Two assumptions have been proposed as the foundation of a neurodevelopmental model of brain pathology in patients with schizophrenia:[95,136] 1) the putative lesion itself occurs prenatally during development of the central nervous system, and 2) the clinical ramifications of the pathological condition vary depending on independent ontogenetic effects occurring during normal brain development, as well as on environmental factors. Several predictions may be derived from such a framework. First, neuropathology should be observed before the onset of symptoms, although theoretically present in asymptomatic patients at risk for the illness. Second, during early childhood these disturbances would be mostly unnoticeable but may involve subclinical deficits of some cognitive functions and social and motor skills.[137–139] Lastly, these changes, being static, will not be correlated with the duration of illness once it is manifested in individual patients or in patient samples.

These assumptions and predictions have been for the most part supported by the results of neuroimaging studies. First-episode and young schizophrenic patients have been found to show ventricular enlargement, temporal cortical changes, and hypofrontality (see preceding discussion), and ventricular size does not appear to covary with the duration of illness. Ventricular size in adult patients predicts premorbid social adjustment during childhood, further suggesting that the pathology responsible for enlarged ventricles existed at that time. Examinations of home movies[140] from families with a child who later became schizophrenic have indicated that the affected sibling can be reliably identified among other children on the basis of soft neurological signs and patterns of social interaction. These studies indicate that the neuropathologic changes associated with schizophrenia are likely to be present long before the onset of debilitating symptoms.

Abnormal Neurodevelopment in Limbic Cortices

Current models of the etiology of schizophrenia generally propose that a subtle abnormality during fetal neurodevelopment,[141–143] possibly occurring in the latter half of pregnancy, affects the development of cortical structures.[33,144] Although only circumstantial evidence currently exists to support this notion, animal data have suggested that developmental cortical lesions, especially involving the limbic cortex, is the best animal model of schizophrenia. Lesions of limbic cortices in newborn rats have been found to uniquely affect dopamine-related behaviors after a developmental delay.[145] Prior to puberty, during an important period of brain development in the rat, lesions of limbic areas show no outward behavioral effects. After puberty, however, the same rats show excessive spontaneous locomotion and increased exploratory behavior after exposure to environmental stress. This effect is presumably due to the oversensitivity of their limbic dopamine response systems.[146] Converging evidence such as this, coming from broad-ranging research areas, lends support to a neurodevelopmental perspective.

Conclusions

In this chapter, we present an overview of several research areas that have been born of neuroimaging studies in which structural and functional techniques have been used. Increased ventricular size, functional hypofrontality, medial temporal lobe pathology, and anomalous cerebral lateralization are findings that have generated new perspectives on the neurobiology of schizophrenia. Although the mechanisms responsible for the etiology and symptomatology of schizophrenia are at present unknown, converging evidence tends to suggest a neurodevelopmental abnormality involving at least limbic and probably other cortical areas. Functionally, such a lesion could be expected to interfere with a network of afferent and efferent connections linking limbic to other cortical structures, in particular the PFC.[147] Proper functioning of the PFC and its connectivity are required during cognitive tasks requiring attention, planning, and processing of error information, functions believed to also require large-scale neurocognitive networks.[148] Dysfunction of areas of the PFC may be secondary to a primary limbic lesion or indicative of a more widespread developmental cortical defect.

At this time, we can only speculate as to the processes underlying schizophrenia, and the scenario presented above is but one of many possibilities.[149] Clearly, as structural image quality has improved and new imaging approaches have become available, evidence of brain anomalies in patients with schizophrenia have themselves become more detailed and will most likely continue to do so with further technological advancements.

References

1. Wigan AL: A New View of Insanity: The Duality of Mind. London, Longman, Brown, Green, and Longman, 1844
2. Wigan AL: Duality of mind, proven by the structure, function, and diseases of the brain. Lancet 1:39–41, 1844

3. Alzheimer A: Beitrage zur pathologishen anatomie der hirnrinde und zur anatomishen grundage einiger psychosen. Monatsschrift fuer Psychiatrie und Neurologie 2:82–120, 1897
4. Kraepelin E: Dementia praecox and paraphrenia. Edinburgh, Churchill-Livingstone, 1919
5. Bleuler EP: The physiogenic and psychogenic in schizophrenia. Am J Psychiatry 87:203–211, 1930
6. American Psychiatric Association: Diagnostic and Statistical Manual for Mental Disorders, 3rd Edition, Revised. Washington, DC, American Psychiatric Association, 1987
7. Huag JO: Pneumoencephalographic studies in mental disease. Acta Psychiatr Scand 38 (suppl 165):1–114, 1962
8. Storey PB: Lumbar air encephalography in chronic schizophrenia: a controlled study. Br J Psychiatry 112:135–144, 1966
9. Weinberger DR, Wagner RL, Wyatt RJ: Neuropathological studies of schizophrenia: a selective review. Schizophr Bull 9:193–212, 1983
10. Johnstone EC, Crow TJ, Frith CD, et al: Cerebral ventricular size and cognitive impairment in chronic schizophrenia. Lancet 2:924–926, 1976
11. Weinberger DR, Torrey EF, Neophytides AN, et al: Lateral cerebral ventricular enlargement in chronic schizophrenia. Arch Gen Psychiatry 36:735–739, 1979
12. Weinberger DR, Bigelow LB, Kleinman JE, et al: Cerebral ventricular enlargement in chronic schizophrenia. Arch Gen Psychiatry 37:11–13, 1980
13. Crow TJ: Molecular pathology of schizophrenia: more than one disease process. Br Med Bull 280:66–68, 1980
14. Crow TJ: A current view of the type II syndrome: age of onset, intellectual impairment, and the meaning of structural changes in the brain. Br J Psychiatry 155:15–20, 1989
15. Daniel DG, Goldberg TE, Gibbons RD, et al: Lack of bimodal distribution of ventricular size in schizophrenia: a gaussian mixture analysis of 1056 cases and controls. Biol Psychiatry 30:887–903, 1991
16. Weinberger DR, DeLisi LE, Perman GP, et al: Computerized tomography in schizophreniform disorder and other acute psychi-

atric disorders. Arch Gen Psychiatry 39:778–783, 1982
17. Schulz SC, Koller MM, Kishore PR, et al: Ventricular enlargement in teenage patients with schizophrenia spectrum disorder. Am J Psychiatry 140:1592–1595, 1983
18. Obiols-Llandrich JE, Ruscelleda J, Masferrer M: Ventricular enlargement in young chronic schizophrenics. Acta Psychiatr Scand 73:42–44, 1986
19. Luchins DJ, Meltzer HY: A comparison of CT findings in acute and chronic ward schizophrenics. Psychiatry Res 17:7–14, 1986
20. Raz N, Raz S, Bigler ED: Ventriculomegaly in schizophrenia: the role of groups and the perils of dichotomous thinking. Psychiatry Res 26:245–248, 1988
21. Smith GN, Iacono WG, Moreau M, et al: Choice of comparison group and findings of computerized tomography in schizophrenia. Br J Psychiatry 153:667–674, 1988
22. Smith GN, Iacono WG: Ventricular size in schizophrenia: importance of choice of control subjects. Psychiatry Res 26:241–243, 1988
23. Raz S, Raz N: Structural brain abnormalities in the major psychoses: a quantitative review of the evidence from computerized imaging. Psychol Bull 108:93–108, 1990
24. Van Horn JD, McManus IC: Ventricular enlargement in schizophrenia: a meta-analysis of studies using the ventricular-brain ratio (VBR). Br J Psychiatry 160:687–697, 1992
25. Reveley AM, Reveley MA, Clifford CA, et al: Cerebral ventricular size in twins discordant for schizophrenia. Lancet 1:540–541, 1982
26. Suddath RL, Christison GW, Torrey EF, et al: Anatomical abnormalities in the brains of monozygotic twins discordant for schizophrenia. N Engl J Med 322:789–794, 1990
27. Bogerts B, Meertz E, Shoenfeldt-Bausch R: Basal ganglia and limbic system pathology in schizophrenia. Arch Gen Psychiatry 42:784–791, 1985
28. Heckers S, Heinsen H, Heinsen Y, et al: Limbic structures and lateral ventricle in schizophrenia: a quantitative postmortem study. Arch Gen Psychiatry 47:1016–1022, 1990
29. Conrad AJ, Scheibel AB: Schizophrenia and the hippocampus:

the embryological hypothesis extended. Schizophr Bull 13:577–587, 1987
30. Conrad AJ, Abebe T, Austin R, et al: Hippocampal pyramidal cell disarray in schizophrenia as a bilateral phenomenon. Arch Gen Psychiatry 48:413–417, 1991
31. Altschuler LL, Conrad A, Kovelman JA, et al: Hippocampal cell orientation in schizophrenia. Arch Gen Psychiatry 44:1094–1098, 1987
32. Christison GW, Casanova MF, Weinberger DR, et al: A quantitative investigation of hippocampal pyramidal cell size, shape, and variability of orientation in schizophrenia. Arch Gen Psychiatry 46:1025–1032, 1989
33. Jakob H, Beckman H: Prenatal developmental disturbances in the limbic allocortex in schizophrenics. Journal of Neural Transmission 65:303–326, 1986
34. Papez JW: A proposed mechanism of emotion. Arch Neurol 38:725–743, 1937
35. Carpenter MB: Core Text of Neuroanatomy. Baltimore, MD, Williams & Wilkins, 1985
36. Suddath RL, Casanova MF, Goldberg TE, et al: Temporal lobe pathology in schizophrenia: a quantitative magnetic resonance imaging study. Am J Psychiatry 146:464–472, 1989
37. Shenton ME, Kikinis R, Jolesz FA, et al: Abnormalities of the left temporal lobe and thought disorder in schizophrenia: a quantitative magnetic resonance imaging study. N Engl J Med 327:604–612, 1992
38. Bogerts B, Ashtari M, Degreef G: Reduced temporal limbic structure volumes on magnetic resonance images in first episode schizophrenia. Psychiatry Res 35:1–13, 1990
39. DeLisi LE, Hoff AL, Schwartz JE, et al: Brain morphology in first-episode schizophrenic-like psychotic patients: a quantitative magnetic resonance imaging study. Biol Psychiatry 29:159–175, 1991
40. Barta PE, Pearlson GD, Powers RE, et al: Auditory hallucinations and smaller superior temporal gyral volume. Am J Psychiatry 147:1457–1462, 1990
41. McCarley RW, Shenton ME, O'Donnell BF, et al: P-300 and tem-

poral lobe structures in schizophrenia. New Research Abstracts 451:158, 1992

42. McKenna PJ, Tamlyn D, Lund CE, et al: Amnesic syndrome in schizophrenia. Psychol Med 20:967–972, 1990
43. Weinberger DR: Anteromedial temporal-prefrontal connectivity: a functional neuroanatomical system implicated in schizophrenia, in Psychopathology and the Brain. Edited by Carroll BJ, Barrett JE. New York, Raven, 1991, pp 25–43
44. Milner B, Petrides M: Behavioral effects of frontal-lobe lesion in man. Trends Neurosci 7:403–407, 1984
45. Crighton-Brown J: On the weight of the brain and its component parts in the insane. Brain 2:42–67, 1879
46. Jackson JH: Selected Writing of John Hughlings Jackson, Vol 2. New York, Basic Books, 1958
47. Zec RF, Weinberger DR: Brain areas implicated in schizophrenia, in The Neurology of Schizophrenia. Edited by Nasrallah HA, Weinberger DR. Amsterdam, Elsevier North-Holland, 1986, pp 175–206
48. Milner B: Some effects of frontal lobectomy in man, in The Frontal Granular Cortex and Behavior. Edited by Warren JM, Akert K. New York, McGraw-Hill, 1964, pp 313–334
49. Milner B: Effects of different brain lesions on card sorting: the role of the frontal lobes. Arch Neurol 9:100–110, 1963
50. Shallice T: From Neuropsychology to Mental Structure. Cambridge, Cambridge University Press, 1986
51. Gold JM, Weinberger DR: Frontal lobe, structure, function, and connectivity in schizophrenia, in Neurobiology and Psychiatry, Vol 1. Edited by Kerwin R. Cambridge, Cambridge University Press, 1991, pp 39–59
52. Weinberger DR: A connectionist approach to the prefrontal cortex. J Neuropsychiatry Clin Neurosci 5:241–253, 1993
53. Goldberg TE, Weinberger DR, Berman KF, et al: Further evidence for dementia of the prefrontal type in schizophrenia? Arch Gen Psychiatry 44:1008–1014, 1987
54. Goldberg TE, Weinberger DR: Probing prefrontal function in schizophrenia with neuropsychological paradigms. Schizophr Bull 14:179–183, 1988

55. Goldberg TE, Weinberger DR, Plishkin NH, et al: Recall memory deficit in schizophrenia: a possible manifestation of prefrontal dysfunction. Schizophr Res 2:251–257, 1989
56. Ingvar DH, Frazen G: Distribution of cerebral activity in chronic schizophrenia. Lancet 2:1484–1486, 1974
57. Ingvar DH, Frazen G: Abnormality of cerebral blood flow distribution in patients with chronic schizophrenia. Acta Psychiatr Scand 50:425–462, 1974
58. Frazen G, Ingvar DH: Abnormal distribution of cerebral activity in chronic schizophrenia. J Psychiatr Res 12:199–214, 1975
59. Frazen G, Ingvar DH: Absence of activation in frontal structures during psychological testing of chronic schizophrenics. J Neurol Neurosurg Psychiatry 38:1027–1032, 1975
60. Berman KF, Weinberger DR: Cerebral blood flow studies in schizophrenia, in The Neurology of Schizophrenia. Edited by Nasrallah H, Weinberger DR. Amsterdam, Elsevier North-Holland, 1986, pp 227–307
61. Weinberger DR, Kleinman JE: Observations of the brain in schizophrenia, in Psychiatry Update: American Psychiatric Association Annual Review, Vol 5. Edited by Hales RE, Frances AJ. Washington, DC, American Psychiatric Press, 1986, pp 42–67
62. Buchsbaum MS, Haier RJ. Functional and anatomical brain imaging: impact on schizophrenia research. Schizophr Bull 13: 115–132, 1987
63. Andreason NC, Resai K, Alliger R: Hypofrontality in neuroleptic-naive patients and in patients with schizophrenia. Arch Gen Psychiatry 49:943–958, 1992
64. Wolkin A, Sanfilipo M, Wolf AP, et al: Negative symptoms and hypofrontality in chronic schizophrenia. Arch Gen Psychiatry 49:959–965, 1992
65. Buchsbaum MS, Haier RJ, Potkin SG, et al: Frontostriatal disorder of cerebral metabolism in never-medicated schizophrenics. Arch Gen Psychiatry 49:935–943, 1992
66. Berman KF, Torrey EF, Daniel DG, et al: Regional cerebral blood flow in monozygotic twins discordant for schizophrenia. Arch Gen Psychiatry 49:927–934, 1992
67. Weinberger DR, Berman KF: Speculation on the meaning of

cerebral metabolic hypofrontality in schizophrenia. Schizophr Bull 14:157–167, 1988

68. Lassen NA, Roland PE: Localization of cognitive function with cerebral blood flow, in Localization in Neuropsychology. Edited by Ketresz A. New York, Academic Press, 1983, pp 141–152
69. Muira SA, Schapiro MB, Grady CL, et al: Effect of gender on glucose utilization rates in healthy humans: a positron emission tomography study. J Neurosci Res 27:500–504, 1990
70. Heaton R: Wisconsin Card Sorting Test. Odessa, TX, Psychological Assessment Resources, 1985
71. Franke P, Maier W, Hain C, et al: Wisconsin Card Sorting Test: an indicator of vulnerability to schizophrenia? Schizophr Res 6:243–249, 1992
72. Weinberger DR, Berman KF, Zec RF: Physiological dysfunction of dorsolateral prefrontal cortex in schizophrenia, I: regional cerebral blood flow (rCBF). Arch Gen Psychiatry 43:1199–1202, 1986
73. Berman KF, Zec RF, Weinberger DR: Physiological dysfunction of dorsolateral prefrontal cortex in schizophrenia, II: role of neuroleptic treatment, attention, and mental effort. Arch Gen Psychiatry 43:126–135, 1986
74. Rubin P, Holm S, Friberg L, et al: Altered modulation of prefrontal and subcortical brain activity in newly diagnosed schizophrenia and schizophreniform disorder: a regional cerebral blood flow study. Arch Gen Psychiatry 48:987–995, 1991
75. Berman KF, Randolph C, Gold J, et al: Physiological activation of frontal lobe studied with positron emission tomography and oxygen-15 water during working memory tasks. J Cereb Blood Flow Metab 11:S851, 1991
76. Berman KF, Illowsky BP, Weinberger DR: Physiological dysfunction of dorsolateral prefrontal cortex in schizophrenia. Arch Gen Psychiatry 45:616–622, 1988
77. Berman KF, Torrey EF, Daniel DG, et al: Regional cerebral blood flow in monozygotic twins discordant for schizophrenia. Arch Gen Psychiatry 49:927–934, 1992
78. Chang WH, Hwu HG, Chen TY, et al: Plasma homovanillic acid and treatment response in a large group of schizophrenic pa-

tients. Schizophr Res 10:259–265, 1993

79. Davidson M, Davis KL: A comparison of plasma homovanillic acid concentrations in schizophrenic patients and normal controls. Arch Gen Psychiatry 45:561–563, 1988
80. Maas JW, Contreras SA, Seleshi E, et al: Dopamine metabolism and disposition in schizophrenic patients. Arch Gen Psychiatry 45:553–559, 1988
81. Shapiro RM: Regional neuropathology in schizophrenia: where are we? where are we going? Psychiatry Res 10:187–239, 1993
82. Crawley JCW, Crow TJ, Johnstone EC, et al: Dopamine D2 receptors in schizophrenia studied in vivo. Lancet ii 26:224–225, 1986
83. Wong DF, Wagner HN, Tune LE, et al: Positron emission tomography reveals elevated D_2 dopamine receptors in drug naive schizophrenics. Science 234:1558–1563, 1986
84. Farde L, Ehrin E, Eriksson L, et al: Substitute benzamines as ligands for visualization of dopamine receptor binding in the human brain by positron emission tomography. Proc Natl Acad Sci U S A 82:3863–3867, 1985
85. Farde L, Hall H, Ehrin E, et al: Quantitative analysis of D_2 dopamine receptor binding in the living human brain by PET. Science 231:258–259, 1986
86. Farde L, Weisel FA, Stone-Elander S, et al: Dopamine receptors in neuroleptic-naive schizophrenic patients: a positron emission tomography study with ^{11}C-raclopride. Arch Gen Psychiatry 47: 213–219, 1990
87. Martinot JL, Peron-Magnan P, Huret JD, et al: Striatal D_2 dopaminergic receptors assessed with positron emission tomography and [^{76}Br]bromospiperone in untreated schizophrenic patients. Am J Psychiatry 147:44–50, 1990
88. Gur RE, Pearlson GD: Neuroimaging in schizophrenia research. Schizophr Bull 19:337–353, 1993
89. Weinberger DR, Berman KF, Illowsky BP: Physiological dysfunction of dorsolateral prefrontal cortex in schizophrenia, III: a new cohort and evidence for a monoaminergic mechanism. Arch Gen Psychiatry 45:609–615, 1988
90. McClelland JL, Rumelhart DE, Hinton GE: The appeal of parallel

distributed processing, in Parallel Distributed Processing: Explorations in the Microstructure of Cognition, Vol 1: Foundations. Edited by Rumelhart DE, McClelland JL, and the Parallel Distributed Processing Research Group. Cambridge, MA, MIT Press, 1986, pp 3–44

91. Liddle PF, Friston KJ, Frith CD, et al: Patterns of cerebral blood flow in schizophrenia. Br J Psychiatry 160:179–186, 1992
92. Friston KJ, Liddle PF, Frith CD, et al: The left medial temporal region and schizophrenia. Brain 115:367–382, 1992
93. Liddle PF: The symptoms of chronic schizophrenia: a re-examination of the positive-negative dichotomy. Br J Psychiatry 151: 145–151, 1987
94. Liddle PF, Barnes TRE: Syndromes of chronic schizophrenia. Br J Psychiatry 157:558–561, 1990
95. Weinberger DR: Implications of normal brain development for the pathogenesis of schizophrenia. Arch Gen Psychiatry 44:660–669, 1987
96. Weinberger DR, Berman KF, Suddath R, et al: Evidence of dysfunction of a prefrontal-limbic network in schizophrenia: a magnetic resonance imaging and regional cerebral blood flow study of discordant monozygotic twins. Am J Psychiatry 149:890–897, 1992
97. Frith CD, Done DJ: Towards a neuropsychology of schizophrenia. Br J Psychiatry 153:437–443, 1988
98. Corballis MC: The Lopsided Ape: Evolution of the Generative Mind. Oxford, Oxford University Press, 1992
99. Hermelin B, O'Conner N: Psychological Experiments with Autistic Children. Oxford, Pergamon, 1970
100. Hauer SL, DeLong GR, Roseman NP: Pneumographic findings in the infantile autism syndrome: a correlation with temporal lobe disease. Brain 98:667–688, 1975
101. Orton ST: Reading, Writing and Speech Problems in Children. London, Chapman and Hall, 1937
102. Hynd GW, Semrud-Clikeman M: Dyslexia and brain morphology. Psychol Bull 106:447–482, 1989
103. Galin D: Implications for psychiatry of left and right specialization. Arch Gen Psychiatry 31:572–583, 1974

104. Galin D, Diamond R, Braff D: Lateralization of conversion syndrome: more frequency of the left. Am J Psychiatry 134:578–583, 1977
105. Harrington A: Nineteenth century ideas on hemisphere differences and "duality of mind." Behavioral and Brain Sciences 8:617–660, 1985
106. Flor-Henry P: Psychosis and temporal lobe epilepsy: a controlled investigation. Epilepsia 10:363–395, 1969
107. Flor-Henry P: Schizophrenia-like reactions and affective psychosis associated with temporal lobe epilepsy: etiological factors. Am J Psychiatry 126:400–404, 1969
108. Crow TJ, Ball J, Bloom SR, et al: Schizophrenia as an anomaly of development of cerebral asymmetry: a postmortem study and a proposal concerning the genetic basis of the disease. Arch Gen Psychiatry 47:213–219, 1990
109. Crow TJ, Colter N, Frith CD, et al: Developmental arrest of cerebral asymmetries in early onset schizophrenia. Psychiatry Res 29:247–253, 1989
110. Crow TJ: Temporal lobe asymmetries as the key to the etiology of schizophrenia. Schizophr Bull 16:433–443, 1990
111. Annett M: Left, Right, Hand and Brain. London, Lawrence Erlbaum, 1985
112. Crow TJ: Neuropathology of schizophrenia: asymmetry as a clue to etiology. Transmissions: Biological Psychiatry in Clinical Practice 1:4–11, 1990
113. Collinge J, DeLisi LE, Boccio A, et al: Evidence for a pseudoautosomal locus for schizophrenia using the method of affected sibling pairs. Br J Psychiatry 158:624–629, 1991
114. Bartley AJ, Jones DW, Torrey EF, et al: Sylvian fissure asymmetries in monozygotic twins: a test of laterality in schizophrenia. Biol Psychiatry 43:853–863, 1993
115. Mesulam MM: Letter to the editor. N Engl J Med 323:548, 1990
116. Luchins DJ, Weinberger DR, Wyatt RJ: Schizophrenia: evidence of a subgroup with reversed cerebral asymmetry. Arch Gen Psychiatry 36:1309–1311, 1979
117. Luchins DJ, Weinberger DR, Wyatt RJ: Schizophrenia and cerebral asymmetry detected by computed tomography. Am J Psy-

chiatry 139:753–757, 1982
118. Andreason NC, Dennert JW, Olsen SA, et al: Hemispheric asymmetry and schizophrenia. Am J Psychiatry 139:427–430, 1982
119. Jernigan TL, Zatz LM, Moses JA, et al: Computed tomography in schizophrenics and normal volunteers, II: cranial asymmetry. Arch Gen Psychiatry 39:771–773, 1982
120. Golden CJ, Graber B, Coffman J, et al: Brain density deficits in chronic schizophrenia. Psychiatry Res 3:179–184, 1981
121. Largen JW, Calderon M, Smith RC: Asymmetries in the density of white and grey matter in the brains of schizophrenic patients. Am J Psychiatry 140:1060–1062, 1983
122. Largen JW, Smith RC, Calderon M, et al: Abnormalities of brain structure and density in schizophrenia. Biol Psychiatry 19:991–1013, 1984
123. Reveley MA, Reveley AM, Baldy R: Left cerebral hemisphere hypodensity in discordant schizophrenic twins. Arch Gen Psychiatry 44:625–632, 1987
124. Johnstone EC, Owens DCG, Crow TJ, et al: Temporal lobe structure as determined by magnetic resonance in schizophrenia and bipolar affective disorder. J Neurol Neurosurg Psychiatry 52: 736–741, 1989
125. Gur RE: Left-hemisphere dysfunction and left-hemisphere overactivation. J Abnorm Psychol 87:226–238, 1978
126. Gur RE, Gur RC, Skonick BE, et al: Brain function in psychiatric disorders, III: regional blood flow in unmedicated schizophrenics. Arch Gen Psychiatry 42:329–334, 1985
127. Gur RE, Resnick SM, Alavi A, et al: Regional brain function in schizophrenia, II: repeated evaluation with positron emission tomography. Arch Gen Psychiatry 44:126–129, 1987
128. Levy AV, Laska E, Brodie JD, et al: The spectral signature method for the analysis of PET images. J Cereb Blood Flow Metab 11: 103–113, 1990
129. DeLisi LE, Buchsbaum MS, Holcomb HH, et al: Increased temporal lobe glucose use in chronic schizophrenic patients. Biol Psychiatry 25:835–851, 1989
130. Brodie JD, Christman DR, Corona JF, et al: Patterns of metabolic activity in the treatment of schizophrenia. Ann Neurol 15:S166–

S169, 1984
131. Kling AS, Metter EJ, Reige WH, et al: Comparison of PET measurement of local glucose metabolism and CAT measurement of brain atrophy in chronic schizophrenia and depression. Am J Psychiatry 143:175–180, 1986
132. Volkow ND, Wolf AP, Van Gelder P, et al: Phenomenological correlates of metabolic activity in 18 patients with chronic schizophrenia. Am J Psychiatry 144:151–158, 1987
133. Buchsbaum MS, Ingvar DH, Kessler R, et al: Cerebral glucography with positron emission tomography use in normal subjects and inpatients with schizophrenia. Arch Gen Psychiatry 39:251–259, 1982
134. Paulman RG, Devous MD, Gregory RR: Hypofrontality and cognitive impairment in schizophrenia: dynamic single-photon tomography and neuropsychological assessment of schizophrenic brain function. Biol Psychiatry 27:377–399, 1990
135. Robertson G, Taylor PJ: Laterality and psychosis: neuropsychological evidence. Br Med Bull 43:634–650, 1987
136. Breslin NA, Weinberger DR: Neurodevelopmental implications of findings from brain imaging studies of schizophrenia, in Fetal Neurodevelopment and Adult Schizophrenia. Edited by Mednick SA, Cannon TD, Barr CE, et al. Cambridge, Cambridge University Press, 1991, pp 199–215
137. Cornblatt BA, Erlenmeyer-Kimling L: Global attentional deviance in children at risk for schizophrenia: specificity and predictive validity. J Abnorm Psychol 94:470–486, 1985
138. Cornblatt BA, Erlenmeyer-Kimling L: Social competence and positive and negative symptoms: a longitudinal study of children and adolescents at risk for schizophrenia and affective disorder. Am J Psychiatry 148:1182–1188, 1991
139. Beatty WW, Jocic Z, Monson N: Memory and frontal lobe dysfunction in schizophrenia and schizoaffective disorder. J Nerv Ment Dis 181:448–453, 1993
140. Dworkin RH, Bernstein G, Kaplansky LM, et al: Prediction of adult-onset schizophrenia from childhood home movies of patients. Am J Psychiatry 147:1052–1056, 1990
141. Kovelman JA, Scheibel AB: A neurohistological correlate of

schizophrenia. Biol Psychiatry 19:1601–1621, 1984
142. Lewis SW, Murray RM: Obstetric complications, neurodevelopmental deviance and risk of schizophrenia. J Psychiatr Res 21: 413–421, 1987
143. Murray RM, Lewis SW, Owen MJ, et al: The neurodevelopmental origins of dementia praecox, in Schizophrenia: The Major Issues. Edited by McGuffin P, Bebbington P. London, Heinemann, 1988, pp 90–107
144. Scheibel AB, Kovelman JB: Disorientation of the hippocampal pyramidal cells and its process in the schizophrenic patient. Biol Psychiatry 16:101–102, 1981
145. Lipska BK, Jaskiw GE, Chrapusta S, et al: Ibotenic acid lesion of the ventral hippocampus differentially affects dopamine and its metabolites in the nucleus accumbens and prefrontal cortex in the rat. Brain Res 585:1–6, 1992
146. Weinberger DR, Lipska BK: Cortical maldevelopment, antipsychotic drugs, and schizophrenia: a neuroanatomical reductionism. Schizophr Res, in press
147. Glowinski J, Tassin JP, Theirry AM: The mesocortico-prefrontal dopaminergic neurons. Trends Neurosci 7:415–418, 1984
148. Mesulam MM: Large-scale neurocognitive networks and distributed processing for attention, language, and memory. Ann Neurol 28:597–613, 1990
149. Berquier A, Ashton R: A selective review of possible neurological etiologies of schizophrenia. Clinical Psychology Review 11:645–661, 1991

CHAPTER

15

Abnormal Frontotemporal Interactions in Patients With Schizophrenia

Karl J. Friston, B.A., M.A.
Sigrid Herold, B.M., B.Ch., M.R.C.Psych.
P. Fletcher, M.B.B.S.
D. Silbersweig, M.D.
C. Cahill, B.Sc.
R. J. Dolan, M.D.
P. F. Liddle, B.M., B.Ch., Ph.D.
R. S. J. Frackowiak, M.A., M.D., F.R.C.P.
C. D. Frith, Ph.D.

The purpose of this work was to use neuroimaging data and the concept of functional connectivity to examine cortico-cortical interactions in patients with schizophrenia. In the context of neuroimaging, functional connectivity is a

---

Dedicated to the memory of Sigrid Herold, our valued friend and colleague, who died during the completion of this work.

Karl Friston was funded by the Wellcome Trust during this work.

relatively new concept and provides a powerful way of characterizing distributed changes in the brain.

The notion that schizophrenia represents a disintegration or fractionation of the psyche is as old as its name, which was introduced by Bleuler[1] to convey a splitting of mental faculties. Many of Bleuler's primary processes, such as "loosening of associations," emphasize a fragmentation and loss of coherent integration. For example, in patients with inappropriate affect, he describes a "tendency of the feelings to work independently of each other."[2] In this chapter, we test the hypothesis that this mentalistic splitting has a physiological basis and, furthermore, that it has a precise and regionally specific character.

Abnormal Frontotemporal Interactions in Patients With Schizophrenia

Abnormal integration of prefrontal neural activity and activity in subcortical, limbic, and temporal structures is a common theme found in many neurobiological accounts of schizophrenia. For example, neurodevelopmental models of schizophrenia[3,4] refer to the concurrent maturation of the frontal lobes in terms of myelination and the emergence of schizophrenic phenomena. Between the ages of 16 and 22, there is evidence for progressive changes in the nature of cortical interactions (as measured by electroencephalography), particularly between the left prefrontal and temporal regions.[5] The pathophysiological basis of abnormal cognitive processing in schizophrenia has been discussed in terms of abnormal frontostriatal and frontotemporal integration.[6,7] Interpretations of (glutaminergic) neurochemical abnormalities in prefrontal and left temporal regions refer to the anatomical connections between these regions.[8]

The evidence for structural and functional abnormalities in both the prefrontal cortices and temporal lobes is strong, particularly in the left hemisphere. This evidence ranges from abnormal quantitative cytoarchitecture[9] to gross morphological changes evident on magnetic resonance imaging (MRI) scans[10] and postmortem examination.[11] Functional abnormalities have been demonstrated with positron-emission tomography (PET)[12] and electrophysiology.[13] Less direct evidence exists, however, for an abnormal integration of prefrontal and temporal cortical activity. The aim of this chapter is to provide such evidence or at least a method for obtaining it and some provisional results.

Functional Connectivity

A single cortical region is implicated in a distributed system by virtue of its functional interactions with other regions. The identification of distributed systems therefore relies on the characterization of neuronal interactions and correlations. In the past two decades, the concepts of functional and effective connectivity have been most thoroughly elaborated in the analysis of multiunit recordings of separable neuronal spike trains obtained simultaneously from different brain areas.[14] Temporal coherence among the activity of different neurons is commonly measured by cross-correlating their spike trains. The resulting correlograms are then interpreted as a signature of functional connectivity.[15,16] In neuroimaging, *functional connectivity* refers to the observed temporal correlation between two electro/neurophysiological measurements from different parts of the brain[17] and can be defined as the temporal correlation between spatially remote neurophysiological events.

This chapter is presented in four sections and concludes with a discussion. The first section describes the nature of the data, the experimental paradigm, and the subjects involved. The second section addresses quantitative differences in the amount of functional connectivity exhibited among different groups of schizophrenic patients and control subjects. The third section characterizes and compares the principal patterns of correlated activity (eigenimages, or spatial modes) for each group. The final section identifies the principal qualitative difference in functional connectivity between patients with schizophrenia and normal subjects in terms of a single distributed pattern of cerebral activity.

The Data

Data Acquisition and Preprocessing

The data were acquired from four groups of six subjects with a PET camera (CTI model 93108/12, Knoxville, Tennessee), using a fast dynamic ^{15}O technique.[18] The reconstructed images had a resolution of about 8.5 mm.[19] Each subject was scanned six times, approximately every 8 minutes, during the performance of three word-production tasks. Each scan lasted for 2 minutes.

The integrated counts per pixel during this time served as an estimate of regional cerebral blood flow (rCBF). The order of the tasks performed was balanced for time effects (A, B, C, C, B, A). Task A was a verbal fluency task requiring subjects to respond to an aurally presented letter with a word that began with that letter. Task B was a semantic categorization task in which the subject responded with "man-made" or "natural," depending on the noun heard. Task C was a word-shadowing task in which the subject simply repeated what was heard. Task C can be thought of as the sensorimotor control for the other two tasks. Words were presented at a rate of one every 5 seconds.

In the context of this analysis, the detailed nature of the tasks is not very important. The tasks were used to introduce variance and covariance that could support an analysis of functional connectivity in terms of cerebral physiology. The choice of tasks is crucial, however, in the sense that they selectively engage specific brain systems and consequently constrain the cortico-cortical interactions that can be examined. The tasks used typically evoke large and widespread rCBF changes in the prefrontal, cingulate, and temporal regions.[20–22]

All the images were stereotactically normalized and mapped into the standard space described by the atlas of Talaraich and Tournoux.[23–25] Voxel differences in rCBF that were due simply to whole-brain or global differences were removed by using analysis of covariance (ANCOVA) for each of the four groups.[26] A mean rCBF estimate for each voxel, for each of the six conditions (scans), and for each group was obtained by averaging the results obtained for six subjects in each group. A subset of voxels was selected for further analysis if the differences between any of the six scans accounted for a significant amount of variance (ANCOVA $F > 3.9$; $P < .001$; df = 5, 24) in one or more of the four groups.

The result was a large matrix of rCBF estimates for each of the four groups, comprising six rows (one for each scan) and 4,802 columns (one for each voxel). The data matrices (*M*) were normalized to a mean of 0 over columns. This subset of voxels is displayed as a statistical parametric map[27] in Figure 15–1. This statistical parametric map is of the average *F* value (from the ANCOVAs) displayed as a maximum-intensity projection, viewing the brain from the side, from above, and from the back. The experimentally introduced physiological variance was evident in a large and distributed set of cerebral regions. As predicted, the left prefrontal and temporal areas were particularly affected.

Subjects

The four groups comprised one group of six control subjects and three groups of six schizophrenic patients (DSM-III-R[28]). The patients were drawn from a cohort of outpatients and inpatients who were under the supervision of a large psychiatric rehabilitation department. The patients all had disease that was relatively chronic and stable and were middle aged to elderly (age range, 45–70 years). All patients were receiving medication.

The schizophrenic groups were categorized according to their performance on a series of verbal fluency tasks. The first group (termed *poverty*) produced fewer than 24 words on a standard (1-minute) FAS verbal fluency task. The other groups all produced more than 24 words. The second schizophrenic group (*odd*) produced neologisms, words not in the semantic category specified, and/or five or more unusual words. *Unusualness* was defined according to the category norms of Battig and Montague.[29] The third group was *unimpaired* according to the above criteria. Although this categorization is explicitly based on performance on psychological

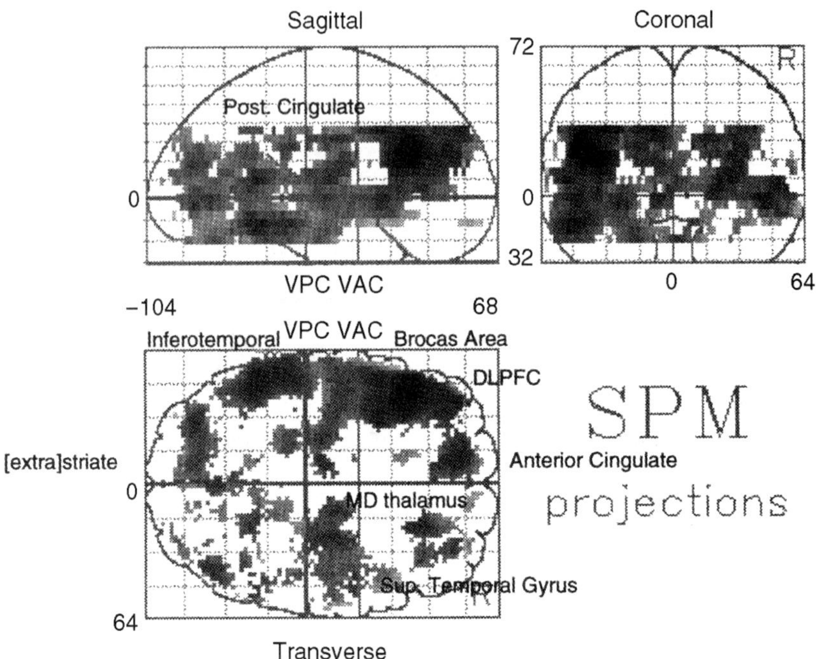

Figure 15–1. Statistical parametric map of the average *F* ratio over all four groups of subjects for each voxel. The *F* ratio reflects the physiological variance introduced by experimental design (relative to the underlying error variance). The display format is standard in statistical parametric mapping and represents a maximum intensity projection from three orthogonal views of the brain (from the right, from behind, and from above). Many brain areas have been engaged, including the prefrontal and temporal regions. VPC, VAC = verticals passing through the posterior and anterior commissures, respectively. DLPFC = dorsolateral prefrontal cortex. MD = mediodorsal.

tests that are germane to the activation paradigm employed, the three groups can be loosely identified with the three dimensions commonly found in clinical ratings of schizophrenia:[30–33]

1. *Psychomotor poverty*, characterized by reduced speech, spontaneous movement, and flattened affect
2. *Disorganization*, associated with inappropriate affect, thought disorder, incoherence, and poverty of content of speech

3. *Reality distortion*, with hallucinations and delusions but less neuropsychological impairment[34]

This categorization of schizophrenic patients is described here for completeness. In this chapter, we address only the differences between schizophrenic and control subjects. The differences among the three schizophrenic groups and their relationship to clinical subsyndromes will be discussed in a further communication.

In what follows, three related examinations of functional connectivity are presented. The first addresses quantitative differences between normal subjects and schizophrenic patients, and the second two address qualitative differences. Because functional connectivity is defined in terms of correlations (or, more generally, covariance), the analyses that follow all pertain to the four covariance matrices (C) associated with the data matrices (M) described above. These covariances are over time (scans) and between different regions (voxels).

Differences in Amount of Functional Connectivity

A useful index of the overall amount of functional connectivity, or covariance, is the Frobenius norm of the covariance matrix, or C. Vector and matrix norms serve the same purpose as absolute values for single scalar quantities. In other words, they furnish a measure of distance. One of the most frequently used norms is the Frobenius norm, $||\cdot||_F$, which is the square root of the sum of the squares of all the matrix elements:

$$||C||_F = \sqrt{\sum_{i,j} C_{ij}^2} \qquad 1$$

where C is a (real symmetric positive definite) covariance matrix ($C = M^T \cdot M$). We will use $|\cdot|$ for vector norms and $||\cdot||$ for matrix norms. From a computational perspective, a useful property of Frobenius norms is that they are invariant under orthogonal transformations. Let the eigenvector (or singular vector) solution of C be denoted by the matrix $U = [u_1, \ldots\ldots, un]$, where $n =$ rank(M):

$$U^T \cdot C \cdot U = \mathrm{diag}(\lambda_i, \ldots\ldots, \lambda_n) \qquad 2$$

where λ_i is the ith largest eigenvalue (or singular value). Therefore:

$$\| C \|_F = \sqrt{\sum_i \lambda_i^2} \qquad 3$$

The importance of the last equation is that the eigenvalues or singular values can be computed directly from M without having to compute the (vast) covariance matrix C. For those familiar with principal-component analysis, the columns of U represent the principal components. Consequently, a covariance structure that is characterized by a small number of principal components with large eigenvalues will have a large Frobenius norm (for a given total variance $= \sum_i \lambda_i$).

Figure 15–2 presents the Frobenius norms for the control group and the three schizophrenic groups. It is immediately obvious that the control subjects and the poverty group have a greater total amount of functional connectivity than do the remaining schizophrenic groups. This finding could mean that the poverty group has a normal amount of connectivity or that the particular disintegration associated with this group (if it exists) is between regions that did not show concurrent activation in the tasks used. There is reason to conjecture that dysfunctional interactions in psychomotor poverty are likely to be found in the frontostriatal system (see "Discussion" in this chapter). If this is the case, we would not expect to see any difference in the present study, which focused on frontotemporal interactions.

Characterizing functional connectivity with the Frobenius norm of the covariance matrix is totally insensitive to the spatial organization of the covariances. This follows from the fact that the Frobenius norm is unchanged by orthogonal rotations. A richer picture is obtained by asking what spatially distributed patterns of correlated activity best account for the observed variance-covariance structure. The identification of these patterns is the subject of the next section.

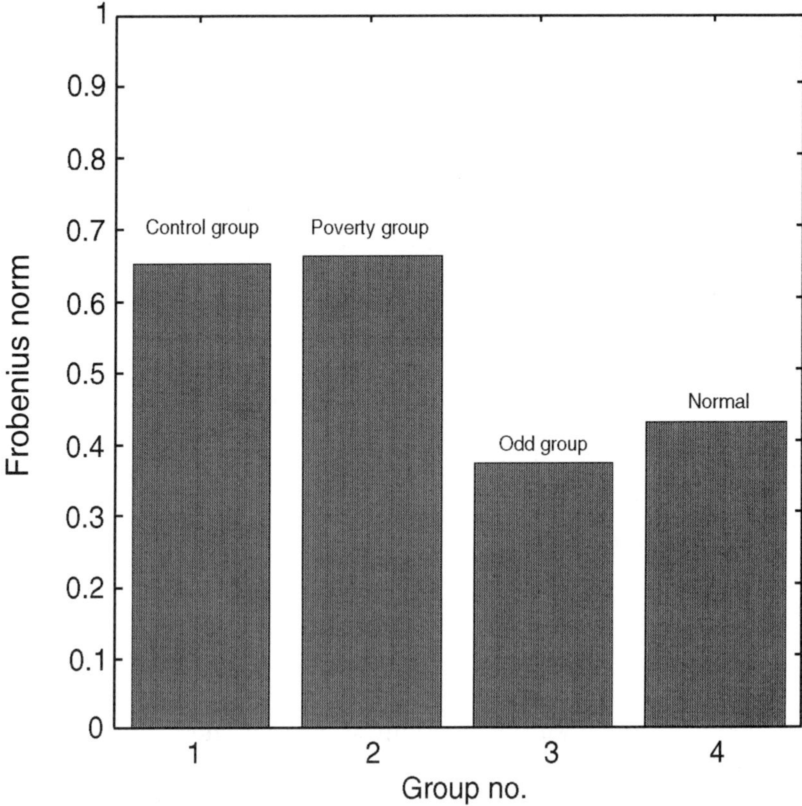

Figure 15–2. Comparison of the total amount of functional connectivity in the four groups of subjects studied. The amount of functional connectivity was measured using the Frobenius norm of the appropriate covariance matrix.

Distributed Patterns of Activity Defined by Functional Connectivity

Functional connectivity is defined in terms of covariance. The point-to-point functional connectivity (covariance) between any one voxel and another is not usually of great interest. The important aspects of the covariance structure are the patterns of correlated activity, which are subtended by individual pairwise covariances. It is useful here to introduce another norm, the 2-norm, which can be used to measure the degree to which a particular pattern of brain activity contributes to the covariance structure. The vector 2-norm is simply the length of the vector in its space. If a pattern is described by a vector (x), with an element for each voxel, then the contribution of that pattern to the covariance structure can be measured by the increase (or decrease) in length it experiences when multiplied by M. This measure is provided by the 2-norm of $M \cdot x = | M \cdot x |_2$. For mathematical expediency, we will work with the square of the 2-norm.

$$| M \cdot x |_2^2 = x^T \cdot M^T \cdot M \cdot x \qquad 4$$

The most prevalent pattern maximizes this 2-norm measure and is simply the eigenvector associated with the largest eigenvalue (u_1). The corresponding eigenvalue is also the *matrix* 2-norm:

$$\max_{|x|_2 = 1} | M \cdot x |_2^2 = || M ||_2^2 = \lambda_1 \qquad 5$$

The pattern of activity defined by u_1 represents a distributed profile that accounts for the most variance-covariance of all possible patterns. The eigenvector can be displayed as an image and is then referred to as an *eigenimage*. Again, note that the first eigenimage is simply the first principal component of the data. It is informative to consider these eigenimages in terms of the Frobenius norm. From equation 3 we can also interpret the (square of the) eigenvalue as the contribution to the (square of the) total amount of functional connectivity due to its corresponding eigenimage or pattern. More generally, the amount of functional connectivity (squared) attributable to a distributed brain system described by x is given by $| M \cdot x |_2^2$. The system that contributes to or accounts for the greatest amount is the first eigenimage.

This approach of decomposing the covariance structure into a small number of important patterns is an extremely powerful way of reorganizing data. It is well established in the electrophysiological literature, where the eigenimages are sometimes referred to as *spatial modes*.

The first eigenimage, based on the data from control subjects, is presented in Figure 15–3. The positive and negative parts are presented at the top left and right, respectively. This pattern involves primarily the left dorsolateral prefrontal cortex and the superior temporal regions, bilaterally, in auditory and periauditory cortex (with some left posterior/occipitotemporal contribution). The corresponding eigenvalue is seen on the lower left and is more than twice the second largest. The first two eigenvectors account for

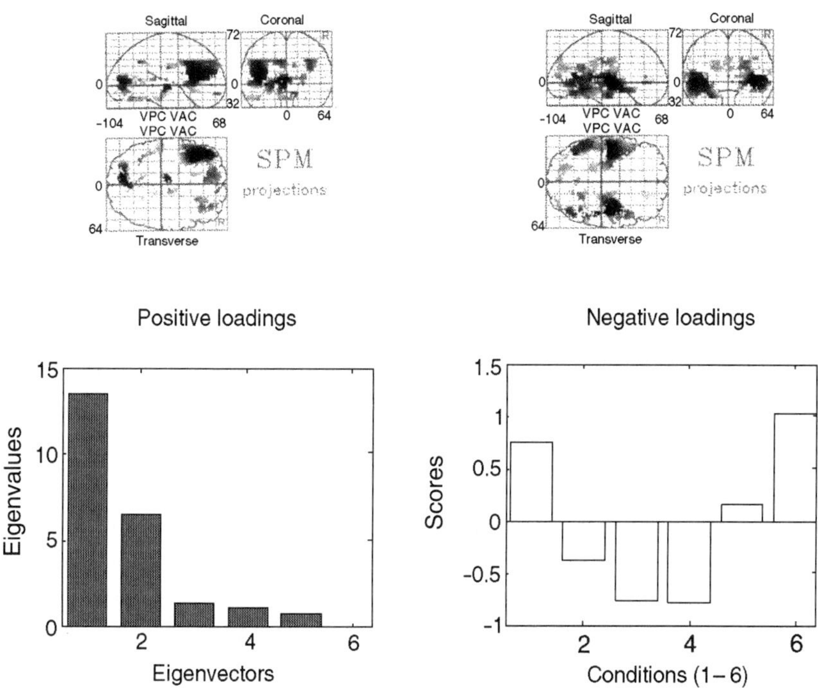

Figure 15–3. Eigenimage analysis of control subjects. *Top left and right:* Positive and negative loadings of the first eigenimage (the most prevalent pattern of correlated activity). The gray scale is arbitrary, and each image has been normalized to the image maximum. The display format is as shown in Figure 15–1. *Bottom left:* Distribution of eigenvalues associated with the first and subsequent eigenimages. *Bottom right:* Degree to which the first eigenimage was expressed during the six scans (as measured by the inner product of the eigenimage and the profile of activity for each condition). The order of tasks was verbal fluency, semantic categorization, word shadowing, word shadowing, semantic categorization, and verbal fluency. SPM = statistical parametric map. VPC, VAC = verticals passing through the posterior and anterior commissures, respectively.

nearly all the variance-covariance observed. This is not uncommon in the analysis of activation studies. The scores on the lower right reflect the degree to which the first eigenimage pattern was expressed during the six scans. It is obvious that this pattern is maximally expressed during the verbal fluency tasks and minimally so in the baseline word-shadowing tasks. In summary, this pattern represented profound negative frontosuperior temporal functional interactions associated with intrinsic word generation. This is almost an exact replication of previous work.[17]

The corresponding first eigenimages from the three schizophrenic groups are presented in Figure 15–4. There are several important observations to be made. First, the three patterns are remarkably similar. This is very pleasing, considering that they were based on completely independent data. Second, they are very different from the normal pattern. Although frontotemporal interactions are the most prominent features of these eigenimages, the correlations are positive, are most evident between left prefrontal and left inferotemporal and middle temporal regions, and the temporal component of this system is not symmetrical. The negative parts of the eigenimages are not shown because most of the substantial values were positive with scant negative components (see Figure 15–4, *bottom right*). In no instance did the negative components involve the temporal lobes. In summary, all three groups of schizophrenic patients exhibited very similar patterns of distributed activity, involving positive interactions between the left prefrontal cortex and the left inferotemporal and middle temporal regions.

Differences Between the Distributed Patterns of Activity

In this, the final section, we present a slightly more formal analysis of the differences between the patterns of correlated activity in control subjects and schizophrenic patients. In the same sense that the (square of the) 2-norm was used as a measure of the prevalence of a particular pattern, it can also be used to identify the pattern ac-

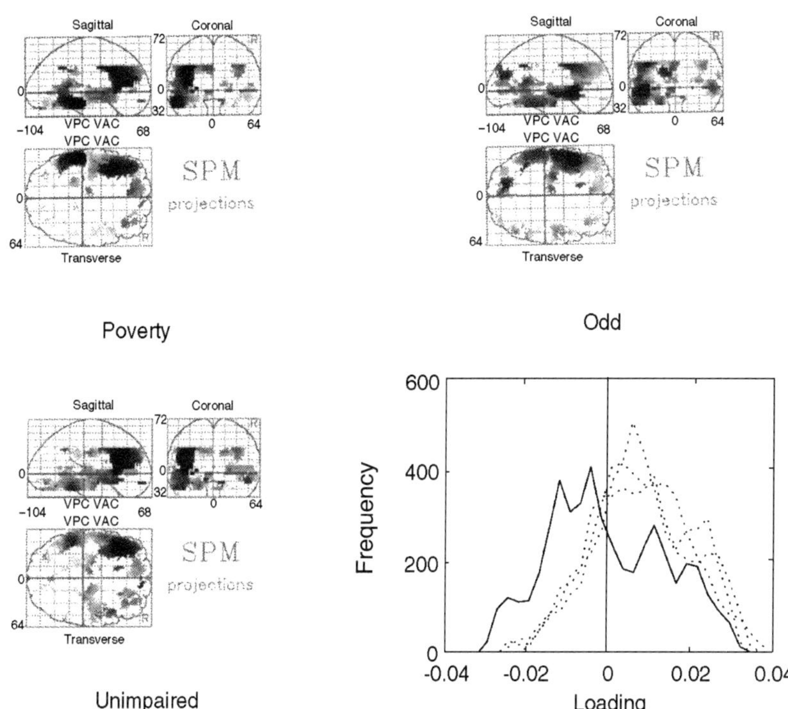

Figure 15–4. First eigenimages for each of the schizophrenic groups. The display format is the same as shown in Figure 15–3. Only positive loadings are shown. *Lower right:* Frequency distribution of the voxel values (loadings) of each of the three eigenimages from the schizophrenic groups *(broken lines)* and the control subjects *(solid line).* These data are presented to show that the negative loadings are poorly represented in the schizophrenia data when compared with the bimodal distribution obtained in normal subjects. SPM = statistical parametric map. VPC, VAC = verticals passing through the posterior and anterior commissures, respectively.

counting for the major differences between two sets of data. More precisely, we want to find the pattern that maximizes:

$$\max_{|x|2=1}(|M_c \cdot x|_2^2 - |M_s \cdot x|_2^2) \qquad 6$$

where M_c and M_s are the data from the control subjects and schizophrenic patients, respectively. The solution to equation 6 is simply the first eigenvector of the covariance matrices due to control subjects minus that from the schizophrenic groups ($C_c - C_s$). C_s

was the average of the three covariance matrices from the three schizophrenic groups. This pooling can be justified given the similarity between the covariance structure of the three groups and, in this chapter, the fact that we are interested in the differences common to all schizophrenic groups.

The results of this analysis are presented in Figure 15–5. It is not surprising to see that the pattern that best captures the differences is very similar to the pattern that is most prevalent in the control subjects, namely, an integrated negative correlation between the left dorsolateral prefrontal cortex and the bilateral superior and left inferotemporal regions. The amount to which this pattern was expressed in each individual group is shown in the lower half of Figure 15–5, using the (square of the) appropriate 2-norm. It is seen that this distributed pattern of activity, although prevalent in the control subjects, is virtually absent in all three of the schizophrenic groups. Equivalently, the substantial frontotemporal functional connectivity within the system portrayed in Figure 15–5 is not found in the schizophrenic data.

It is worth considering this approach to discriminating between data from two sets of subjects in terms of multivariate linear regression. The problem of discerning between neurophysiological patterns of activity in control subjects and schizophrenic patients can be reformulated in terms of prediction, namely, given a set of measures (predictors), what linear combination best predicts group membership (predicted variable). Normally in multivariate regression the linear combination of measures, whose mean (first-order moment) best predicts group membership, is identified. In the current approach, one finds the linear combination of predictors whose sum of squares, or second-order characteristics, are the best predictor. This second-order characteristic (square of the 2-norm) can be directly interpreted in terms of functional connectivity.

Discussion

We have analyzed cortical interactions in control subjects and schizophrenic subjects by using the concept of functional connec-

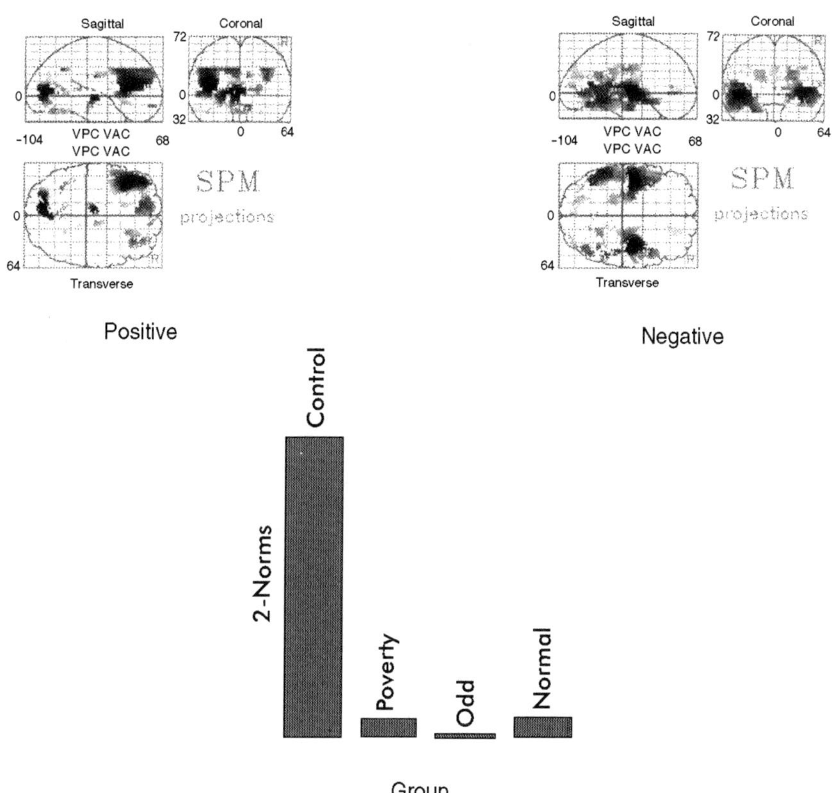

Figure 15–5. Eigenimage analysis of the covariance differences between normal subjects and (pooled) schizophrenic patients *(top)*. The statistical parametric maps (SPMs) depict positive and negative components of the eigenimage or pattern that represents the largest difference between the two covariance structures. In fact, this difference is attributable to its virtual absence in the schizophrenic data. This point is made by expressing the amount of functional connectivity attributable to this system in each of the four groups, using the appropriate 2-norm *(bottom)*. VPC, VAC = verticals passing through the posterior and anterior commissures, respectively.

tivity. In comparison with normal subjects, the schizophrenic groups were characterized by an overall reduction in the amount of functional connectivity (with some qualifications) and a very different pattern of distributed cerebral physiology. The nature of this difference was remarkably consistent among the groups of schizophrenic patients analyzed. The main differences between control subjects and schizophrenic patients was a double dissociation in terms of regionally specific frontotemporal functional connectivity: profound left prefrontosuperior temporal interactions were seen in normal subjects but not in schizophrenic patients, and marked left prefronto-left infero/middle temporal correlations were marked in the schizophrenic groups but less so in normal subjects. A further qualitative difference was that the frontotemporal covariances were measured as negative in normal subjects but as positive in schizophrenic patients.

These results indicate not only regionally specific and consistent differences in functional connectivity, but also a complete reversal in the nature of the large-scale frontotemporal interactions. This reversal might be viewed as a failure of the prefrontal cortex to suppress activity in the temporal lobes (or vice versa). We now discuss several aspects of abnormal cortico-cortical interactions in patients with schizophrenia, with an emphasis on frontotemporal integration. The neuropsychological arguments presented here are based on a more wide-ranging and complete analysis that can be found in the monograph by Frith.[35]

Intrinsically and Extrinsically Cued Behavior

Underlying our thinking about the nature of frontotemporal interactions is an assumption that the prefrontal cortices are necessary for intrinsically generated behavior and that the temporal cortices (in the context of word generation) are necessary for extrinsically generated responses. The evidence for this association derives from studies of patients with neurological problems, unit recording studies in behaving primates, and functional imaging studies during cognitive activation.

Psychomotor poverty in patients with schizophrenia is closely related to psychomotor retardation,[36] which includes decreased spontaneous movement, decreased communication, flatness of vocal inflection, unchanging facial expression, and social withdrawal.

Among the most common causes of psychomotor retardation is damage to the frontal lobes and Parkinson's disease. In particular, patients with damage to the anterior cingulate and/or the supplementary motor area tend to become mute and show decreased spontaneous movement.[37] Passingham et al.[38] demonstrated that lesions in the supplementary motor area and anterior cingulate in monkeys impair responses when the movement is self-initiated but have little effect when the movement is extrinsically cued. Largely akinetic patients with Parkinson's disease can show a dissociation between movements that are self-initiated and those that are extrinsically cued (e.g., paradoxical kinesis[39]).

Clearly, the pathophysiology of Parkinson's disease and prefrontal cortical damage are different, and yet there are some behavioral homologies. A parsimonious explanation is that normal frontostriatal integration is necessary for intrinsically generated behavior. Robbins[6] has reviewed the case for frontostriatal dysfunction in patients with schizophrenia. He comes down in favor of such a hypothesis and concludes that the pathophysiological basis of schizophrenia is unlikely to be found in a single area but is more likely to be associated with dysfunctional integration in the corticostriatal loops.

These observations are very consistent with some of our own findings with PET. The fact that the prefrontal cortices of control subjects are activated by tasks that involve intrinsic generation of representations and that are, by implication, mnemonic is now well established.[20,40] An even more specific and relevant finding was presented in our cross-sectional study of regional physiology in patients with schizophrenia:[12] rCBF was correlated with symptom severity in 30 patients with schizophrenia as defined by DSM-III-R criteria.[28] Significant negative correlations where found in the dorsolateral prefrontal cortex (with a left-sided emphasis). Significant positive correlations were found in, and only in, the heads of caudate. This pattern of regionally specific correlations were found only for symptom severity corresponding to psychomotor poverty.

In conclusion, psychomotor poverty in patients with schizophrenia is possibly associated with dysfunctional interactions between the prefrontal cortex and the striatum. In this regard, it is worth noting that in the present study we implicitly examined frontotemporal integration in the sense that the tasks employed introduced experimental variance-covariance into these regions. The poverty group (loosely identifiable with psychomotor poverty) was comparable to the control group in terms of the amount of functional connectivity, whereas the remaining two groups were deficient. One might conjecture that an alternative paradigm (that activated both the prefrontal cortex and striata) would be more potent in revealing differences between a psychomotor poverty group and normal subjects. At present, this remains a hypothesis.

Although the above observations address negative signs (psychomotor poverty), they do not directly relate to the positive signs (disorganization syndrome) and experiential symptoms (reality distortion) of schizophrenia. Below we discuss the role of abnormal frontolimbic and frontotemporal interactions in the genesis of positive symptoms.

The distinction between intrinsically and extrinsically generated behavior can be expressed in terms of the temporal relationship between cues and the contingent behavior. Extrinsically cued behavior is specified by cues extant at the time of responding or some short time beforehand. Intrinsically generated behavior is predicated on cues experienced in the recent or distant past. In this sense, intrinsically generated behavior is necessarily mnemonic. The ways in which cues affect future behavior can be broadly divided into 1) those that do so by an enduring effect on neural activity and 2) those in which the effect is mediated by long-lasting changes in synaptic efficacy associated with learning and memory.

Clear-cut examples of the first sort of intrinsically generated behavior are visuospatial delayed-response tasks, which are associated with unit activity of the dorsolateral prefrontal cortex during the delay period.[41] Delay period activity is a ubiquitous brain phenomenon and reflects a potential mechanism whereby cues can influence behavior that occurs after the cue has disappeared. In the sense that intrinsically generated action depends, at some level, on previous perceptual experience, it would be a mistake to assume that intrinsically generated acts appear de novo with magical spontaneity. The generation of intrinsically cured behavior is, under normal circumstances, one aspect of a coherent integration of perception and action that is dictated by the history of the individual (the history may be recent and reflected in neural dynamics or embedded in associative changes in neural connectivity).

The essential point being made is that intrinsically generated action cannot be divorced from perception. Intrinsically generated behavior corresponds to an adaptive response to concurrent stimuli that is informed by past events. In responding, the individual operates on the environment and causes (expected) sensorial changes, if only at the level of proprioception. The coherent temporal succession of self-initiated action and perception depends on a continuous dialogue between the neural systems responsible for executing motor behavior and the sensory systems that register the consequences. This dialogue is probably mediated by connections between the prefrontal cortex and the appropriate sensory systems to integrate the sensed and expected consequences of acting. An extremely useful metaphor for this sort of neuronal interaction is found in the occulomotor system.

Self-Monitoring and Corollary Discharge

Helmholtz[42] pointed out that, when we move our eyes, the image slips across the retina, and yet we perceive the world as stationary. This phenomenon can be accounted for by corollary discharge[43] or reafference copy.[44] Robinson and Wurtz[45] identified cells in the superficial layers of the superior colliculus that respond to moving stimuli but do not respond when the eye is moved across a stationary target. At that time, they tentatively identified the frontal eye fields in the prefrontal cortex as the source of modulating corollary discharge.

Similar selectivity of unit response for extrinsically and intrinsically caused sensory changes is found in the auditory system. Muller-Preuss and Jurgens[46] identified cells in the auditory cortex of squirrel monkeys that respond to extrinsically generated sounds but not to self-generated vocalization. Ploog[47] concluded that the inhibition of these cells is caused by corollary discharges associated with vocalization, possibly from the anterior cingulate (in the prefrontal cortex). The anterior cingulate projects not only to Broca's area but also auditory areas, including Brodmann's area 22.

Two sequelae might follow disruption of this sort of corollary discharge: 1) impairment of intrinsically generated behavior secondary to disintegration between (prefrontal and premotor) intentional and (discriminative and proprioceptive) sensory systems and 2) aberrant perception. The latter would follow from misattribution of a self-induced sensory change to the external agencies. We now discuss how this might relate to schizophrenia and why frontotemporal interactions could be central.

Schizophrenia and Frontotemporal Integration

The argument presented above is that intrinsically generated behavior depends on coherent interactions between prefrontal cortices and those devoted to perceptual representations. Of the many interactions among these systems, we have focused on efferents from the prefrontal cortex to sensory systems and their role in modulating unit activity in their targets. This modulatory role may be as simple as suppressing responsiveness to self-induced sensory changes (for which electrophysiological evidence exists[46]), or they may reflect dynamic interactions that are less easy to characterize.

Schizophrenia is primarily a disorder of intrinsically generated behavior, and furthermore, this disorder is confined to a relatively limited sphere. Many signs and experiential symptoms of schizophrenia impinge on the relationship of self to others, as mediated by language and expression or their absence (e.g., poverty of speech, inappropriate or flat affect, incoherent speech, decreased content of speech, auditory hallucinations, and paranoid delusions).[48] The perceptual representations that are implicated are relatively circumscribed, both categorically and in terms of functional anatomy. They include semantic and syntactical representations, the prosodic or emotional tone of someone else's speech, and representations of facial expressions and expressive gestures. The corresponding functional anatomy probably includes the superior temporal regions, the inferotemporal cortex, and the superior temporal sulcus—in short, the temporal lobe. It follows that there might be something quite specific about frontotemporal disconnection and schizophrenia.

In this regard, structural MRI studies of schizophrenic brains have found, with some consistency, abnormalities in the superior temporal gyrus and underlying white matter.[13,49,50] A few symptoms are now considered in terms of defective frontotemporal reentry. The term *representation,* used frequently in the discussion that follows, refers to a pattern of neuronal activity that can be directly associated with some attribute in the sensorium or some component of behavior.

Auditory hallucinations. Consider the effects of a failure to modulate neuronal activity associated with intrinsically generated (speech-related) semantic and syntactical representations in posterior superior temporal regions and related cortex. This might result in the perception of formed utterances and words that are experienced as extrinsic. The activation of semantic representations (in the absence of properly functioning afferents from prefrontal and cingulate cortices) is a likely concomitant of neural activity in premotor speech areas (e.g., Broca's area, or BA 44) associated with sub- or prevocal speech, or just the intention to speak. (Profound changes in neural dynamics are observed many hundreds of milliseconds before actual movement in other motor systems.[51])

Evidence for concomitant neural activity in Broca's area and the temporal cortex during speech can be found in the disconnection syndromes that result in jargon aphasia.[52] Jargon aphasia is associated with damage to the arcuate fasciculus (a conspicuous frontotemporal white-matter tract connecting Broca's area and the temporal cortex) and the parietotemporal junction.[53] In this model, the reentrant projections in the arcuate fasciculus are not dysfunctional, but the patterns of coherent neural activity they mediate are not properly modulated by afferents from, for example, the anterior cingulate. It is perhaps easy to see how the precursor of a spoken thought may, if inadequately suppressed in some distant and sensory form, be reexperienced as not belonging to one's self[54]—a possible substrate for thought insertion. These examples are far removed from corollary discharge and retinal slip and presuppose the existence of unitary representations (at a neural level) that correspond to a spoken phrase or proposition. Although unitary in the sense that they can be (or fail to be) modulated neurophysiologically, they could be distributed in space and time. Evidence for high-level but unitary representations is presented below in terms of circumscribed psychological deficits in neurological patients.

Delusional misinterpretations. A similar disintegration can be envisaged in terms of (putative) inferotemporal[55] or inferior parietal lobule activity evoked by particular facial expressions. A failure to integrate responses elicited in others with the intentional act eliciting that response might result in the experience of inappropriate (and impolite) expressions on the part of the listener. Not only would this lend itself to a malignant interpretation, but it would disrupt any coherent discourse. This example furnishes an entertaining explanation for psychodynamic constructs like reaction formation and projection (e.g., "I like him"—a reaction formation; "I hate him"—a projection; "he hates me"). In this example, the sensory representation evoked by an intrinsically generated behavior has been mediated by the patent acting on the world. In the example above, the semantic representations were mediated directly by neural interactions. In both cases, they were not properly integrated and were experienced as being caused by another.

Inappropriate affect. Signs such as inappropriate affect and incoherent speech have meaning only in the context of interaction with someone else. Abnormal emotional constructs underlying inappropriate and incoherent social expression could result from a failure to modulate representations of a prosodic or emotional nature that were a result of the patient's own behavior. These representations could derive from the patient's own speech, subvocal or articulated, or indeed, from the responses of another that were caused (and would normally be predicted) by the patient himself or herself. Note that the patient could readily and correctly represent the tempo and prosody of someone else's speech to the extent that these attributes were not expected. The deficit proposed here is that affective reactions elicited in the listener are experienced as being produced by the listener without any apparent cause. The secondary reaction to this confusing and disruptive sort of listener could predispose to the sort of behavior that would be interpreted as inappropriate.

Delusions of control and passivity experiences. Although not easily framed in terms of frontotemporal interactions, delusions of control and "made acts" are related to the above by noting that proprioceptive input could be subject to the same dysfunctional reentrant modulation as neural activity in the cortex concerned with the discriminative senses. In this case, failure to suppress proprioceptive input directly resulting from volitional acts might be wrongly attributed to an extrinsic cause.

Neuronal Basis of Sensory Representations

Many of the examples above are predicated on the assumption that there is some unitary abstract representation (e.g., prosody and familiarity) that is separable from other attributes of communication (in terms of neuronal interactions and functional anatomy). There is ample evidence that simple attributes of sensory input can be associated with stereotyped and reproducible patterns of electro- and neurophysiology in regionally specific cortical areas.[56] Indeed, the concept of functional specialization as a principle of brain organization is based on such evidence (e.g., functional specialization in extrastriate cortex).[57,58] There is also evidence for similarly separable or dissociable representations of more abstract aspects of the sensory stream, for example, the double dissociation between identification of faces and the recognition that they are familiar that is evident in prosopagnosia and delusional misidentification. Capgras's syndrome is probably the best-known delusion of misidentification.[59] Alexander et al.[60] considered that a combination of prefrontal and posterior right hemisphere damage is present in all types of misidentification syndrome. Ellis and Young[61] discussed delusional misidentification in terms of cognitive processes that underlie face and object recognition. The premise is that the identification of a face and the recognition that it is familiar are dissociable, both psychologically and in terms of functional anatomy. The evidence for this separable processing comes in part from studies of prosopagnosic patients, in whom there is a complementary failure of identification but a preserved sense of familiarity. Bauer[62] has suggested that a ventral stream underlies the identification of faces, whereas the sense of familiarity depends on a dorsal pathway from extra-striate areas to the inferior parietal regions.

Two qualifications are relevant to the present work. First, the finding of abnormal prefrontotemporal interactions in this small group of schizophrenic subjects does not necessarily reflect the fact that this is the only or the most important abnormality in large-scale interactions. The finding was deliberately highly constrained by using tasks that targeted the prefrontal and temporal cortices. Second, the patients were medicated, and the control subjects were not. One aspect of our current work is the hypothesis that some components of altered functional connectivity between the prefrontal and temporal cortex is sensitive to pharmacological manipulation of dopamine neurotransmission.[63]

Conclusions

The results presented here are provisional but point to an important (frontotemporal) axis of disintegration in cerebral interactions that may be common to some schizophrenic subjects. Clearly, there is much empirical evidence from schizophrenia research that could be brought to bear on this issue. A observation of particular relevance is that psychotic symptoms, including complex auditory hallucinations and delusions, are a prominent feature of metachromatic leukodystrophy presenting between the ages of 12 and 30 years. The pathology of metachromatic leukodystrophy is demyelination affecting many systems but particularly the subfrontal white matter.[64]

References

1. Bleuler E: Dementia praecox or the group of schizophrenias (1913), in The Clinical Routes of the Schizophrenia Concept. Edited by Cutting J, Shepherd M. Cambridge, Cambridge Uni-

versity Press, 1987

2. Bleuler E: Physiogenic and psychogenic in schizophrenia. Am J Psychiatry 10:203–211, 1930
3. Weinberger DR: Implications of normal brain development for the pathogenesis of schizophrenia. Arch Gen Psychiatry 44:660–669, 1987
4. Murray RM, Lewis SR: Is schizophrenia a developmental disorder? Br Med J 295:681–682, 1987
5. Buchsbaum MS, Mansour CS, Teng DG, et al: Adolescent developmental changes in topography of EEG amplitude. Schizophr Res 7:101–107, 1992
6. Robbins TW: The case for frontostriatal dysfunction in schizophrenia. Schizophr Bull 16:391–402, 1990
7. Frith CD: The positive and negative symptoms of schizophrenia reflect impairments in the initiation and perception of action. Psychol Med 134:225–235, 1987
8. Deakin JFW, Slater P, Simpson MDC, et al: Frontal cortical and left temporal glutaminergic dysfunction in schizophrenia. J Neurochem 52:1781–1786, 1989
9. Benes FM, Davidson J, Bird ED: Quantitative cytoarchitectural studies of the cerebral cortex of schizophrenics. Arch Gen Psychiatry 43:31–35, 1986
10. Bogerts B, Ashtari M, Degreef GJ, et al: Reduced temporal limbic structure volumes on magnetic resonance images in first episode schizophrenia. Psychiatry Res 35:1–13, 1991
11. Brown R, Colter N, Coreslis JAN, et al: Postmortem evidence of structural brain changes in schizophrenia: differences in brain weight, temporal horn area, and parahippocampal gyrus compared with affective disorder. Arch Gen Psychiatry 43:36–42, 1986
12. Liddle PF, Friston KJ, Frith CD, et al: Patterns of cerebral blood flow in schizophrenia. Br J Psychiatry 160:179–186, 1992
13. McCarley RW, Shenton ME, Odonnell BF, et al: Auditory P300 abnormalities and left posterior superior temporal gyrus volume reduction in schizophrenia. Arch Gen Psychiatry 50:190–197, 1993
14. Gerstein GL, Perkel DH: Simultaneously recorded trains of ac-

tion potentials: analysis and functional interpretation. Science 164:828–830, 1969

15. Aertsen A, Preissl H: Dynamics of activity and connectivity in physiological neuronal networks, in Nonlinear Dynamics and Neuronal Networks. Edited by Schuster HG. New York, VCH Publishers, 1991, pp 281–302
16. Gerstein GL, Bedenbaugh P, Aertsen AMHJ: Neuronal assemblies IEEE. Trans Biomed Eng 36:4–14, 1989
17. Friston KJ, Frith CD, Liddle PF, et al: Functional connectivity: the principal component analysis of large (PET) data sets. J Cereb Blood Flow Metab 15:5–14, 1993
18. Lammertsma AA, Cunningham VJ, Deiber MP, et al: Combination of dynamic and integral methods for generating reproducible functional CBF images. J Cereb Blood Flow Metab 10:675–686, 1990
19. Spinks TJ, Jones T, Gilardi MC, et al: Physical performance of the latest generation of commercial positron scanner. IEEE Transactions on Nuclear Science 35:721–725, 1988
20. Frith CD, Friston KJ, Liddle PF, et al: Willed action and the prefrontal cortex in man. Proc R Soc Lond B Biol Sci 244:241–246, 1991
21. Frith CD, Friston KJ, Liddle PF, et al: A PET study of word finding. Neuropsychologia 28:1137–1148, 1991
22. Friston KJ, Frith CD, Liddle PF, et al: Investigating a network model of word generation with positron emission tomography. Proc R Soc Lond B Biol Sci 244:101–106, 1991
23. Friston KJ, Passingham RE, Nutt JG, et al: Localization in PET images: direct fitting of the intercommissural (AC-PC) line. J Cereb Blood Flow Metab 9:690–695, 1989
24. Friston KJ, Frith CD, Liddle PF, et al: Plastic transformation of PET images. J Comput Assist Tomogr 15:634–639, 1991
25. Talaraich J, Tournoux P: A Co-planar Stereotaxic Atlas of a Human Brain. Stuttgart, Germany, Thieme, 1988
26. Friston KJ, Frith CD, Liddle PF, et al: The relationship between local and global changes in PET scans. J Cereb Blood Flow Metab 10:458–466, 1990
27. Friston KJ, Frith CD, Liddle PF, et al: Comparing functional

(PET) images: the assessment of significant change. J Cereb Blood Flow Metab 11:690–699, 1991

28. American Psychiatric Association: Diagnostic and Statistical Manual of Mental Disorders, 3rd Edition, Revised. Washington, DC, American Psychiatric Association, 1987
29. Battig WF, Montague WE: Category norms of verbal items in 56 categories: a replication and extension of the Connecticut norms. J Exp Psychol 80:1–46, 1969
30. Bilder RM, Mukherjee S, Reider RO, et al: Symptomatic and neuropsychological components of defect states. Schizophr Bull 11:409–419, 1985
31. Liddle PF: The symptoms of chronic schizophrenia: a re-examination of the positive-negative dichotomy. Br J Psychiatry 151: 145–151, 1987
32. Mortimer AM, Lund CE, McKenna PJ: The positive-negative dichotomy in schizophrenia. Br J Psychiatry 157:41–49, 1990
33. Arndt S, Alliger RJ, Andreasen NC: The distinction of positive and negative symptoms: the failure of a two dimensional model. Br J Psychiatry 158:317–322, 1991
34. Liddle PF, Morris DL: Schizophrenic syndromes and frontal lobe performance. Br J Psychiatry 158:340–345, 1991
35. Frith CD: The Cognitive Neuropsychology of Schizophrenia. Sussex, England, Lawrence Erlbaum, 1992
36. Benson DF: Psychomotor retardation. Neuropsychiatry, Neuropsychology and Behavioral Neurology 3:36–47, 1990
37. Damasio AR, Van Hoesen GW: Emotional disturbances associated with focal lesions of the frontal lobe, in Neuropsychology of Human Emotion. Edited by Heilman K, Satz P. New York, Plenum, 1983
38. Passingham RE, Chen YC, Thaler D: Supplementary motor cortex and self initiated movement, in Neural Programming. Edited by Ito M. Tokyo, Japan Scientific Societies Press, 1989, pp 13–24
39. Marsden CD, Parkes JD, Quinn N: Fluctuations of disability in Parkinson's disease: clinical aspects, in Movement Disorders. Edited by Marsden CD, Fahn S. London, Butterworth, 1982, pp 459–467
40. Friston KJ, Grasby P, Bench C, et al: Measuring the neuromodu-

latory effects of drugs in man with positron tomography. Neurosci Lett 141:106–110, 1992

41. Goldman-Rakic PS: Circuitry of primate prefrontal cortex and regulation of behavior by representational memory, in Handbook of Physiology, Vol 5. Edited by Mountcastle VB, Bloom FE, Geiger SR. Philadelphia, PA, American Physiological Society, 1986, pp 373–417
42. Helmholtz H: Handbuch der Physiologischen Optik. Leipzig, Germany, Voss, 1866
43. Sperry RW: Neural basis of the spontaneous opticokinetic response produced by visual inversion. Journal of Comparative and Physiological Psychology 43:482–489, 1950
44. von Holst E, Mittelstaedt H: Das reafferenzprinzip. Naturwissenschaften 37:464–476, 1950
45. Robinson DL, Wurtz RH: Use of an extraretinal signal by monkey superior colliculus neurons to distinguish real from self induced movement. J Neurophysiol 39:832–870, 1976
46. Muller-Preuss P, Jurgens U: Projections from the "cingular" vocalization area in the squirrel monkey. Brain Res 103:29–43, 1976
47. Ploog D: Phonation, emotion, cognition: with reference to the brain mechanisms involved, in Brain and Mind. CIBA Foundation symposium 69. Amsterdam, Elsevier North-Holland, 1979, pp 79–86
48. Andreasen NC: Comprehensive assessment of symptoms and history. Iowa City, University College of Iowa, College of Medicine, 1986
49. Williamson P, Pelz D, Merskey H, et al: Frontal, temporal and striatal proton relaxation times in schizophrenic patients and normal comparison subjects. Am J Psychiatry 149:549–551, 1992
50. Shenton ME, Kikinis R, Jolesz FA, et al: Abnormalities of the left temporal lobe and thought disorder in schizophrenia: a quantitative magnetic resonance imaging study. N Engl J Med 327: 604–612, 1992
51. Thatcher RW, Toro C, Pflieger M, et al: Human neural network dynamics using multimodal registration of EEG, PET and MRI, in Functional Neuroimaging: Technical Foundations. Edited by

Thatcher RW, Hallett M, Zeffiro T, et al. San Diego, CA, Academic Press, 1994, pp 269–278

52. Butterworth B: Jargon aphasia: process and strategies, in Current Perspective in Dysphasia. Edited by Newman S, Epstein R. New York, Churchill Livingstone, 1985, pp 61–97
53. McCarthy RA, Warrington EK: Cognitive Neuropsychology. London, Academic Press, 1990
54. Feinberg I: Efference copy and corollary discharge: implications for thinking and its disorders. Schizophr Bull 4:636–640, 1978
55. Perret DI, Mistlin AJ, Potter DD, et al: Functional organization of visual neurones processing face identity, in Aspects of Face Processing. Edited by Ellis H, Jeeves MA, Newcombe F, et al. Dordrecht, Netherlands, Martinus Nijhoff, 1986, pp 187–198
56. Phillips CG, Zeki S, Barlow HB: Localization of function in the cerebral cortex: past, present, and future. Brain 107:327–361, 1984
57. Zeki S, Watson J, Lueck C, et al: A direct demonstration of functional specialization in human visual cortex. J Neurosci 11:641–649, 1991
58. Zihl J, von Cramon D, Mai N: Selective disturbance of movement vision after bilateral brain damage. Brain 106:313–340, 1983
59. Capgras J, Reboul-Lachaux J: L'illusion de "sosies" dans un dlire systmatise chronique. Bulletin de la Societe Clinique de Medecine Mentale 2:6–16, 1923
60. Alexander MP, Struss DT, Benson DF: Capgras' syndrome: a reduplicative phenomenon. Neurology 29:334–339, 1978
61. Ellis HD, Young AW: Accounting for delusional mis-identifications. Br J Psychiatry 157:239–248, 1990
62. Bauer RM: Autonomic recognition of names and faces in prosopagnosia: a neuropsycholgical application of the guilty knowledge test. Neuropsychologia 22:457–469, 1984
63. Friston KJ, Grasby P, Bench C, et al: Measuring the neuromodulatory effects of drugs in man with positron tomography. Neurosci Lett 141:106–110, 1992
64. Hyde TM, Ziegler JC, Weinberger DR: Psychiatric disturbances in metachromatic leukodystrophy: insights into the neurobiology of psychosis. Arch Neurol 49:401–406, 1992

CHAPTER

16

Mechanism of Action of Atypical Antipsychotic Drugs: An Update

Herbert Y. Meltzer, M.D.
Bryan Yamamoto, Ph.D.
Martin T. Lowy, Ph.D.
Craig A. Stockmeier, Ph.D.

A basic tenet of biological psychiatry and neuropsychopharmacology for well over three decades has been the concept that the effectiveness of antipsychotic drugs is based on blockade of dopamine (DA), subtype 2 (D_2), receptors in the mesolimbic system, with subsequent decreases in the firing rate of ventral tegmental (A10) DA neurons by the process of depolarization inactivation.[1–4] The primary evidence for this hypothesis

This research was supported in part by U.S. Public Health Service Grant MH 41684, GCRC MO1RR00080, and the National Alliance for Research on Schizophrenia and Depression, as well as by grants from the Elisabeth Severance Prentiss and John Pascal Sawyer Foundations. H.Y.M. is the recipient of U.S. Public Health Service Research Career Scientist Award MH 47808.

The secretarial assistance of Ms. Lee Mason is greatly appreciated.

is 1) the evidence that all effective antipsychotic drugs have affinities for D_2 receptors that are proportional to their average clinical dose,[5,6] and 2) electrophysiological evidence that chronic administration of antipsychotic drugs produces nearly complete inhibition of the firing of ventral tegmental (A10) DA neurons.[7] However, clozapine, now established as the prototypical atypical antipsychotic drug, also satisfies both criteria.[5,8] The subsequent demonstration that clozapine is more effective than other antipsychotic drugs for the treatment of schizophrenic patients who are responsive to typical neuroleptics,[9] as well as those who are neuroleptic resistant,[10] constitutes prima facie evidence that the DA hypothesis of neuroleptic drug action is at best insufficient because it cannot explain the superior efficacy of clozapine and is at worst wrong. Recent evidence from positron-emission tomography (PET) studies (see below) indicates that, at clinically effective doses, clozapine achieves less D_2 receptor occupancy and, hence, less antagonism of D_2 receptors in the striatum, and probably the limbic system as well, than do typical neuroleptic drugs. This further challenges the adequacy of the DA hypothesis to explain the effectiveness of clozapine, a view we have discussed previously.[11–13]

The basis for the greater effectiveness of clozapine as an antipsychotic drug has become one of the most exciting areas of research in neuroscience. It is part of a broader effort to identify other drugs that have antipsychotic efficacy at least comparable to that of clozapine but that do not have its nearly 1% risk of agranulocytosis[14] and to clarify their mechanism of action. Beyond the clinical benefit to be obtained from a safer clozapine-like drug, determining the mechanism of action of clozapine and other antipsychotic drugs with advantages over typical neuroleptics could lead to a greater understanding of the etiology of schizophrenia. Of course, understanding the mechanism of action of a drug does not necessarily indicate the pathogenesis of the disease for which it is efficacious. This is particularly true for a disorder such as schizophrenia, for which no drug yet discovered, including clozapine, can produce a complete recovery or entirely prevent relapses.

In this chapter, we briefly discuss the concept of atypical antipsychotic drugs and then review some recent advances in understanding their mechanism of action. Of necessity, we focus on clozapine, on drugs with a possible related method of action (e.g., risperidone, olanzapine, ziprasidone, seroquel, and sertindole), and on remoxipride, a different type of atypical antipsychotic drug, because most is known about their actions.

Atypical Antipsychotic Drugs

An atypical antipsychotic drug is one that produces an antipsychotic effect at least equal to that of the classical neuroleptics, such as haloperidol, fluphenazine, and thiothixene, but with fewer extrapyramidal symptoms (EPS). Improved efficacy for treating positive, negative, and disorganization symptoms is not a defining characteristic of an atypical antipsychotic drug. Some typical antipsychotic drugs (e.g., thioridazine and remoxipride) meet the criteria of having low EPS, yet there is no published evidence to indicate that their efficacy is superior to that of typical antipsychotics. This is not a trivial consideration, because EPS may contribute to negative symptoms (e.g., withdrawal, flat affect) and consequently to noncompliance, which almost invariably leads to major relapses. On the other hand, there is definite evidence that the efficacy of clozapine is superior to those of typical neuroleptics in the short and long term[9,10] and increasing evidence that, at least at some lower doses and for the short term, that this may also be true of risperidone.[15] Although low EPS is the core concept of atypicality in our view, the scope of this chapter is not confined to considering the basis for low EPS of the various atypical drugs. Possible explanations for the greater effectiveness of clozapine for treating positive, negative, and disorganization symptoms and cognitive function in patients with schizophrenia and Parkinson's disease are also considered.

Mesolimbic and Mesocortical Versus Nigrostriatal Selectivity

There is considerable evidence that atypical antipsychotic drugs generally affect the nigrostriatal system with a lower potency than that with which they affect the mesolimbic and mesocortical dopaminergic systems, whereas the typical neuroleptic drugs affect all three systems with equivalent potencies. In particular, the low incidence of EPS with many atypical antipsychotic drugs appears to be related to the inability of these drugs during chronic administration to decrease the firing rate of A9 DA neurons. This has been demonstrated for clozapine,[8,16,17] olanzapine,[18] sertindole[19] tiospirone,[20] and seroquel.[21] However, it has recently been reported that chronic administration of risperidone may not have a major effect on the firing rate of either A9 or A10 DA neurons (T. Skarsfeldt, personal communication, December 1993). In contrast, typical neuroleptic drugs inactivate both the A9 and A10 DA neurons after chronic administration.[7,17] The inhibition of firing of both A9 and A10 DA neurons by typical neuroleptic drugs and of A10 DA neurons by clozapine has been attributed to depolarization inactivation,[7,22–24] but there is some evidence that is inconsistent with this explanation, as discussed elsewhere.[13,25] The reason for the selective effect of some, if not all, atypical drugs to cause depolarization inactivation of only the A10 DA neurons is not known.

In addition to not interfering with the firing rate of A9 neurons, the ability of chronic clozapine to maintain DA release in the striatum has been suggested to be important to its incidence of low EPS. We have reported that chronic treatment with clozapine (21 days at 20 mg/kg per day in drinking water) had no effect on the extracellular concentrations of DA or of its major metabolite, dihydroxyphenylacetic acid (DOPAC), in the striatum. Administration of a subsequent dose of clozapine, 20 mg/kg, to rats that had received clozapine chronically still increased DA release in the striatum.[26,27] Invernizzi et al.[28] also reported no changes in basal DA release and metabolism in either the striatum or the nucleus accumbens after chronic treatment with clozapine by in vivo microdialysis. These results in the striatum were also confirmed by Chen et al.[29] However, studies in which in vivo voltammetry was used to measure DA levels indicate that chronic administration of clozapine decreases basal DA release in the accumbens but not the striatum.[30,31] Finally, levels of 3-methoxytyramine, a metabolite of DA that is thought to be a measure of DA release,[32] are increased only in limbic regions by clozapine but in the striatum and accumbens by typical neuroleptics.[33,34]

There is some evidence that chronic haloperidol decreases extracellular DA efflux in the striatum.[26,27] Because DA efflux may be independent of the firing of DA neurons,[35] the finding that haloperidol impairs DA efflux but clozapine does not may be an important contribution to determining why clozapine produces fewer EPS than haloperidol. In all, these studies suggest that clozapine may not decrease DA levels in the striatum as compared with typical neuroleptics.

The pharmacologic basis for the inability of clozapine to inactivate A9 DA neurons may be its 5-hydroxytryptamine$_{2A}$ (5-HT$_{2A}$) receptor–blocking properties, because at least three other drugs—seroquel, sertindole, and tiospirone—that also selectively inactivate A10 DA neurons and spare A9 neurons are relatively potent 5-HT$_{2A}$ receptor antagonists in comparison with their D$_2$ antagonism.[36] Chronic administration of MDL 100939, a 5-HT$_{2A}$ antagonist with atypical antipsychotic-like profile with regard to blockade of amphetamine-induced behaviors and with no significant ability to block D$_2$ receptors in vivo, has also been reported to selectively inactivate A10 DA neurons.[37]

There is additional evidence that bears on the hypothesis that 5-HT$_{2A}$ receptor blockade accounts for the limbic selectivity of clozapine. Rivest et al.[38] and Rivest and Marsden,[39] using in vivo voltammetry, pretreated rats with amfonelic acid, an indirect DA agonist that inhibits DA uptake and facilitates the transfer of DA in the storage pool to the vesicular and hence releasable DA pool.[40] Their approach enhanced the increase in striatal and accumbens DOPAC produced by typical neuroleptics (haloperidol and perphenazine). The effect of the atypical antipsychotics on DOPAC, however, was blocked. Brougham et al.[41] also found that the effect of the combination of haloperidol and ritanserin or clozapine on striatal DOPAC was suppressed in rats pretreated with amfonelic acid. MDL 100907, a selective 5-HT$_{2A}$ antagonist with a preclinical profile of potential antipsychotic activity and low EPS, similarly had no effect alone or in combination with amfonelic acid on striatal DOPAC.[37] The results of Brougham et al.[41] and of Sorensen et al.[37] suggest that the ability of some antipsychotic drugs to affect the transfer of DA in the storage pool to a releasable pool in the striatum may be modulated by 5-$HT_{2A/2C}$ antagonism. Gudelsky et al.,[42] however, using in vivo microdialysis, reported that the haloperidol-induced increase in DOPAC was potentiated in both the striatum and nucleus accumbens in rats pretreated with amfonelic acid, whereas amfonelic acid decreased the clozapine-induced increase in DOPAC in both regions. Amfonelic acid also potentiated the increase in DOPAC produced by the combination of ritanserin, a 5-$HT_{2A/2C}$ antagonist, and haloperidol. These authors suggested that 5-$HT_{2A/2C}$ receptor antagonism did not influence the interaction of D_2 receptor blocker with amfonelic acid. The discrepancy between their results and those of Brougham et al.[41] requires further study.

The limbic selectivity of clozapine and thioridazine is also evident in the difference in potency with which these two drugs block the ability of injections of the γ-aminobutyric $acid_A$ ($GABA_A$) agonist muscimol into the A9 and A10 regions to selectively stimulate nigrostriatal and mesolimbic pathways. These two antipsychotic drugs were much more potent in blocking locomotor activity and stereotypy from muscimol injected into the A10 than the A9 area, whereas haloperidol and fluphenazine had the same effect in both regions.[43]

Several studies show that clozapine has a potent ability to stimulate the release of DA in rat medial prefrontal cortex.[29,44] Tolerance to the ability of clozapine to increase extracellular mesocortical DA does not appear to develop.[45] These results are important because they raise the possibility that the ability of clozapine to improve cognitive function and negative symptoms may be due in part to this increased mesocortical dopaminergic activity.

Clozapine, Atypical Antipsychotic Drugs, and Serotonin

The role of 5-HT in the mechanism of action of atypical antipsychotic drugs, and of clozapine in particular, was first studied in 1974.[46] We reviewed the early literature concerning the 5-HT antagonist properties of clozapine elsewhere[12,13,47] and briefly comment here on more recent literature.

The evidence for an effect of clozapine on 5-HT turnover in rat brain is conflicting. Csernansky et al.[48] reported that acute treatments with clozapine and two other putative atypical antipsychotic drugs, sulpiride or (−)-3-PPP, but not the typical antipsychotic haloperidol, produced significant increases in 5-HT turnover in the nucleus accumbens. The three atypical drugs caused a decrease in 5-HT turnover in the accumbens after 28 days of treatment. In the striatum, the acute treatment with each of the three drugs also produced increases in 5-HT turnover that were followed by subsequent decreases.

The basis for these surprising findings is not apparent. Because sulpiride has been thoroughly studied clinically and has few, if any, of the advantages of clozapine, it is doubtful that, if these effects on 5-HT turnover were to be produced in humans under clinical conditions, they would have an important bearing on the clinical profile of clozapine. There are numerous studies, however, in which behavioral, endocrine and temperature end points were used and that show that clozapine is an effective in vivo antagonist of the actions of 5-HT at what are now known to be 5-HT_{2A} or 5-HT_{2C} receptors.[12,47,49–52]

There is also evidence that clozapine is an effective antagonist at 5-HT_3 receptors.[53,54] Most other atypical antipsychotic drugs (e.g., risperidone, *l*-sulpiride, thioridazine), however, are ineffective in this regard.[53] Blockade of 5-HT_3 receptors would be expected to inhibit the release of DA.[55] In support of the possible importance of 5-HT_3 antagonism to the action of clozapine, however, it has recently been reported that clozapine and the 5-HT_3 antagonist DAV 6215 were both able to inhibit the ability of the psychotomimetic sigma agonist (+)-SKF 10,087 to increase DA release in the rat nucleus accumbens. Each of these drugs was shown to be more potent in the accumbens than in the striatum. Haloperidol had no inhibitory effect in this paradigm.[56]

Clozapine has been reported to block the activity of 5-HT or DA to inhibit 5-[^{3}H]HT release stimulated by K^+ from synaptosomes prepared from accumbens.[57] Chen et al.,[45] using in vivo microdialysis, demonstrated that clozapine had an equivalent ability to enhance endogenous DA release in the accumbens and striatum in awake, freely moving rats. Pretreatment with 5,7-dihydroxytryptamine (5,7-DHT) pretreatment to induce lesions in the 5-HT system, however, preferentially increased the ability of clozapine to increase extracellular DA in the accumbens. These authors proposed that 5-HT inhibits DA release in both forebrain regions but that the 5-HT_2 receptors in the accumbens undergo greater development of supersensitivity than those in the striatum after 5,7-DHT lesions because the accumbens has a denser 5-HT innervation, leading to the greater effect of clozapine in the accumbens.

Several recent reports have suggested the importance of 5-HT_{1A} receptors to the action of clozapine. Mason and Reynolds[58] studied the 5-HT_{1A} affinity of nine antipsychotics in human hippocampus and reported that clozapine had the highest affinity (630 ± 72 nM, pK_i = 6.46). However, an earlier, more comprehensive study of the affinity of antipsychotic drugs for 5-HT_{1A} receptors in human cortex showed seven antipsychotics with greater 5-HT_{1A} affinity than clozapine, including chlorprothixene, thioridazine, mesoridazine, and molindone.[59]

A recent behavioral study in which a putative animal model of negative symptoms was used[60] has suggested that a higher ratio of D_1 to 5-HT_{1A} affinities distinguishes some atypical antipsychotics, including clozapine, from typical neuroleptic drugs. These authors proposed a 5-HT_{1A} agonist action for these atypical agents, but no direct evidence in support of the 5-HT_{1A} agonist action was provided.

Recently, two methoxynaphthylpiperazine 5-HT_{1A} agonists with moderate D_2 and D_3 and weak D_1 antagonist properties (S14506 and S14671) were reported to have an antipsychotic profile and minimal efficacy as striatal D_2 receptor antagonists in vivo.[61,62] Therefore, further study of 5-HT_{1A} agonist effects on the antipsychotic or EPS profile of atypical antipsychotic drugs is indicated.

Buspirone, a 5-HT_{1A} agonist, has been reported to have some beneficial effects on both psychosis and EPS when added to neuroleptics, but the results of studies are mixed.[63] The 5-HT_{1A} agonist 8-OH-DPAT has also been found to reverse haloperidol-induced catalepsy.[64]

Two new 5-HT receptors have been cloned, the 5-HT_6 and 5-HT_7 receptors, both of which have high affinities for clozapine.[65,66] The

5-HT_6 receptor is enriched in the striatum, whereas the 5-HT_7 receptor is found in the hypothalamus and other limbic areas. There is a variable pattern for clozapine-like putative atypical antipsychotics to bind to 5-HT_6 and 5-HT_7 receptors.[67] Thus, risperidone has a high affinity for the 5-HT_7 but not the 5-HT_6 receptor, whereas the reverse is true for olanzapine.[67] It is likely that antagonist effects at these receptors contribute in some way to the action of clozapine and related drugs, but it is impossible to assess the importance of these effects at this time.

The 5-HT_{2C} receptor (formerly called the 5-HT_{1C} receptor) has also been implicated in the action of clozapine and other atypical antipsychotic drugs. Clozapine and some other atypical antipsychotic drugs bind with high affinity to the 5-HT_{2C} receptor.[68,69] Of particular interest is that the 50% inhibitory concentration (IC_{50}) of *N*-desmethylclozapine, the major metabolite of clozapine, to inhibit 5-HT_{1C} receptor-mediated phosphoinositide hydrolysis in rat choroid plexus was 29.4 nM, as compared with 110 nM for clozapine. *N*-Desmethylclozapine also bound with higher affinity to the 5-HT_{1C} binding site than did clozapine ($K_i = 2.9 \pm 0.1$ versus 13.2 ± 2.1 nM).[70] However, a comparison of 22 antipsychotic drugs with typical and atypical properties suggests that neither a high affinity for the 5-HT_{2C} receptor nor a high $5\text{-HT}_{2C}/D_2$ affinity ratio is essential for clozapine-like atypical properties.[69] This does not rule out the possibility that binding to 5-HT_{2C} receptors, which are highly concentrated in the choroid plexus but are also widely distributed in other areas of the brain (e.g., the striatum, substantia nigra, and nucleus accumbens[71]), may contribute to the effects of some atypical and typical neuroleptics. Chronic clozapine administration decreased 5-HT_{2C} receptor density in rat choroid plexus.[72] Also of interest is that only compounds with a high affinity for both 5-HT_{2A} and 5-HT_{2C} receptor sites, but not compounds with a high affinity for only one of these receptors, substituted for clozapine in a two-key operant discrimination procedure in pigeons.[73] These latter results suggest that blockade of both 5-HT_{2A} and 5-HT_{2C} receptors is important to produce the clozapine-like discriminative stimulus.[73] Wiley and Porter,[74] however, found that ritanserin, a $5\text{-HT}_{2A/2C}$ antagonist, had no effect as a substitute for clozapine in rats trained to discriminate clozapine using a two-lever discrimination procedure under an FR30 schedule of food reinforcement.

The greatest interest in the role of 5-HT in the action of atypical antipsychotic drugs has focused on possible influences on the 5-HT_{2A} receptor. The background for this has been reviewed by us elsewhere.[36,75] Briefly, the 5-HT_{2A} receptor may be involved in, among other effects, perception, mood regulation, and motor control and serves to regulate the release of DA either by effects on firing rates of DA neurons or via heteroreceptors on DA nerve terminals or both. Serotonin acting on 5-HT_2 receptors appears to promote the synthesis and release of DA.[76–79] 5-HT_{2A} receptor antagonists can diminish the effect of amphetamine to decrease the firing of A10 DA neurons[37,80,81] and can reduce amphetamine-induced DA efflux in the striatum and accumbens.[76,82] These results suggest that 5-HT_{2A} antagonists may decrease EPS while decreasing stimulated DA release in the mesolimbic and mesocortical DA systems, thus contributing to an antipsychotic action.[37]

As previously mentioned, there is evidence from in vitro binding studies that clozapine and other related drugs that produce little catalepsy in rodents and fewer EPS in humans have a higher affinity for 5-HT_{2A} than for D_2 receptors.[36,83] Absolute affinity for 5-HT_{2A} receptors is not the key feature that distinguishes typical from atypical antipsychotic drugs. Rather, it is the fact that these drugs produce stronger 5-HT_{2A} than D_2 receptor antagonism both in vitro and in vivo. The evidence in support of this is now briefly reviewed.

Groups of clozapine-like atypical and haloperidol-like typical antipsychotic drugs (classified on the basis of preclinical and clinical data of catalepsy and EPS) do not differ in their average ability in vitro to displace [^{3}H]ketanserin binding in the frontal cortex.[36] The clozapine-like atypical antipsychotic drugs are about 13-fold less potent as a group than the typical antipsychotic drugs in displacing [^{3}H]spiperone binding in vitro to D_2 receptors in striatum.[36] However, there are several drugs, such as loxapine and amoxapine, both of which are members of the same dibenzazepine family as is clozapine, that are typical neuroleptics but that were more potent in vitro as 5-HT_{2A} than as D_2 antagonists. This study provided no evidence that D_1 antagonist properties are important to the distinction between typical and atypical antipsychotic drugs. However, there is other evidence for the importance of D_1 receptor blockade in the action of clozapine.[47] Recently, Wadenberg et al.[84] again suggested that the D_1 antagonist effect of clozapine may be important because it more closely resembles the D_1 antagonist SCH 23390 than the D_2 antagonist raclopride with regard to dose effects on conditioned avoidance behavior and induction of catalepsy. These authors also noted that the effect of clozapine to block 5-hydroxytryptophan accumulation (after inhibition of cerebral aromatic L-amino acid decarboxylase) in the striatum occurred at low, behaviorally active doses but that it had no such effect on levodopa accumulation. They suggested that this effect on 5-HT neurotransmission might contribute to these behaviors.

To further clarify the importance of 5-HT_{2A} and D_2 receptor antagonism to the distinction between typical and atypical antipsychotics, in vivo studies of rat brain occupancy have been done. The $pED_{50}s$ (the negative log 10 of the dose that produces 50% blockade of $[^3H]$NMSP) of 10 typical and 10 atypical antipsychotic drugs were reported not to differ in their average ability to prevent the accumulation of ^3H-labeled *N*-methylspiperone (NMSP) in a measure of receptor 5-HT_2 occupancy in the frontal cortex.[85] The atypical antipsychotic drugs, however, were about eightfold less potent than the group of typical antipsychotic drugs in preventing the accumulation of $[^3H]$NMSP in striatum, a measure of D_2 occupancy. Individual exceptions to the latter generalization include risperidone and tiospirone, atypical antipsychotic drugs whose potencies to occupy D_2 receptors in vivo are not unlike those of trifluoperazine, perphenazine, and *cis*-flupentixol. Both of the atypical drugs, however, have more potent effects on cortical 5-HT_2 receptors in vivo, by 1.2 and 1.3 log units, respectively.

The atypical antipsychotic drugs as a group have a significantly greater average affinity in vivo for the 5-HT_2 than the D_2 receptor, by 1.14 log units. The typical antipsychotic drugs (e.g., haloperidol), however, tend to be either more potent in occupying D_2 than 5-HT_2 receptors or nearly equipotent in occupying both types of receptors. In agreement with the in vitro data, amoxapine was a conspicuous exception among typical antipsychotic drugs in that it is more potent, by 0.8 log units, in blocking 5-HT_2 than D_2 receptors. However, loxapine was similar to other typical neuroleptic drugs in vivo. Chlorpromazine was also an exception among the typical antipsychotic drugs in having a fourfold greater potency to occupy 5-HT_{2A} than D_2 receptors. Melperone, an atypical antipsychotic drug, resembled the typical antipsychotic drugs, having only a twofold preference for 5-HT_{2A} versus D_2 receptors. Zotepine, which has been classified as an atypical antipsychotic, had a relationship between ED_{50} for 5-HT_{2A} and D_2 binding in vivo that was characteristic of the atypical antipsychotics. The in vitro pK_i values for zotepine were characteristic of those for atypical neuroleptics. Similar in vivo binding data have been reported by Matsubara et al.[86] and Sumiyoshi et al.[87]

Some (e.g., clozapine, fluperlapine, setoperone) but not all (e.g., melperone, amperozide, tiospirone) clozapine-like atypical antipsychotics can produce an acute downregulation of cortical 5-HT_2 receptors.[88,89] Chronic clozapine administration also downregulated cortical 5-HT_2 receptors[89,90,91] without increased D_2 receptor density in striatum,[90,91] but clozapine did increase D_1 receptor density in striatum.[91]

Thus, the group of typical antipsychotic drugs examined (from five different classes) can be distinguished from the group of atypical antipsychotic drugs that are clozapine-like on the basis of the atypical antipsychotic drugs having a relatively higher ratio of occupancy at 5-HT_{2A} versus D_2 receptors, as measured either in vitro or in vivo. Results of recent PET studies are consistent with this.[92,93] The average relative potency of the groups of typical but not atypical antipsychotic drugs at 5-HT_{2A} versus D_2 receptors was essentially equivalent when examined either in vivo or in vitro. The average clinical dose of only the typical antipsychotic drugs was significantly correlated with their in vivo occupancy of D_2 receptors.

These data may provide assistance in choosing clozapine-like atypical antipsychotic drugs for further study and may suggest appropriate ranges for clinical doses. The hypothesis that strong blockade of 5-HT_{2A} receptors and weak blockade of D_2 receptors may identify clozapine-like atypical antipsychotic drugs can be tested when the effectiveness of blockade of 5-HT_{2A} versus D_2 receptors can be verified in humans under clinical conditions.

Some of the clinical advantages of the atypical antipsychotic drugs, such as clozapine (as opposed to haloperidol), may be the result of a higher occupancy of 5-HT_{2A} receptors than of D_2 receptors. Haloperidol causes catalepsy in rats, whereas clozapine only weakly induces catalepsy in rats and results in fewer EPS in humans.[10,94] The ability of clozapine to block 5-HT_{2A} receptors may be related to its weak induction of EPS, because drugs with antagonist properties at 5-HT_{2A} receptors, such as ketanserin, block haloperidol-induced catalepsy in rats and dystonia and parkinsonism in monkeys.[95–97] Ritanserin, a selective antagonist at 5-HT_{2A} and 5-HT_{2C} receptors with little activity at D_2 receptors in vivo,[98,99] decreases EPS induced by haloperidol.[100] In addition, mianserin, also a 5-HT_{2A} and 5-HT_{2C} receptor antagonist, significantly decreased negative and global symptoms in hospitalized patients with chronic schizophrenia who were treated with neuroleptic drugs.[101] These data therefore suggest that a preferential blockade of 5-HT_{2A} receptors, together with blockade of D_2 receptors, may contribute to the favorable side effect profile and efficacy of some novel antipsychotic drugs.

The in vivo occupancy of D_2 receptors was not significantly correlated with the clinically effective dose for clozapine-like atypical antipsychotic drugs. This lack of correlation for atypical antipsychotic drugs may therefore indicate that 1) the in vivo occupancy of D_2 receptors alone is not the critical factor in their antipsychotic action, 2) there are species differences in receptor occupancy, or 3) reliable information on clinically effective doses for some of the atypical antipsychotic drugs is not available. The latter possibility is suggested by the absence of studies with fixed doses to establish the minimum and optimal clinical doses and by recent evidence with risperidone, for which such data are available. The dose-response data available for risperidone suggest that doses of 6–8 mg per day[102,103] produce fewer EPS and may be more effective than haloperidol at doses of 10–20 mg per day. At lower and higher doses of risperidone, these advantages may not be present.[15] These findings have led to the strong recommendation to use doses of risperidone within the range of 6–8 mg per day[103] (R. Meibach, personal communication, September 1992). The clinical advantages of risperidone may be due to its relatively greater occupancy of 5-HT_{2A} than D_2 receptors in the range of 6–8 mg per day. In contrast, at higher doses, risperidone may similarly occupy both 5-HT_{2A} and D_2 receptors.

The hypothesis that clozapine acts via D_2 and 5-HT_{2A} receptor blockade was challenged by Wadenberg et al.,[84] who found no evidence for D_2 receptor blockade in vivo and evidence for 5-HT receptor stimulation (type not specified), rather than antagonism, on the basis of studies of 5-HT and DA synthesis rates after inhibition of L-amino acid decarboxylase. Their findings with regard to D_2 and 5-HT_{2A} antagonism produced by clozapine are in disagreement with the very large body of evidence from human and animal studies and thus are very difficult to integrate.

The literature summarized here suggests a broad array of effects of clozapine on, at least, the 5-HT_{1A}, 5-HT_{2A}, 5-HT_{2C}, 5-HT_3, 5-HT_6, and 5-HT_7 subtypes of serotonin receptors. At clinically effective doses, it is likely that 5-HT_{2A}, 5-HT_{2C}, 5-HT_6, and 5-HT_7 antagonism takes place, along with decreases in the density of 5-HT_{2A} and 5-HT_{2C} receptors. Much greater occupancy of 5-HT_{2A} than D_2 receptors is likely to occur. The net effect of these influences on serotonergic receptors and availability is apparently to maintain DA efflux in the limbic and striatum system and possibly to increase it in the cortex. These effects are mediated by a variety of actions on DA cell bodies and heteroreceptors on DA terminals, as we have reviewed elsewhere.[75] Some of these effects of clozapine, especially those mediated by 5-HT_{2A} blockade and downregulation, are shared by most, if not all, clozapine-like atypical drugs, suggesting that the relative blockade of 5-HT_{2A} receptors may be the most critical factor in the action of clozapine on the serotonergic system. Effects on the other receptor subtypes, however, may also be of importance. To the extent that these effects are not shared by clozapine, these other atypical drugs will be unable to provide all of the advantages (and possibly may cause fewer side effects). The complex interaction of clozapine and these other agents with other receptors and transporters and their effects, in turn, on 5-HT will influence the clinical profile of these drugs.

Clozapine and the Cholinergic System

Centrally acting anticholinergic drugs decrease EPS due to neuroleptic drugs or in Parkinson's disease by restoring the balance between DA and acetylcholine in the striatum. The limited ability of thioridazine and clozapine, both of which are potent anticholinergic drugs, to cause EPS has therefore been attributed to their antimuscarinic properties.[104] Both clozapine and the anticholinergic trihexyphenidyl decrease acetylcholine content in the striatum and block the increase in acetylcholine turnover produced by haloperidol.[105] The discriminative cue provided by clozapine is mimicked by anticholinergic drugs.[106] Recent studies have established that clozapine is a very potent antagonist of the muscarinic m_1 receptor subtype (K_d = 3.1 nM), followed by the m_4 and m_5 subtypes (K_d = 11.0 and 11.2, respectively) and the m_3 and m_2 subtypes (K_d = 20.1 and 48 nM, respectively). Thioridazine has a virtually identical profile with regard to antagonism of muscarinic receptor subtypes.[107,108] Fluperlapine, a morphanthradine analogue of clozapine with atypical antipsychotic properties, also has a similar profile but can cause acute dystonic reactions.[109] It has been proposed that high m_1 affinity and selectivity are required for clozapine-like profiles.[108] This has been linked to blockade of the activity of cholinergic neurons, which may be increased in number in the pedunculopontine nucleus of patients with schizophrenia.[110]

There is, however, considerable evidence against the hypothesis that the low EPS of clozapine are primarily due to its anticholinergic properties. First, thioridazine, which shares many of the properties of clozapine as an anticholinergic agent, nevertheless produces more EPS in both patients with schizophrenia and those with Parkinson's disease than does clozapine, and there is no evidence that it has any advantages over typical neuroleptics with regard to its likelihood to cause tardive dyskinesia. A number of studies show that combined treatment with a typical neuroleptic plus an anticholinergic does not produce the same effects on rat brain DA metabolism or behavior as does treatment with clozapine alone.[111–113] Furthermore, it has been reported that the ability of clozapine, but not haloperidol, to increase extracellular DOPAC concentrations in the striatum and nucleus accumbens is blocked by pretreatment with atropine or scopolamine, both potent anticholinergic drugs, in rats anesthetized with chloral hydrate.[39] Neither of these agents alone had any effect on extracellular DOPAC concentrations. Thus, the important effect of clozapine in the striatum to enhance dopaminergic activity depends on the availability of intact muscarinic receptors, possibly located on DA nerve terminals. It has been suggested that m_2 receptors, which are blocked by scopolamine and atropine but not clozapine, located on DA nerve terminals can increase DA metabolism.[114] According to this model, clozapine produces effective blockade of only m_1 muscarinic receptors.

Using in vivo microdialysis in awake freely moving rats, we have studied the effect of scopolamine on DA, DOPAC, and homovanillic acid (HVA) efflux in the striatum and nucleus accumbens, as well as the effect of clozapine on extracellular DA in the cortex.[115] Scopolamine itself (1 mg/kg administered intraperitoneally) had no effect on extracellular DA, DOPAC, or HVA concentrations in the striatum or nucleus accumbens or on DA in the prefrontal cortex. However, scopolamine inhibited the ability of clozapine to increase extracellular DA and HVA concentrations in the striatum and nucleus accumbens but not those produced by haloperidol or thioridazine. Clozapine increased DOPAC in the striatum only, an effect that was also blocked by pretreatment with scopolamine.

These results are in partial agreement with those of Rivest and Marsden,[114] with the exception that clozapine did not increase extracellular DOPAC concentrations in the nucleus accumbens. These results indicate that cholinergic stimulation is essential for clozapine, administered acutely, to increase extracellular DA in the striatum, but not in the accumbens or prefrontal cortex, and that clozapine, despite its potent antimuscarinic properties, does not by itself produce complete anticholinergic blockade. This is consistent with other evidence indicating that clozapine can increase brain acetylcholine release, although only at very high doses.[116] There is also behavioral evidence that clozapine is an indirect cholinomimetic agent (S. Ögren, personal communication, November 1994). These data are consistent with the clinical evidence that the hypersalivation produced by clozapine can be blocked by anticholinergic drugs. It is possible that an indirect effect of clozapine on the cholinergic system in the striatum, an effect not shared by thioridazine, could be relevant to its lack of ability to produce EPS and possibly tardive dyskinesia.

Clozapine and Activation of Immediate-Early Genes

Because the onset of action of clozapine in ameliorating psychotic symptoms may be delayed for prolonged periods, it is of interest to consider the possible effects on genetic mechanisms that might contribute to the development and maintenance of long-term changes in the brain. The immediate-early gene c-*fos* is a marker of metabolic activation of neurons by a variety of stimuli.[117] The regional specificity of c-*fos* activation by antipsychotic drugs has been used to study the differences between typical and atypical antipsychotic drugs.

Haloperidol increases c-*fos* expression mainly in the striatum and nucleus accumbens[118–121] but does not affect the prefrontal cortex in this regard.[120,122] Clozapine is without effect on c-*fos* in the striatum but increases c-*fos* in the nucleus accumbens, medial prefrontal cortex, and lateral septal nucleus. The effect of clozapine on the lateral septal nucleus and prefrontal cortex was not affected by 6-hydroxydopamine–induced lesions of the median forebrain bundle, whereas the effects of clozapine on c-*fos* in the nucleus accumbens were blocked by 6-hydroxydopamine–induced lesions. Deutch et al.[122a] reported that the effect of clozapine on c-*fos* in the accumbens was confined to the shell region, sparing the core. The effect of clozapine was like that of remoxipride but different from that of haloperidol, which also increased c-*fos* in the core. Neither 5-HT nor norepinephrine depletion with 5,7-DHT or 6-hydroxydopamine, respectively, affected clozapine-induced c-*fos* induction in the medial prefrontal cortex in rats.

Clozapine, but not haloperidol, in a single dose produced increased c-*fos* immunoreactivity in the deep but not the superficial layers of the medial prefrontal cortex (Oh, Meltzer, and Lowy, unpublished data). c-*fos* was increased in both pyramidal cells and GABAergic, calbindin-positive neurons. It was suggested that these results on the cortical effects of clozapine may be relevant to why clozapine is not effective in patients with extensive frontal cortical atrophy (Oh, Meltzer, and Lowy, unpublished data).

Differential effects of clozapine and haloperidol on neuropeptide concentrations or messenger RNA (mRNA) levels have been reported. Haloperidol increased neurotensin/neuromedian mRNA in the dorsal lateral striatum, but clozapine was without effect. Both haloperidol and clozapine, however, increased the mRNA levels of both peptides in the shell of the nucleus accumbens.[123] Chronic treatment with haloperidol but not clozapine increased neurotensin mRNA in the substantia nigra and the ventral tegmentum.[124] Other differential effects for specific regions have been reported for chronic administration of clozapine and haloperidol on preprosomatostatin mRNA.[125] Chronic haloperidol administration decreases preprosomatostatin mRNA in neurons of the nucleus accumbens and frontal cortex but not in the lateral striatum. Clozapine, on the other hand, increased levels of preprosomatostatin mRNA in the nucleus accumbens but not in the striatum or frontal cortex. Ennulat and Cohen,[126] using polymerase chain reaction amplification, reported increased expression of three unidentified mRNAs in the brains of rats. Synthesis of the tachykinins substance P and neurokinin A in the striatum are tonically stimulated by DA. Protachykinin mRNA concentrations were suppressed by a variety of typical neuroleptic drugs but not by clozapine.[127]

It was previously reported that the muscarinic receptor antagonist scopolamine can attenuate the haloperidol-increase in c-*fos* expression in the striatum and lateral septum but not in the nucleus accumbens.[128] Because the effect of scopolamine on clozapine induction of c-*fos* was not reported, we studied the effect of scopolamine on clozapine-induced c-*fos* in several brain regions (Oh et al., manuscript in preparation). Scopolamine (1 mg/kg) attenuated the clozapine induction of c-*fos* in the medial prefrontal cortex and medial septum but was without effect in the olfactory tubercle and arcuate nucleus. These results are in partial agreement with the in vivo microdialysis studies discussed above, which suggest that clozapine may have cholinomimetic properties that could be relevant to its unique therapeutic profile.

The differential effects of clozapine and typical neuroleptics on the expression of various genes are of considerable interest, especially the selective activation of various genes in the cortex and the nucleus accumbens by clozapine by a mechanism that does not depend on an intact dopaminergic or serotonergic system. This does not rule out the possibility that the effect of clozapine may depend on postsynaptic 5-HT or DA receptors, however. It will be of interest to determine whether these effects of clozapine are shared with other putative atypical antipsychotics, such as risperidone, olanzapine, and remoxipride, to clarify whether these effects are relevant to the efficacy or the side effect profile of clozapine, both, or neither.

Role of Glutamate in the Action of Clozapine

There has been increasing interest in the role of excitatory amino acids in the pathogenesis of schizophrenia, antipsychotic drug efficacy, and/or the motor side effect liability of typical neuroleptics. Several studies have implicated excitatory amino acids in the pathophysiology of schizophrenia. Phencyclidine, a noncompetitive *N*-methyl-d-aspartate (NMDA) receptor antagonist, can elicit symptoms of schizophrenia. Consistent with this observation, there appears to be decreased glutamate release[129] and low cerebrospinal fluid levels of glutamate in the brains of schizophrenic patients.[130] Furthermore, postmortem studies have shown increases in [^{3}H]MK-801 and [^{3}H]kainate binding in the frontal cortex of schizophrenic brains.[129,131,132] It is conceivable that the increase in postsynaptic binding in the frontal cortex may be due to the development of receptor supersensitivity in response to a loss of glutamatergic terminals. Collectively, these data are consistent with the theory that schizophrenia is a glutamatergic deficiency disorder.[133]

The interaction and colocalization of glutamate and DA terminals within nigrostriatal and mesolimbic regions are further suggestive of a possible glutamatergic dysfunction in patients with schizophrenia. If a glutamatergic hypofunction is present in these patients, it follows that the antipsychotic effect of neuroleptic drugs could be due in part to an augmentation of glutamate transmission. Previous studies in which the effects of neuroleptics on glutamate levels were examined have yielded variable results but generally support this hypothesis. Glutamate receptor antagonists, such as MK-801 and phencyclidine, have been used in behavioral assays to determine the profile and mechanism of action of antipsychotic drugs.[134,135] Clozapine, haloperidol, and the D_2 receptor–selective antagonist eticlopride decrease MK-801–induced locomotor activity.[135] Similar results have been reported by Verma and Kulkarni.[136] Clozapine was less effective in blocking sniffing than haloperidol or eticlopride. The significance of this difference must be further studied with other atypical antipsychotic drugs, such as risperidone and olanzapine. In vitro application of haloperidol but not chlorpromazine, clozapine, or sulpiride to rat cortical slices increased glutamate release.[133] Others have reported that chronic but not acute sulpiride administration increased glutamate levels in cerebrospinal fluid.[137] In contrast, the addition of haloperidol to synaptosomes prepared from frozen schizophrenic brain tissue increase GABA but not glutamate release.[133] Squires and Saederup[138] proposed a general theory of schizophrenia and depression in which both were due to excessive GABAergic/deficient glutamatergic neurotransmission and proposed that clozapine may act in part by decreasing $GABA_A$ receptor stimulation and enhancing glutamatergic activity.

A more recent study examining the effects of both neuroleptic and putative atypical antipsychotic drugs (clozapine, 3-PPP, and sulpiride) on amino acid concentrations in tissue showed that all three putative atypical drugs acutely reduced tissue concentrations of glutamate in the nucleus accumbens, whereas haloperidol had no significant effect.[139] Chronic administration of clozapine increased glutamate levels in the left but not the right striatum, whereas (–)-3-PPP and sulpiride did not have this effect. One interpretation of the reduced glutamate concentrations in the accumbens may be enhanced synthesis, release, and metabolism. Because there is no clinical evidence indicating that 3-PPP and sulpiride have antipsychotic effects comparable to those of clozapine, however, the significance of this observation is unclear. In any event, after chronic treatment, glutamate levels in the accumbens in clozapine-treated animals returned to control levels, whereas those of (–)-3-PPP and sulpiride were slightly higher than in control subjects.

Similarly, acute administration of clozapine[140–142] and the putative atypical antipsychotic drug amperozide, but not haloperidol,[143] selectively increased extracellular glutamate and DA concentrations in the medial prefrontal cortex when measured in vivo. It is possible that this greater propensity of amperozide and clozapine to enhance glutamate transmission in the medial prefrontal cortex may contribute to the ability of these drugs to alleviate the negative symptoms of schizophrenia. Comprehensive studies of the effect of chronic treatment with clozapine and other atypical antipsychotic drugs, such as risperidone and olanzapine, on glutamate synthesis and release in medial prefrontal cortex, accumbens, and striatum are needed before the results of the studies cited here can be reliably interpreted.

Recent neurochemical models of schizophrenia implicate an important role for glutamate in the pathogenesis of schizophrenia. Carlsson[144] and Carlsson and Carlsson[145] have suggested that a dysfunction in corticostriatal glutamatergic input, combined with an increase in mesostriatal dopaminergic tone, can alter the ability of the thalamus to filter incoming sensory information to the cortex. This subsequently results in the symptoms of schizophrenia. In this model, a striatothalamocortical loop serves to filter and focus incoming sensory information. The thalamic filtering process is dependent on two parallel pathways (inhibitory and excitatory) involving the balance between excitatory glutamate input and either a stimulatory or an inhibitory effect of DA on striatal function. A loss of excitatory glutamatergic input and/or an increase in inhibitory dopaminergic activity would then decrease the striatally mediated inhibitory pathway to the thalamus. This decrease in thalamic filtering capacity would then be manifested as the positive symptoms of schizophrenia. Conversely, a decrease in the excitatory effects of glutamate, combined with an increase in the stimulatory effect of DA on striatal activity, would activate the parallel striatothalamic excitatory path and increase the capacity of the thalamus to filter incoming sensory information to the cortex. This deficit in sensory input to the cortex would then result in the negative symptoms of schizophrenia.

Grace[22] also hypothesized a decrease in corticostriatal glutamatergic function as an etiologic factor in schizophrenia. This model focuses on a direct interaction between glutamate and DA within the striatum. Specifically, it is proposed that schizophrenia is the result of an imbalance between the phasic and tonic components of DA release. The excitatory actions of glutamate enhance tonic DA efflux. Removal of this excitatory effect, such as that hypothesized to occur due to the hypoactivity of the frontal cortex in patients with schizophrenia, results in the reduction of tonic DA release. This eventually could result in a homeostatic compensatory upregulation of DA function mediated by enhanced phasic or impulse-mediated dopaminergic activity. Recently, Baskys et al.[146] reported that haloperidol and loxapine facilitated excitatory postsynaptic potentials in the CA1 area of rat hippocampal slices, whereas clozapine induced a transient depression followed by a small augmentation. Studies of the effect of chronic administration of clozapine and other atypical antipsychotic drugs on excitatory synaptic transmission in various brain regions are needed. Even then, however, the results must be interpreted with caution, because they might not apply to schizophrenia if there is, in fact, one or more abnormalities in the glutamate system in that disorder.

As noted by the above studies, attention has been limited to the restoration and/or elevation of glutamatergic function as a goal for the therapeutic efficacy of antipsychotic drugs. Underlying this objective, however, is the increased possibility of side effects resulting from persistently high concentrations of glutamate. In particular, striatal glutamate may be involved in the EPS of the typical antipsychotic drugs. Glutamate is the primary transmitter of the projections from motor and premotor cortices to the striatum.[147] Chronic elevation of glutamate produces striatal neurodegeneration.[148,149] Consequently, glutamate has been implicated in a number of neurodegenerative movement disorders,[149–153] including Huntington's disease.[154] Rao et al.[155] reported that clozapine was able to block an effect of NMDA receptor activation (increased cyclic guanosine monophosphate [cGMP]) levels in mouse cerebellum and showed that this might be related to its central α_1-adrenergic–blocking properties. These authors relate this effect to a neuroprotective action in ischemia-induced neuronal cell action. Clozapine, loxapine, and amoxapine were protective against MK-801–induced neurotoxicity.[156] Clozapine was the most effective of the three drugs, but because all three were active, it is not clear whether this effect is relevant to the specific clinical advantages of clozapine.

Clozapine but not haloperidol delays the rate at which kindling of the limbic system develops.[157] This effect of clozapine was partially blocked by pilocarpine, a cholinergic agonist, but it was suggested that its antiglutamate properties, evidenced by its ability to displace [^{3}H]MK-801 binding to striatal glutamate receptors, might be involved as well.[157]

Although most studies have focused on the stimulatory effects of glutamate on nigrostriatal DA neurons,[158,159] less is known about the effects of DA on corticostriatal glutamatergic function. Studies of cortical lesions indicate that up to 50% of striatal D_2 receptors are localized on corticostriatal terminals.[160–163] Although these anatomical studies are somewhat controversial,[164–166] more recent evidence indicates that corticostriatal terminals possess D_2 receptors.[167] Corresponding results indicate that the nigrostriatal DA path inhibits in vitro glutamate release and high-affinity uptake.[168,169] It has been demonstrated that DA inhibits striatal glutamate release in vivo via the D_2 receptor.[170] It is therefore possible that changes in dopaminergic transmission, through presynaptic or postsynaptic mechanisms after acute and/or chronic D_2 antagonism with typical neuroleptic administration, can increase striatal glutamate concentrations and subsequently influence motor function through stimulatory or perhaps excitotoxic mechanisms. A more recent study that partially addressed this hypothesis showed that chronic treatment with haloperidol increases basal extracellular concentrations of glutamate in the striatum by fivefold.[171] In contrast, chronic clozapine treatment had no effect on striatal glutamate. This lack of effect of clozapine on striatal glutamate, in combination with its various direct and indirect effects on NMDA receptor complex,[135,172] may contribute to the absence of EPS after chronic treatment with this drug.

Differences in pharmacological effects on glutamate transmission after chronic clozapine and haloperidol administration may contribute to the absence of morphological changes with chronic clozapine versus haloperidol treatment. A reversible increase in the number of "perforated" synapses has been reported in the dorsolateral caudate but not the accumbens 24 hours after chronic haloperidol but not chronic clozapine treatment.[173–175] Perforated synapses show a discontinuous density in electromicroscopic sections along the contact region with the nerve terminals. The perforated synapse has been hypothesized to be an indicator of more efficient transmitter release, possibly relevant to learning and memory.[176] It also has been speculated that the haloperidol-induced increases in these synapses are due to activation of the excitatory corticostriatal pathway.[173,175] Support for this notion is indicated by the ability of the NMDA antagonist MK-801 to reverse the haloperidol-induced increase in perforated synapses.[177] A possible role of 5-HT_2 receptor blockade by clozapine in the effect of clozapine not to increase perforated synapses has been discussed by Meshul et al.[174]

Overall, there is mounting evidence that glutamate transmission in cortical and subcortical structures may be involved in both the therapeutic effects of clozapine drugs and the side effect profile of typical neuroleptic agents. Future studies with a more extensive array of clozapine-like drugs are needed to further elucidate the interactions between glutamate and DA in mesolimbic and mesostriatal systems and their possible clinical significance.

Conclusions

The mechanism of action by which atypical antipsychotic drugs produce low EPS undoubtedly differs among drugs. It is clear that a minimal effect on striatal DA function is a final common pathway for low EPS. Atypical antipsychotic drugs produce less inhibition of dopaminergic input into the striatum and less disruption of the striatal-cholinergic/ dopaminergic balance. How these drugs achieve this is highly variable. With remoxipride, differences between the drug's effects on D_2 and postsynaptic receptors in the striatum and its effects on the mesolimbic and mesocortical dopaminergic systems, as well as an effect on sigma receptors, may be involved. It is possible that 5-HT_{2A} antagonism serves to enhance dopaminergic activity for a variety of drugs (e.g., olanzapine, sertindole, seroquel, clozapine, and risperidone) with a stronger affinity for the 5-HT_{2A} receptor than for the D_2 receptor. For clozapine, melperone, and possibly other clozapine-like drugs, D_4 receptor antagonism may also be relevant. Indeed, for clozapine and other atypical compounds, a wide variety of other effects, such as 5-HT_6 and 5-HT_7 antagonism, anticholinergic properties, increase in neurotensin-like immunoreactivity, induction of various genes, and D_1 receptor blockade, may contribute to their atypical properties, namely, their low EPS. The mechanism of clozapine's ability to improve positive, negative, and disorganization symptoms is more obscure than are its effects on extrapyramidal function. All of these mechanisms, in addition to others, such as the ability to inhibit neurotoxicity, may participate in this effect.

References

1. Matthysse S: Dopamine and the pharmacology of schizophrenia: the state of the evidence. J Psychiatr Res 11:107–113, 1974
2. Meltzer HY, Stahl SM: The dopamine hypothesis of schizophrenia: a review. Schizophr Bull 2:19–76, 1976
3. Bunney BS, Chiodo LA, Grace AA: Midbrain dopamine system electrophysiological functioning: a review and hypothesis. Synapse 9:79–94, 1991
4. Davis KL, Kahn RS, Ko G, et al: Dopamine and schizophrenia: a review and reformulation. Am J Psychiatry 148:1474–1476, 1991
5. Seeman P, Lee T: Antipsychotic drugs: direct correlation be-

tween clinical potency and presynaptic action on dopamine neurons. Science 188:1217–1219, 1975

6. Creese I, Burt DR, Snyder SH: Dopamine receptor binding predicts clinical and pharmacological potencies of anti-schizophrenic drugs. Science 192:481–483, 1976
7. Chiodo LA, Bunney BS: Typical and atypical neuroleptics: differential effects of chronic administration on the activity of A9 and A10 midbrain dopaminergic neurons. J Neurosci 3:1607–1619, 1983
8. Chiodo LA, Bunney BS: Possible mechanisms by which repeated clozapine administration differentially affects the activity of two subpopulations of midbrain dopamine neurons. J Neurosci 5:2539–2544, 1985
9. Meltzer HY. Treatment of the neuroleptic non-responsive schizophrenic patient. Schizophr Bull 18:515–542, 1992
10. Kane J, Honigfeld G, Singer J, Meltzer HY (Clozaril Collaborative Study Group): Clozapine for the treatment-resistant schizophrenic. Arch Gen Psychiatry 45:789–796, 1988
11. Meltzer HY: Clinical studies on the mechanism of action of clozapine: the dopamine-serotonin hypothesis of schizophrenia. Psychopharmacology 99:S18–S27, 1989
12. Meltzer HY. Clozapine: mechanism of action in relation to its clinical advantages, in Recent Advances in Schizophrenia. Edited by Kales A, Stefanos GN, Talbott JA. New York, Springer-Verlag, 1990, pp 237–246
13. Meltzer HY. The mechanism of action of novel antipsychotic drugs. Schizophr Bull 17:263–287, 1991
14. Krupp P, Barnes P: Leponex-associated granulocytopenia: a review of the situation. Psychopharmacology 99 (suppl):S118–S121, 1989
15. Chouinard G, Jones B, Remington G, et al: A Canadian multicenter placebo-controlled study of fixed doses of risperidone and haloperidol in the treatment of chronic schizophrenic patients. J Clin Psychopharmacol 13:25–40, 1993
16. White FJ, Wang RY: Differential effect of classical and atypical antipsychotic drugs on A9 and A10 dopamine cells. Science 221:1054–1057, 1983

17. White FJ, Wang RY: Comparison of the effects of chronic haloperidol treatment on A9 and A10 dopamine neurons in the rat. Life Sci 32:983–993, 1983
18. Stockton ME, Rasmussen K: A comparison of olanzapine and clozapine effects of dopamine neuronal activity: an electrophysiological study. Society of Neuroscience Abstracts 19:383, 1993
19. Skarsfeldt T, Perregaard J: Sertindole, a new neuroleptic with extreme selectivity on A10 versus A9 dopamine neurons in the rat. Eur J Pharmacol 182:613–614, 1990
20. White FJ, Wang RY: Electrophysiological evidence for the existence of both D_1 and D_2 dopamine receptors in the rat nucleus accumbens. J Neurosci 6:274–280, 1986
21. Goldstein JM, Litwin LC, Sutton EB, et al: Seroquel: electrophysiological profile of a potential atypical antipsychotic. Psychopharmacology 112:293–299, 1993
22. Grace AA: Phasic versus tonic dopamine release in the modulation of dopamine system responsivity: a hypothesis for the etiology of schizophrenia. Neuroscience 41:1–24, 1991
23. Lane RF, Blaha CD: Electrochemistry in vivo: application to CNS pharmacology. Ann N Y Acad Sci 473:50–69, 1986
24. Chen J, Paredes W, Gardner EL: Chronic treatment with clozapine selectively decreases basal dopamine release in nucleus accumbens but not in caudate-putamen as measured by in vivo microdialysis: further evidence for depolarization block. Neurosci Lett 122:127–131, 1991
25. Ichikawa J, Meltzer HY: Apomorphine does not reverse basal dopamine release in rat striatum and nucleus accumbens after chronic haloperidol treatment. Brain Res 507:738–742, 1990
26. Ichikawa J, Meltzer HY: The effect of chronic clozapine and haloperidol on basal dopamine release and metabolism in rat striatum and nucleus accumbens studied by in vivo microdialysis. Eur J Pharmacology 176:371–374, 1990
27. Ichikawa J, Meltzer HY: Differential effects of repeated treatment with haloperidol and clozapine on dopamine release and metabolism in the striatum and the nucleus accumbens. J Pharmacol Exp Ther 256:348–357, 1991
28. Invernizzi R, Morali F, Pozzi L, et al: Effects of acute and chronic

clozapine on dopamine release and metabolism in the striatum and nucleus accumbens of conscious rats. Br J Pharmacol 100: 774–778, 1990

29. Chen J, Ruan D, Paredes W, et al: Effect of acute and chronic clozapine on dopaminergic function in medial prefrontal cortex of awake, freely moving rats. Brain Res 571:235–241, 1992
30. Blaha CD, Lane RF: Chronic treatment with classical and atypical antipsychotic drugs differentially decreases dopamine release in striatum and nucleus accumbens in vivo. Neurosci Lett 78:188–204, 1987
31. Lane RF, Blaha CD, Rivest JM: Selective inhibition of mesolimbic dopamine release following chronic administration of clozapine involvement of α_1-noradrenergic receptors demonstrated by in vivo voltammetry. Brain Res 460:398–401, 1988
32. Kehr W: 3-Methoxytyramine as an indicator of impulse-induced dopamine release in rat brain in vivo. Naunyn Schmiedebergs Arch Pharmacol 293:209–215, 1988
33. Wood PL, Nair NPV, Lal S, et al: Buspirone: a potential atypical neuroleptic. Life Sci 33:269–273, 1983
34. Egan MF, Karoum F, Wyatt RJ: Effects of acute and chronic clozapine and haloperidol administration on 3-methoxytyramine accumulation in rat prefrontal cortex, nucleus accumbens and striatum. Eur J Pharmacol 199:191–199, 1991
35. Abercrombie EC, Zigmond MJ: Striatal DA release: in vivo evidence for local initiation, in Presynaptic Receptors and the Question of Autoregulation of Neurotransmitter Release, Vol 604. Edited by Kalsner S, Westfall TC. New York, The New York Academy of Sciences, 1990, pp 575–578
36. Meltzer HY, Matsubara S, Lee, J-C: Classification of typical and atypical antipsychotic drugs on the basis of dopamine D-1, D-2 and serotonin$_2$ pKi values. J Pharmacol Exp Ther 251:238–246, 1989
37. Sorensen SM, Kehne JH, Fadayel GM, et al: Characterization of the 5-HT$_2$ receptor antagonist MDL 100907 as a putative atypical antipsychotic: behavioral, electrophysiological and neurochemical studies. J Pharmacol Exp Ther 266:684–691, 1993
38. Rivest R, Jolicoeur FB, Marsden CA: Use of amfonelic acid to

discriminate between classical and atypical neuroleptics and neurotensin: an in vivo voltammetric study. Brain Res 544:86–93, 1991

39. Rivest R, Marsden CA: Differential effects of amfonelic acid on the haloperidol- and clozapine-induced increase in extracellular DOPAC in the nucleus accumbens and the striatum. Synapse 10:71–78, 1992
40. Miller HH, Shore PA: Effects of amphetamine and amfonelic acid on the disposition of striatal newly synthesized dopamine. Eur J Pharmacol 78:33–44, 1982
41. Brougham LR, Cornway PG, Ellis DB: Effect of ritanserin on the interaction of amfonelic acid and neuroleptic-induced striatal dopamine metabolism. Neuropharmacology 30:1137–1140, 1991
42. Gudelsky FA, Nwajei EE, DeFife K, et al: Interaction of amfonelic acid with antipsychotic drugs on dopaminergic neurons. Synapse 12:304–311, 1992
43. Oakley NR, Hayes AG, Sheehan MJ: Effects of typical and atypical neuroleptics on the behavioral consequences of activation by muscimol of mesolimbic and nigrostriatal dopaminergic pathways in the rat. Psychopharmacology 105:204–208, 1991
44. Imperato A, Angelucci L: The effects of clozapine and perlapine on the in vivo release and metabolism of dopamine in the striatum and in the prefrontal cortex of freely moving rats. Psychopharmacol Bull 25:383–389, 1989
45. Chen J, Paredes W, van Praag HM, et al: Serotonin denervation enhances responsiveness of presynaptic dopamine efflux to acute clozapine in nucleus accumbens but not in caudate-putamen. Brain Res 583:173–179, 1992
46. Maj J, Sowinska H, Baran L, et al: The central action of clozapine. Polish Journal of Pharmacology and Pharmacy 26:425–435 1978
47. Meltzer HY: Dopaminergic and serotonergic mechanisms in the action of clozapine, in Advances in Neuropsychiatry and Psychopharmacology, Vol 1: Schizophrenia Research. Edited by Schulz SC, Tamminga CA. New York, Raven Press, 1991, pp 333–340
48. Csernansky JG, Wrona CT, Bardgett ME, et al: Subcortical dopa-

mine and serotonin turnover during acute and subchronic administration of typical and atypical neuroleptics. Psychopharmacology 110:145–151, 1993

49. Meltzer HY: Clozapine: clinical advantages and biological mechanisms, in Schizophrenia: A Scientific Focus. International Conference on Schizophrenia. Edited by Schulz SC, Tamminga C. New York, Oxford Press, 1988, pp 302–309
50. Meltzer HY, Maes M, Lee MA: The cimetidine-induced increase in prolactin secretion in schizophrenia: effect of clozapine. Psychopharmacology 112:S95–S104, 1993
51. Kahn RS, Siever L, Davidson M, et al: Haloperidol and clozapine treatment and their effect on m-chlorophenylpiperazine-mediated responses in schizophrenia: implications for the mechanism of action of clozapine. Psychopharmacology 12: S90–S94, 1993
52. Owens RR Jr, Gutierrez-Esteinou R, Hsaio J, et al: Effect of clozapine and fluphenazine treatment on responses to m-chlorophenylpiperazine infusions in schizophrenia. Arch Gen Psychiatry 50:636–644, 1993
53. Ashby CR Jr, Minabe Y, Edwards I, et al: Comparison of the effects of various typical and atypical antipsychotic drugs on the suppressant action of 2-methylserotonin on medial prefrontal cortical cells in the rat. Synapse 8:155–161, 1991
54. Watling KJ, Beer MS, Stanton JA, et al: Interaction of the atypical neuroleptic clozapine with 5-HT_3 receptors in the cerebral cortex and superior cervical ganglion of the rat. Eur J Pharmacol 182:465–472, 1990
55. Blandina P, Goldfarb J, Craddock-Royal B, et al: Release of endogenous dopamine by stimulation of 5-$hydroxytryptamine_3$ receptors in rat striatum. J Pharmacol Exp Ther 251:803–809, 1989
56. Volonté M, Ceci A, Borsini F: Effect of haloperidol and clozapine on (+)SKF 10,047-induced dopamine release: role of 5-HT_3 receptors. Eur J Pharmacol 213:2163–164, 1992
57. Drescher K, Hetey L: Influence of antipsychotics and serotonin antagonists on presynaptic serotonin receptors modulating the release of serotonin in synaptosomes of the nucleus accumbens

of rats. Neuropharmacology 27:31–36, 1988

58. Mason SL, Reynolds GP: Clozapine has sub-micromolecular affinity for 5-HT_{1A} receptors in human brain tissue. Eur J Pharmacol 221:397–398, 1992
59. Wander TJ, Nelson A, Okazaki H, et al: Antagonism by neuroleptics of serotonin 5-HT_{1A} and 5-HT_2 receptors of normal human brain in vitro. Eur J Pharmacol 143:279–282, 1987
60. Corbett R, Hartman H, Klerman LL, et al: Effects of atypical antipsychotic agents on social behavior in rodents. Pharmacol Biochem Behav 45:9–17, 1993
61. Rivest JM, Audenot V, Gobert A, et al: Actions of the potent methoxynaphthylpiperazine 5-HT_{1A} receptor agonists S14506 and S14671 at dopamine D_1, D_2 and D_3 receptors in vitro and in vivo. Society of Neuroscience Abstracts 10:597, 1993
62. Millan MJ, Gobert A, Laurelle G, et al: Potential antidepressive and antipsychotic properties of the high efficacy methoxynaphthylpiperazine 5-HT_{1A} agonists, S14506 and S14671. Society of Neuroscience Abstracts 19:597, 1993
63. Goff DC, Midha KK, Brotman AW, et al: An open trial of buspirone added to neuroleptics in schizophrenic patients. J Clin Psychopharmacol 11:193–197, 1991
64. Neal-Beliveau BS, Joyce JN, Lucki I: Serotonergic involvement in haloperidol-induced catalepsy. J Pharmacol Exp Ther 265: 207–217, 1993
65. Monsma FJ Jr, Shen Y, Ward RR, et al: Cloning and expression of a novel serotonin receptor with high affinity for tricyclic psychotropic drugs. Mol Pharmacol 43:320–327, 1993
66. Shen Y, Monsma FJ Jr, Metcalf MA, et al: Molecular cloning and expression of a 5-hydroxytryptamine serotonin receptor subtype. J Biol Chem 7:18200–18204, 1993
67. Roth BL, Craigo SC, Choudhary MS, et al: Binding of typical and atypical antipsychotic agents to 5-$hydroxytryptamine_6$ (5-HT_6) and 5-$hydroxytryptamine_7$ (5-HT_7) receptors. J Pharmacol Exp Ther 268:1406–1410
68. Canton H, Verrièle L, Colpaert FC: Binding of typical and atypical antipsychotics to 5-HT_{1C} and 5-HT_2 sites: clozapine potently interacts with 5-HT_{1C} sites. Eur J Pharmacol 191:93–96, 1990

69. Roth BL, Ciaranello RD, Meltzer HY: Binding of typical and atypical antipsychotic agents to transiently expressed 5-HT$_{1C}$ receptors. J Pharmacol Exp Ther 260:1361–1365, 1992
70. Kuoppamäki M, Seppälä T, Syvälahti E, et al: Clozapine and *N*-desmethylclozapine are potent 5-HT$_{1C}$ receptor antagonists. Eur J Pharmacol 245:179–182, 1993
71. Molineaux SA, Jessell TM, Axel R, et al: 5-HT$_{1C}$ receptor in a prominent serotonin receptor subtype in the central nervous system. Proc Natl Acad Sci U S A 88:6793–6797, 1989
72. Kuoppamäki M, Seppälä T, Syvälahti E, et al: Chronic clozapine treatment decreases 5-hydroxytryptamine$_{1C}$ receptor density in the rat choroid plexus: comparison with haloperidol. J Pharmacol Exp Ther 264:1262–1267, 1993
73. Hoenicke EM, Vanecek SA, Woods JH: The discriminative stimulus effects of clozapine in pigeons: involvement of 5-hydroxytryptamine$_{1C}$ and 5-hydroxytryptamine$_2$ receptors. J Pharmacol Exp Ther 263:276–284, 1992
74. Wiley JL, Porter JH: Serotonergic drugs do not substitute for clozapine in clozapine-trained rats in a two-lever drug discrimination procedure. Pharmacol Biochem Behav 43:961–965, 1992
75. Meltzer HY, Nash JF: Effects of antipsychotic drugs on serotonin receptors. Pharmacol Rev 43:587–604, 1991
76. Nash JF: Ketanserin pretreatment attenuates MDMA-induced dopamine release in the striatum as measured by in vivo microdialysis. Life Sci 47:2401–2406, 1990
77. Schmidt CJ, Abbate GM, Black CK, et al: Selective 5-hydroxytryptamine$_2$ receptor antagonists protect against the neurotoxicity of methylenedioxymethamphetamine in rats. J Pharmacol Exp Ther 478–483, 1990
78. Schmidt CJ, Black CK, Taylor VL: Antagonism of the neurotoxicity due to a single administration of methylenedioxymethamphetamine. Eur J Pharmacol 181:59–70, 1990
79. Schmidt CJ, Taylor VL, Abbate GM, et al: 5-HT$_2$ antagonists stereoselectively prevent the neurotoxicity of 3,4-methylenedixymethamphetamine. J Pharmacol Exp Ther 256:230–235, 1991
80. Goldstein JM, Litwin LC, Sutton EB, et al: Effects of ICI

169,369, a selective serotonin antagonist in electrophysiological tests predictive of antipsychotic activity. J Pharmacol Exp Ther 249:673–680, 1989

81. Sorensen SM, Humphreys TM, Taylor VI, et al: 5-HT_2 antagonists reverse amphetamine-induced slowing of dopaminergic neurons by interfering with stimulated dopamine synthesis. J Pharmacol Exp Ther 260:872–878, 1992
82. Schmidt CJ, Fadayel GM, Sullivan CK, et al: 5-HT_2 receptors exert a state dependent regulation of dopaminergic function: studies with MDL 100,907 and the amphetamine analogue, 3,4-methylenedioxymethamphetamine. Eur J Pharmacol 223:65–74, 1992
83. Altar CA, Wasley AM, Neale RF, et al: Typical and atypical antipsychotic occupancy of D_2 and S_2 receptors: an autoradiographic analysis in rat brain. Brain Res Bull 16:517–525, 1986
84. Wadenberg M-L, Ahlenius S, Svensson TH: Potency mismatch for behavioral and biochemical effects by dopamine receptor antagonist: implications for the mechanism of action of clozapine. Psychopharmacology 110:273–279, 1993
85. Stockmeier CA, DiCarlo JJ, Zhang Y, et al: In vivo characterization of typical and atypical antipsychotic drugs based on in vivo occupancy serotonin-2 and dopamine-2 receptors. J Pharmacol Exp Ther 266:1374–1384, 1993
86. Matsubara S, Kusumi I, Koyama T, et al: Dopamine D_1, D_2 and serotonin$_2$ receptor occupation by typical and atypical antipsychotic drugs in vivo. J Pharmacol Exp Ther 265:498–503, 1993
87. Sumiyoshi T, Kido H, Sakamoto H, et al: Time course of dopamine-D_2 and serotonin-5-HT_2 receptor occupancy rates by haloperidol and clozapine in vivo. Jpn J Psychiatry Neurol 47: 131–137, 1993
88. Lee T, Tang SW: Loxapine and clozapine decrease serotonin (S_2) but do not elevate dopamine (D_2) receptor numbers in the rat brain. Psychiatr Res 12:277–285, 1984
89. Matsubara S, Meltzer HY: Effect of typical and atypical antipsychotic drugs on 5-HT_2 receptor density in rat cerebral cortex. Life Sci 45:1397–1406, 1989
90. Wilmot CA, Szczepanik AM: Effects of acute and chronic treatments with clozapine and haloperidol on serotonin (5-HT_2) and

dopamine (D_2) receptors in the rat brain. Brain Res 487:288–298, 1989

91. O'Dell S, La Hoste GJ, Widwark CB, et al: Chronic treatment with clozapine or haloperidol differentially regulates dopamine and serotonin receptor in rat brain. Synapse 6:146–153, 1990
92. Fardé L, Nordström A-L, Wiesel FA, et al: Positron emission tomographic analysis of central D_1 and D_2 dopamine receptor occupancy in patients treated with classical neuroleptics and clozapine. Arch Gen Psychiatry 49:538–544, 1992
93. Goyer PF, Berridge MS, Semple QE, et al: Dopamine$_2$ and serotonin$_2$ receptor indices in clozapine treated schizophrenic patients. Schizophr Res 9:199, 1993
94. Costall B, Naylor RJ: Neuroleptic interactions with the serotonergic-dopaminergic mechanisms in the nucleus accumbens. J Pharm Pharmacol 30:257–259, 1973
95. Balsara JJ, Jaelhav JH, Chandorkar AG: Effect of drugs influencing central serotonergic mechanisms or haloperidol-induced catalepsy. Psychopharmacology 22:67–69, 1979
96. Korsgaard S, Gerlach J, Christensson E: Behavioral aspects of serotonin-dopamine interactions in the monkey. Eur J Pharmacol 118:245–252, 1985
97. Hicks PB: The effect of serotonergic agents on haloperidol-induced catalepsy. Life Sci 47:1609–1615, 1990
98. Schotte A, de Bruychere K, Janssen PFM, et al: Receptor occupancy by ritanserin and risperidone measured using ex vivo autoradiography. Brain Res 500:295–301, 1989
99. Meltzer HY, Zhang Y, Stockmeier CA: Effects of amperozide on rat cortical 5-HT$_2$ and striatal and limbic dopamine D_2 receptor occupancy: implications for antipsychotic action. Eur J Pharmacol 216:67–71, 1992
100. Bersani G, Grispini A, Marini S, et al: Neuroleptic-induced extrapyramidal side effects: clinical perspectives with ritanserin (R35667), a new selective 5-HT$_2$ receptor blocking agent. Current Therapeutic Research 40:492–499, 1986
101. Rogue A, Rogue P: Mianserin in the management of schizophrenia, in Schizophrenia 1992, an International Conference Abstract Book. Vancouver, British Columbia, 1992, p 135

102. Gelders YG, Heylen SL, Vanden BG, et al: Pilot clinical investigation of risperidone in the treatment of psychotic patients. Pharmacopsychiatry 23:206–211, 1990
103. Borison RL, Diamond BI, Pathiraja AP, et al: Clinical overview of risperidone, in Novel Antipsychotic Drugs. Edited by Meltzer HY. New York, Raven Press, 1992, pp 233–239
104. Miller RJ, Hiley CR: Anti-muscarinic properties of neuroleptics and drug-induced parkinsonism. Nature 248:596–597, 1974
105. Racagni G, Cheney DL, Trabucchi M, et al: In vivo actions of clozapine and haloperidol on the turnover rate of acetylcholine in rat striatum. J Pharmacol Exp Ther 196:323–332, 1976
106. Nielsen EB: Cholinergic mediation of the discriminative stimulus properties of clozapine. Psychopharmacology 94:115–118, 1988
107. Bolden C, Cusack B, Richelson E: Clozapine is a potent and selective muscarinic antagonist at the five cloned human muscarinic cholinergic receptors expressed in CHO-K1 cells. Eur J Pharmacol 192:205–206, 1991
108. Bolden C, Cusack B, Richelson E: Antagonism by antimuscarinic and neuroleptic compounds at the five cloned human muscarinic cholinergic receptors expressed in Chinese hamster ovary cells. J Pharmacol Exp Ther 260:576–580, 1992
109. Scholz E, Dichgans J: Treatment of drug-induced exogenous psychosis in Parkinsonism with clozapine and fluperlapine. European Archives of Psychiatry and Neurological Sciences 235:60–61, 1985
110. Karson CN, Garcia-Rill E, Biedermann J, et al: The brain stem reticular formation in schizophrenia. Psychiatr Res 40:31–48, 1991
111. Ljunberg T, Ungerstedt U: Evidence that the different properties of haloperidol and clozapine are not explained by differences in anticholinergic potency. Psychopharmacology 60:303–307, 1979
112. Boyson SJ, McGonigle P, Luthin GR, et al: Effects of chronic administration of neuroleptic and anticholinergic agents on densities of D_2 dopamine and muscarinic cholinergic receptors in rat striatum. J Pharmacol Exp Ther 244:987–993, 1988

113. de Belleroche J, Neal MJ: The contrasting effects of neuroleptics on transmitter release from the nucleus accumbens and corpus striatum. Neuropharmacology 21:529–537, 1982
114. Rivest R, Marsden CA: Muscarinic antagonists attenuate the increase in accumbens and striatum dopamine metabolism produced by clozapine but not by haloperidol. Br J Pharmacol 104:234–238, 1991
115. Meltzer HY, Chai BL, Thompson PA, et al: Effect of scopolamine on the efflux of dopamine and its metabolites following clozapine, haloperidol or thioridazine. J Pharmacol Exp Ther, 1994, pp 1452–1461
116. Stadler H, Lloyd KG, Bartholini G: Dopaminergic inhibition of striatal cholinergic neurons: synergistic blocking action of gamma-butyrolactone and neuroleptic drugs. Naunyn Schmiedebergs Arch Pharmacol 283:129–134, 1974
117. Sheng M, Greenberg ME: The regulation and function of c-*fos* and other immediate early genes in the nervous system. Neuron 4:477–485, 1990
118. Miller JC: Induction of c-*fos* mRNA expression in rat striatum by neuroleptic drugs. J Neurochem 54:1453–1455, 1990
119. Gradunow M, Robertson GS, Faull RLM, et al: D_2 dopamine receptor antagonists induce *fos* and related protein in rat striatal neurons. Neuroscience 37:287–294, 1990
120. Robertson GS, Fibiger HC: Neuroleptic increase on c-*fos* expression in the forebrain: contrasting effects of haloperidol and clozapine. Neuroscience 46:315–318, 1992
121. Nguyen TV, Kosofsky BE, Birnbaum R, et al: Differential expression of c-*fos* and Zif268 in rat striatum after haloperidol, clozapine, and amphetamine. Proc Natl Acad Sci U S A 89:4270–4274, 1992
122. Cameron DS, Duman RS, Deutsch AY: Clozapine induces *fos* expression in pyramidal cells and interneurons in the prefrontal cortex in a regionally specific manner. Society of Neuroscience Abstracts 19:1213, 1993
122a. Deutch AY, Lee MC, Iadarola MJ: Regionally specific effects of atypical antipsychotic drugs on striatal fos expression: the nucleus accumbens shell as a locus of antipsychotic action. Mo-

lecular Cellular Neural Science 3:332–341, 1992

123. Merchant KM, Dobner PR, Dorsa DM: Differential effects of haloperidol and clozapine on neurotensin gene transcription in rat neostriatum. J Neurosci 12:652–663, 1992
124. Bolden-Watson C, Watson MA, Murray KD, et al: Haloperidol but not clozapine increases neurotensin receptor mRNA levels in rat substantia nigra. J Neurochem 61:1141–1143, 1993
125. Salin P, Mercugliano M, Chesselet M-F: Differential effects of chronic treatment with haloperidol and clozapine on the level of preprosomatostatin mRNA in the striatum, nucleus accumbens, and frontal cortex of the rat. Cell Mol Neurobiol 10:127–143, 1990
126. Ennulat DJ, Cohen BM: Differential display of mRNAs following neuroleptic treatment. Society of Neuroscience Abstracts 19: 384, 1993
127. Angulo JA, Cadet JL, McEwen BS: Effect of typical and atypical neuroleptic treatment on protachykinin mRNA levels in the striatum of the rat. Neurosci Lett 113:217–221, 1990
128. Guo N, Robertson GS, Fibiger HC: Scopolamine attenuates haloperidol-induced c-*fos* expression in the striatum. Brain Res 588: 164–167, 1992
129. Deakin JFW, Slater P, Simpson MDC, et al: Frontal cortical and left temporal glutamatergic dysfunction in schizophrenia. J Neurochem 52:1781–1786, 1989
130. Kim JS, Kornhuber HH, Schmic-Burgk W, et al: Low cerebrospinal fluid glutamate in schizophrenic patients and a new hypothesis on schizophrenia. Neurosci Lett 20:379–382, 1980
131. Kornhuber J, Mack-Burkhardt F, Rieferer P, et al: [^{3}H]MK-801 binding sites in postmortem brain regions of schizophrenia patients. Journal of Neural Transmission 77:231–236 1989
132. Harrison PJ, McLaughlin D, Kerwin RW: Decreased hippocampal expression of a glutamate receptor gene in schizophrenia. Lancet 337:450–452, 1991
133. Sherman AD, Davidson AT, Baruah S, et al: Evidence of glutamatergic deficiency in schizophrenia. Neurosci Lett 121:77–80, 1991
134. Tiedtke PI, Bischoff C, Schmidt WJ: MK-801-induced stereotypy

and its antagonism by neuroleptic drugs. Journal of Neural Transmission 81:173–182, 1990

135. Hoffman DC: Typical and atypical neuroleptics antagonize MK-801-induced locomotion and stereotypy in rats. J Neural Transm Gen Sect 89:1–10, 1992
136. Verma A, Kulkarni SK: Modulation of MK-801 response by dopaminergic agents in mice. Psychopharmacology 107:431–436, 1992
137. Kim JS, Clause D, Kornhuber HH: Cerebral glutamate, neuroleptic drugs and schizophrenia: increase of cerebrospinal fluid glutamate levels and decrease of striate body glutamate levels following sulpiride treatment in rats. Eur Neurol 22:367–370, 1983
138. Squires RF, Saederup E: A review of evidence for GABA-ergic predominance/glutamatergic deficit as a common etiological factor in both schizophrenia and affective psychoses: more support for a continuum hypothesis of "functional" psychosis. Neurochem Res 16:1009–1111, 1991
139. Bardgett ME, Wrona CT, Newcomer JW, et al: Subcortical excitatory amino acid levels after acute and subchronic administration of typical and atypical neuroleptics. Eur J Pharmacol 230:245–250, 1993
140. Moghaddam B, Bunney BS: Acute effects of typical and atypical antipsychotic drugs on the release of dopamine from prefrontal cortex, nucleus accumbens, and striatum of the rat: an in vivo microdialysis study. J Neurochem 54:1755–1760, 1990
141. Pehek EA, Yamamoto BK, Meltzer HY: The effects of clozapine on dopamine, 5-HT, and glutamate release in the rat medial prefrontal cortex. Schizophr Res 4:323, 1991
142. Daly DA, Moghaddam B: Actions of clozapine and haloperidol in the extracellular levels of excitatory amino acids in the prefrontal cortex and striatum of conscious rats. Neurosci Lett 152:61–64, 1993
143. Pehek EA, Meltzer HY, Yamamoto BK: The atypical drug amperozide enhances rat cortical and striatal dopamine efflux. Eur J Pharmacol 240:107–109, 1993
144. Carlsson A: The current status of the dopamine hypothesis of

schizophrenia. Neuropsychopharmacology 1:179–186, 1988

145. Carlsson M, Carlsson A: Systems within the basal ganglia: implications for schizophrenia and Parkinson's disease. Trends Neurosci 13:272–276, 1990
146. Baskys A, Wang S, Remington G, et al: Haloperidol and loxapine but not clozapine increase synaptic responses in the hippocampus. Eur J Pharmacol 235:305–307, 1993
147. Hassler R, Haug P, Nitsch C, et al: Effect of motor and premotor cortex ablation on concentrations of amino acids, monoamines, and acetylcholine, and on the ultrastructure in the rat striatum: a confirmation of glutamate as the specific corticostriatal transmitter. J Neurochem 38:1087–1098, 1982
148. Mangano RM, Schwarcz R: Chronic infusion of endogenous excitatory amino acids into rat striatum and hippocampus. Brain Res Bull 10:47–51, 1983
149. McBean GJ, Roberts PJ: Chronic infusion of L-glutamate causes neurotoxicity in rat striatum. Brain Res 290:372–375, 1984
150. Coyle JT: Excitotoxins, in Psychopharmacology: A Third Generation of Progress. Edited by Meltzer HY. New York, Raven Press, 1987, pp 333–340
151. Ellison DW, Beal MF, Mazurek MF, et al: Amino acid neurotransmitter abnormalities in Huntington's disease and the quinolinic acid animal model of Huntington's disease. Brain 11:1657–1673, 1987
152. Donzanti BA, Uretsky NJ: Magnesium selectively inhibits N-methyl-aspartic acid-induced hypermotility after intra-accumbens injection. Pharmacol Biochem Behav 20:243–246, 1984
153. Martin JB: Huntington's disease: new approaches to an old problem. Neurology 34:1059–1072, 1984
154. Schwarcz R, Foster A, French ED, et al: Excitotoxic models for neuro-degenerative disorders. Life Sci 35:19–32, 1984
155. Rao TS, Contreras PC, Cler JA, et al: Clozapine attenuates *N*-methyl-d-aspartate receptor complex-mediated responses in vivo: tentative evidence for a functional modulation by a noradrenergic mechanism. Neuropharmacology 30:557–565, 1991
156. Farber NB, Price MT, Labrugere J, et al: Protection against NMDA antagonist neurotoxicity by clozapine and repeated analog cor-

relates with antipsychotic efficacy. Society of Neuroscience Abstracts 19:384, 1993

157. Graham SR, Kokkindis L: Clozapine inhibits limbic system kindling: implications for antipsychotic action. Brain Res Bull 30:-597–605, 1993
158. Snell LD, Johnson KM: Characterization of the inhibition of excitatory amino acid-induced neurotransmitter relapse in the rat striatum by phencyclidine-like drugs. J Pharmacol Exp Ther 238:938–946, 1986
159. Krebs MO, Desce JM, Kemel ML, et al: Glutamatergic controls of dopamine release in the rat striatum: evidence for a presynaptic *N*-methyl-d-aspartate receptor on dopaminergic terminals. J Neurochem 56:81–85, 1991
160. Garau L, Govini S, Stefanini E, et al: Dopamine receptors: pharmacological and anatomical evidences indicate that two distinct populations are present in rat striatum. Life Sci 23:1745–1750, 1978
161. Schwarcz R, Creese L, Coyle JT, et al: Dopamine receptors localized on cerebral cortical afferents to rat striatum. Nature 271: 766–768, 1978
162. Spano PF, Mamo M, Stefanni E, et al: Detection of multiple receptors for dopamine, in Receptors of Neurotransmitters and Peptide Hormones. Edited by Pepeu G, Kuhar MJ, Enna SJ. New York, Raven Press, 1980, pp 243–251
163. Theodorou A, Reaveill C, Jenner P, et al: Kainic acid lesions of striatum and decortication reduce specific [^{3}H]sulpiride binding in rats, so D-2 receptors exist post-synaptically on corticostriate afferents and striatal neurons. J Pharm Pharmacol 33: 439–444, 1981
164. Trugman JM, Geary WA, Wooten GF: Localization of D-2 dopamine receptors on intrinsic striatal neurons by quantitative autoradiography. Nature 322:267–269, 1986
165. Joyce JN, Loeschen SK, Marshall JF: Dopamine D-2 receptors in rat caudate-putamen: the lateral to medial gradient does not correspond to dopaminergic innervation. Brain Res 338:209–218 1985
166. Beckstead RN: Association of dopamine D_1 and D_2 receptors

with specific cellular elements in the basal ganglia of the cat: the uneven topography of dopamine receptors in the striatum is determined by intrinsic striatal cells, not nigrostriatal axons. Neuroscience 27:852–863, 1988

167. Filloux R, Liu TH, Hsu CY, et al: Selective cortical infarction reduces [^{3}H]sulpiride binding in rat caudate-putamen: autoradiographic evidence for presynaptic D_2 receptors on corticostriate terminals. Synapse 2:251–531, 1988
168. Kornhuber J, Kornhuber ME: Presynaptic dopaminergic modulation of cortical input to the striatum. Life Sci 39:669–674, 1986
169. Kerkerian L, Nieoullon A: Supersensitivity of presynaptic receptors involved in the dopaminergic control of striatal high affinity glutamate uptake after 6-hydroxydopamine lesions of the nigrostriatal dopaminergic neurons. Exp Brain Res 69:424–430, 1988
170. Yamamoto BK, Davy S: Dopaminergic modulation of glutamate release in striatum as measured by microdialysis. J Neurochem 58:1736–1742, 1992
171. Yamamoto BK, Cooperman MA: Effect of chronic antipsychotic treatment of extracellular dopamine and glutamate concentrations in the rat striatum. Society of Neuroscience Abstracts 18:379, 1992
172. Lidsky TI, Alter E, Banerjee SP: Effects of clozapine on glutamatergic transmission. Society of Neuroscience Abstracts 17:686, 1991
173. Meshul CK, Casey DE: Regional reversible ultrastructural changes in rat brain with chronic neuroleptic treatment. Brain Res 489:338–346, 1989
174. Meshul CK, Janowsky A, Casey DR, et al: Effect of haloperidol and clozapine on the density of "perforated" synapses in caudate, nucleus accumbens, and medial prefrontal cortex. Psychopharmacology 106:45–52, 1992
175. Meshul CK, Janowsky A, Casey DE, et al: Coadministration of haloperidol and SCH-23390 prevents the increase in "perforated" synapses due to either drug alone. Neuropsychopharmacology 7:285–293, 1992
176. Greenough WT, West RW, De Voogd TJ: Subsynaptic plate perfo-

rations: changes with age and experiences in the rat. Science 202:1096–1098, 1978

177. Meshul CK, Janowsky A, Casey DE, et al: Haloperidol-induced synaptic changes in rat caudate nucleus are prevented by prior treatment with MK-801 or lesioning of the thalamus. Society of Neuroscience Abstracts 16:419, 1990

CHAPTER

17

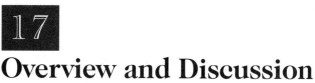

Overview and Discussion

Steven Matthysse, Ph.D.

When I first became interested in schizophrenia, people were still pursuing will-o'-the-wisps like ceruloplasmin and taraxein. We are not chasing ceruloplasmin and taraxein any more, nor are we studying wasting cells, double binds, or synaptic slippage. Schizophrenia research is no longer an embarrassment, because it has achieved a healthy relationship with basic science. In 1959, in his famous articles appearing in *Science*, Seymour Kety[1] showed that the fault in the old biochemical approaches was that there was no logical connection between the abnormalities reported in patients with schizophrenia and established principles of brain function, but rather "the extremely small chance of selecting this particular and heretofore unknown substance from the thousands of substances which occur in blood and which might have been chosen" (p. 1592).

Seymour Kety's critique marked the watershed. We have come a long way in these 35 years, as Charles Nemeroff's graph of the cascade of brain peptides dramatically illustrated. We know many of the "molecular actors," to use Huda Akil's nice phrase. Joseph Coyle put it exactly when he said, "How close the walk is, between the lab bench and the patient's bed." Who would have guessed that restriction enzymes in bacteria would provide a key to human genetic linkage? Or that electron-positron annihilation would make possible the powerful imaging techniques that Marcus Raichle showed us? In the present period, there will be those who want the fruits of science but are such bad gardeners that they kill the tree. We know that basic science is the wellspring of clinical research, but we are going to have to say it again and again.

Perhaps it is less obvious, but equally important, that basic science can prosper from the stimulus of clinical problems. David Housman gave the excellent example of *anticipation*, a puzzling clinical phenomenon that geneticists were reluctant to take seriously but turned out to be fully explicable in terms of unstable DNA repeats, which now prove to be important in the genetics of several neuropsychiatric diseases. It is no accident that clinical problems stimulate basic science. Our practical needs spring from the same universe described by scientific law; disease manifests the processes of Nature, as their dark side. Life turns against itself: the immune mechanisms that protect us from invaders make antibodies against our own cells; viruses subvert the DNA transcriptional mechanism to reproduce themselves; recurrent neuronal excitation, without which signal propagation would be impossible, goes out of control and causes seizures; the limitless capacity of cell division turns into cancer. The powers of the body are the source of its diseases. So it will be with schizophrenia and affective illness: they will help us to understand higher mental functions, just as autoimmune disease, virus replication, and cancer help us to understand molecular biology.

In 1856, when the brewers of Lille asked the dean of the local university to figure out what had gone wrong in their distilleries, no one could guess that he would discover the biochemistry of fermentation. Pasteur insisted on the stimulating value of the applied problem: "No, a thousand times no; there does not exist a category of science to which one can give the name applied science," he said[2] (p. 74). Of course, we must not forget one ingredient in his success: after the brewers gave him the problem, they left him alone. "Louis is now up to his neck in beet juice," his wife wrote.[3] We need to immerse our scientists up to their necks in schizophrenia, and leave them alone.

If we really accept the idea that disease is a great teacher, we have to learn to listen. Sometimes what I heard over the last 2 days sounded as though we were rushing out, armed with our new techniques, to slay this dragon, schizophrenia, but it could have been any dragon at all—a sort of generic dragon—not this particular foe, schizophrenia. We would section it, link it, image it, record from it, double-label it—whatever it was—but would we take the time to look at it? Would our methods apply equally well to any disease at all? We need to get to know our enemy:[4]

> "*A fish can live in water because. . . .*" Because it's learned to swim. "*What if it couldn't swim?*" Not naturally, he couldn't. Why do certain gods have effects on seas like that? What does the earth have such an effect to break their backs? The fishes near home come to the surface and break. "*Why?*" I think it is due to bodies that people lose. A body becomes adapted to the air. Think thoughts and break the fishes. (p. 25)

Patricia Goldman-Rakic stressed the role of loose associations in schizophrenia. The patient is dominated by immediate impressions, "the here and now," and the train of thought gets derailed because "the patient can't keep in mind where he is going." To explain loosening of associations by defective working memory is a nice hypothesis, but our view would be too limited if we regarded loose associations as the whole story of thought pathology in schizophrenia. The failure of logic and pragmatics goes beyond loosening of associations. Consider the example cited; schizophrenic thinking just does not come out right.

In nonpsychotic people, by contrast, thinking not only comes out right, but it comes out right without apparent effort. Our language must conform to rules of syntax, semantics, logic, and pragmatics, but there is no sign that we calculate before we speak. Ordinary thinking demands no special concentration and takes hardly any time. We do not have to sift through a mixture of logical and illogical, appropriate and inappropriate thoughts. We do not form our thoughts by a process of trial and error.

There is not even any sign that as children we were clumsy in our thinking but have practiced the skill to the point where it has become automatic; we do not learn to think the way we learn to ride a bicycle. The child's thoughts occur as abundantly as the adult's, and they spontaneously obey rules of form appropriate to his age. Indeed, on the basis of clever habituation experiments, E. S. Spelke[5] has been able to characterize the logical structure of the infant's spatial world. Infants appear to endow the world with entities that are:

- Cohesive: "When objects move freely, they move as wholes."
- Bounded: "Objects do not blend into other objects when they are freely displaced."
- Substantial: "When objects move freely, they do not pass through one another."
- Spatiotemporally continuous: "An object does not move from one place to another without tracing a continuous path between them."

From the earliest ages on, thought seems to operate as though it had available an intrinsically well-behaved raw material. Well-formed elements of thought come to the thinker, prior to any active work on his or her part, in abundance and with an inherent tendency to combine in ways that are logically appropriate. In those with schizophrenia, this natural preconditioning of thought is lost. The thoughts that come to mind combine in perverse ways that violate logic and common sense. Through conscious mental effort, thought can be redirected into normal channels, and indeed some schizophrenic patients, in the early stages, try to regain control over their thinking, but eventually they fail. I do not think that this disability is a loss of normal "filtering." Nonpsychotic people do not need to filter out ill-formed thoughts. They choose among good candidates. Like an orchestra, Marcus Raichle observed, the brain has an "immense capacity to produce a wide variety of behaviors . . . drawn from a larger pool in many combinations and ways." To pursue his metaphor, the orchestra's conductor can count on each of the musicians to obey the rules of musical form. Schizophrenic individuals, on the other hand, seem to be offered possibilities for ideation that just would not occur to nonpsychotic people.[6]

Let us take as our starting point Patricia Goldman-Rakic's postulate that "the cortex evolved to establish internal representations of the external world." Can we imagine a form of representation that would embed the formal structure that Spelke observed in children's conceptions of space into the raw material of imagination and action? The task of representation is difficult. The laws of the mind are jurisprudential (like the laws of a commonwealth)—constraining, but not dictating, choice—but the laws of neurons are mechanical. Translating jurisprudential law to mechanical law is the fundamental problem of cerebral representation.

Long before "representation" became part of the vocabulary of cognitive science, it was an honored term in mathematics, and if we look closely at the mathematical concept we shall discover that the mathematicians had the idea we need. As an example, here are the axioms for "groups of dihedral type." The symbol ∀ means "for all," and the symbol ∃ means "there exists." Λ is short for "and."

Associativity:	$\forall xyz(x \cdot (y \cdot z) = (x \cdot y) \cdot z)$
Identity:	$\forall x(x \cdot 1 = x \wedge 1 \cdot x = x)$
Inverse:	$\forall x \exists y(x \cdot y = 1 \wedge y \cdot x = 1)$
Noncommutativity:	$\exists xy(x \cdot y \neq y \cdot x)$
Generating involutions:	$\exists xy[x \cdot x = 1 \wedge y \cdot y = 1 \wedge \forall z \exists m_1, n_1, \ldots, m_r, n_r(z = x^{m_1} y^{n_1} \ldots x^{m_r} y^{n_r})]$

The axioms state "a few things that must be" (for example, the last one states that every element z in the group is expressible as a product of a sequence of the two generators x and y), but they do not define completely "everything that may be." Indeed, there are an infinite number of finite groups satisfying these axioms, as well as one group with an infinite number of members[7] (pp. 115–118).

Now I will show you a *representation* of these axioms, that is, a concrete realization in a definite mathematical system. The particular representation consists of eight 2 × 2 matrices of complex numbers. Ignore, for the moment, the letters *R* and *F* appearing under the matrices:

$$\begin{bmatrix}1&0\\0&1\end{bmatrix}\begin{bmatrix}0&1\\1&0\end{bmatrix}\begin{bmatrix}\sqrt{-1}&0\\0&-\sqrt{-1}\end{bmatrix}\begin{bmatrix}-1&0\\0&-1\end{bmatrix}\begin{bmatrix}-\sqrt{-1}&0\\0&\sqrt{-1}\end{bmatrix}\begin{bmatrix}0&\sqrt{-1}\\-\sqrt{-1}&0\end{bmatrix}\begin{bmatrix}0&-1\\-1&0\end{bmatrix}\begin{bmatrix}0&-\sqrt{-1}\\\sqrt{-1}&0\end{bmatrix}$$

$C \quad F \quad R \quad R^2 \quad R^3 \quad RF \quad R^2F \quad R^3F$

The operation · in the list of axioms is interpreted as matrix multiplication, which is a way of taking two matrices and combining them to get a third (the details of how matrices are multiplied do not matter for this discussion, just the concept that there is a way to do it). You can multiply these eight matrices to your heart's content, and the axioms will always be satisfied. The axioms are, so to speak, built in to the structure of the matrices, so that operations on the matrices will never fail to satisfy them.

Matrices are a little more concrete than axioms but still are rather abstract, so now let us consider a very concrete representation of the same axioms. It is one very close to the hearts of public speakers. Imagine a slide put into the projector backwards. You take it out and put it back into the projector, only this time it is upside down. A third try gets you upside down and backwards. There are seven ways to get it wrong, and only one way to get it right.

In fact, what we have here is a representation of the same group, the dihedral group with eight members. Let C stand for "correct," R for "rotate a quarter turn clockwise," and F for "flip." The two "generators" referred to in the last axiom can be chosen as "flip" and "flip and then rotate," F and FR. They are called "involutions" because doing either of them twice in succession gets you back where you started from. (Try it with a book, starting right side up: two flips get you back to right side up, and so do two "flip-and-then-rotate-a-quarter-turn.")

We have, as you see, two very different representations of the same set of axioms: matrices and ways of arranging lantern slides. In this case, the objects in the two representations correspond to each other; the letter under each matrix, like "R^3F," indicates the corresponding alignment of the lantern slide ("R^3F" means "rotate a quarter turn three times, then flip").

Now I will show you what use all this is. Suppose we set out to prove a theorem about the dihedral group with eight elements, such as "$RFR^2F = R^3$." That theorem is true, and you can prove it by multiplying the matrices R and F, but that is the hard way. The easy way is just to take out a lantern slide and carry out the indicated actions: rotate, flip, rotate twice more, and flip again, and compare the result with the right-hand side of the equation, rotating three times in succession. You end up with the same alignment, whichever set of actions you carry out. Proving the theorem was easy the second way, because the axioms of the dihedral group are directly built into the motions of lantern slides. Jurisprudential laws (what the axioms allow) are expressed by mechanical laws (how rotations and flips of real objects combine). The right choice of representation makes proving the theorem easy.

In the normal brain, it may be that the axioms of cognition are directly built into the physiology of local neuronal circuits so that, however complex their interactions, they never fail to be governed by rule. In the schizophrenic brain, the corresponding neuronal circuits are not capable of physiologically "representing" the axioms, so their outputs are free to combine in ways that violate the laws of thought.

This proposal has two obvious weaknesses, which unfortunately cannot be remedied at the present time, even if in broad outline it turns out to be true. First, we cannot write down a set of "axioms of cognition" as we can axioms for groups of dihedral type, even though we have a general intuition that cognition has lawful properties. Second, we know far too little about the physiology of neuronal circuits to state precisely what it would mean for local neuronal circuits to serve as a realization of a set of axioms. Nevertheless, we can put some flesh on these philosophical bones. Let us talk about Josephson junctions. Granted, they are not neurons, but at least they are closer to neurons than matrices and lantern slides.

Josephson junctions are solid state devices in which an electron pair tunnels through a very thin insulating barrier between superconductors. They are very useful in electronic circuits, for example, in the ultrasensitive magnetic field detectors used in magnetoencephalography.

Typically, such arrays oscillate in a fully symmetric mode; all the units oscillate at the same frequency, and all in phase. In that way their signals add and the array can be used, for example, as a voltage-tuned radiofrequency source. It can happen, however, that the symmetry is broken and the individual junctions no longer are completely synchronized. When the symmetry breaks, the array becomes multistable. A large number of patterns emerge, but they are always of two reproducible types:[9]

1. The junctions divide into two approximately equal groups, oscillating with half the original frequency. Within each group, the waveform is constant and the oscillations are synchronized, but between the two groups the waveform differs. Because the assignments of the individual junctions to the two groups are not determined, approximately $2N$ different patterns are possible if there are N junctions.
2. All the junctions continue to oscillate with the same waveform and frequency, but their phases are regularly staggered, each one leading the next by an approximately constant interval (this is called the "ponies on a merry-go-round" solution[8]). Because the order of phase lags (i.e., who goes first on the merry-go-round) is not determined, approximately $(N - 1)!$ patterns are possible.

In short, the symmetry can break in a very large number of ways [$\approx 2N + (N - 1)!$], but there are definite rules constraining the patterns that emerge. To pursue our earlier analogy, the constraints on the patterns are the jurisprudential laws of the Josephson junction array, whereas the equations of the electronic circuit are the mechanical laws by which they are realized. The array satisfies two of the requirements that we have set out for cerebral representation: 1) natural satisfaction of constraints and 2) fertility of combinations. Of course, it remains only an analogy, but it gives us a different way of looking at the behavior of neuronal circuits, one that may bridge the gap between cognition and neurophysiology more effectively than traditional methods of analysis.

Stanley Watson charged each of the speakers with pointing out new experimental methods that may be useful in understanding the biology of schizophrenia and affective disorders in the years ahead. The major obstacle to the analyses I have described is the fact that we can record from only one, or at most a few, neurons at the same time. Conventional analyses of single-neuron behavior cannot tell us anything about the array as a whole, any more than examining the immediate environment of one H_2O molecule can tell us whether we are looking at water or ice. Nevertheless, one neuron can serve as a probe of the whole array, thanks to an ingenious method invented by David Ruelle and Floris Takens that (so to speak) turns space into time. Interspike interval (ISI), the time between action potentials, is the standard indicator of neuronal activity; the shorter the interval, the greater the firing rate. In our context, the idea is to take as data not the simultaneous ISIs of many cells, but the successive ISIs of one cell.

Imagine a multidimensional space describing one cell in which the most recent ISI is represented along the z-axis, the next most recent ISI on the x-axis, and the ISI before that on the y-axis. More axes could be used if necessary. As time goes on, the neuron being recorded emits more and more action potentials. For each firing, one more point is added, with the new "most recent ISI" on the z-axis, the new "next most recent" on the x-axis, and so on. The history of the neuron is represented by a succession of points tracing out a path in the multidimensional space. The path will wind around itself in a complicated fashion, not forming a closed loop, as it would if the circuit containing the neuron were strictly periodic, but (probably) not a random tangle, either.

In a well-studied example, the Beluzhov Zhabotinski reaction, although there are many components in the reaction, recording the trajectory of just one component (bromide) does not lead to a hopeless tangle, because the present bromide potential depends on the past bromide potentials in an orderly, although nonperiodic, fashion. As a function of time, the bromide potential winds around a thin band in the "time-lagged" space.[10]

R. Hoffman, B. S. Bunney, and I are applying similar techniques to ISIs recorded from midbrain dopamine cells. Our working hypothesis is that changes in behavioral state will be reflected by changes in the band that winds around the multidimensional ISI space. We are looking for changes that are "topological" as well as "geometrical." For example, if the band twisted into a knot or curled up into a torus (inner tube), the change would be topological, whereas if it elongated or became more angular, the change would be geometrical. Topological changes are interesting because, if they occur in a neural circuit, they probably will be independent of which neuron is being recorded from, whereas the geometrical properties of the trajectory in ISI space are likely to be dependent on the neuron selected to represent the population.

Let us retrace our steps. The mysterious quality of thought disorder in schizophrenia led us to reflect on the facility of normal thinking, by which I mean its fertility (the abundance of ideas) and its natural tendency to conform to rules of competence. We found that abundant combinations that naturally satisfy rules can be readily found in systems of mathematical objects. Perhaps more to the point, some electronic circuits have the same remarkable properties, for example, Josephson junction arrays that break symmetry into thousands of oscillation patterns but only into patterns conforming to a few simple rules. Even though neurophysiologists are ordinarily restricted to recording from one or a few neurons at a time, there is a method of plotting the response of one neuron with sequential time lags that might nevertheless be able to reveal global changes in the network pattern.

These ideas lead to a particular way of thinking about schizophrenic thought pathology. If the resistive or capacitative load in the Josephson junction array is changed, the symmetry may not break, or the outcomes when it does break may not conform to the simple rules that we discussed before. In other words, the performance of these arrays depends very much on *tuning*. Detuning leads to stereotypical or underconstrained behavior. The same may be true in schizophrenia. "Tipping the balance" between excitatory (glutamate) and inhibitory (*N*-acetyl-aspartyl-glutamate [NAAG]) actions at *N*-methyl-D-aspartate (NMDA) receptors, as Joseph Coyle conjectured, could affect the tuning of local circuits. So could developmental disruption of prefrontal cortex connectivity, as in Daniel Weinberger's model, or changes in the levels of our old friend dopamine (as reviewed by René Kahn). Indeed, dopamine blockers might restore the balance of a local circuit detuned by decreased γ-aminobutyric acid (GABA)-ergic inhibition, as Francine Benes suggested. One clinical phenomenon that is consistent with this circle of ideas is *intermittency* in the behavior of some schizophrenic patients: their thinking is not constantly and uniformly abnormal, but fluctuates in and out of pathology from moment to moment. It is a hopeful view, because circuits that fail because their parameters are outside the proper operating ranges might be tuned up again.

To sum up, although we have reason to take pride in our new technologies, let us also allow ourselves to be genuinely puzzled by the phenomena of schizophrenia—by the woman who could say, and somehow mean, "think thoughts and break the fishes." Our reward may be not only understanding schizophrenia, but—because it is the dark side of the thought process—understanding the marvel that, for the rest of us, thinking is so easy.

References

1. Kety SS: Biochemical theories of schizophrenia: a two-part critical review of current theories and of the evidence used to support them. Science 129:1528–1532, 1590–1596, 1959
2. Pasteur L: Why France lacked superior men at the moment of peril. La Revue Scientifique de la France et de l'Etranger 1:73–77, 1871
3. Vallery-Radot R: The Life of Pasteur. New York, Doubleday, 1923
4. Cameron N: Reasoning, regression and communication in schizophrenics. Psychological Monographs 50:1–34, 1938
5. Spelke ES: Where perceiving ends and thinking begins: the apprehension of objects in infancy, in Minnesota Symposium on Child Psychology, Vol 20. Edited by Yonas A. Hillsdale, NJ, Erlbaum, 1988, pp 197–234
6. Matthysse S: Why thinking is easy, in Philosophy and Psychopathology. Edited by Spitzer M, Maher BA. New York, Springer-Verlag, 1990, pp 178–186
7. Rose JS: A Course on Group Theory. Cambridge, Cambridge University Press, 1978
8. Aronson DG, Golubitsky M, Mallet-Paret J: Ponies on a merry-

go-round in large arrays of Josephson junctions. Nonlinearity 4: 903–910, 1991
9. Hadley P, Beasley MR, Wiesenfeld K: Phase locking of Josephson-junction series arrays. Physical Review B 38:8712–8719, 1988
10. Swinney HL: Geometry and dynamics in experiments on chaotic systems. Contemporary Mathematics 28:349–355, 1984

Index

Page numbers printed in **boldface** *type refer to tables or figures.*

A

ACTH. *See* Adrenocorticotropic hormone (ACTH)
Adenovirus major late promoter, **54**
Adenylosuccinate lyase deficiency, 132
ADI. *See* Autism Diagnostic Interview (ADI)
Adoption studies
  of schizophrenia, 171–172
    schizoid personality disorder, 184–185
    schizotypal personality disorder, 183
ADOS. *See* Autism Diagnostic Observation Schedule (ADOS)
Adrenal glands
  glucocorticoids synthesis in, 17
  volume of in affective disorder patients, 266–267, **268**
α-Adrenergic function, of noradrenergic system, 211–212
α_2-Adrenergic function, antidepressant action mechanism and, 313
β-Adrenergic function
  antidepressant action mechanism and, 310–312
  of noradrenergic system, 210–211
Adrenergic system. *See* Suicide postmortem studies
Adrenocortical steroids. *See* Glucocorticoids
Adrenocorticotropic hormone (ACTH). *See also* Corticotropin-releasing factor (CRF)
  stress response role of
    circadian rhythm function of, 22–24
    derivation of, 17–19
    function of, 19–21
    LHPA dysregulation in aged rats and, 35–36
    LHPA negative regulation and, 26–29
    LHPA positive regulation and, 30–31

Affective disorders. *See also* Bipolar disorder; Neuropeptides, affective disorders and; Schizoaffective disorder
adrenal gland volume and, 266–267, **268**
pituitary gland volume and, 266–267, **268**
schizoaffective disorder and, 182
SRIF and, 270–277, **273**
TRH and, 277–282
Agranulocytosis, 452
Alcoholism suicide, 197
Allelic heterogeneity, 131–132
Alzheimer's disease
CRF concentrations and, 265, 269
SRIF concentrations and, 272, 275
γ-Aminobutyric acid (GABA). *See also* Antidepressant action mechanism, other neurotransmitter systems
atypical antipsychotics and, 456
dysfunction in neurotransmission of
in schizophrenia, 92–93, **94**
in layer II of anterior cingulate region, 93–95
prenatal abnormalities affecting, 95, 102
systems level schizophrenia model and, 98–102, **100–101**
in familial pure depressive disease (FPDD), 251
GAT/NET gene family relationships and, 57, **58**
glutamatergic dysfunction and, 470
suicide postmortem studies of, 198
Amitriptyline, 52
Amoxapine
glutamatergic dysfunction and, 473
serotonergic system and, 461–462
Amperozide
glutamatergic dysfunction and, 471
serotonergic system and, 462
Amphetamines, 59, 68
Amygdala
brain circuitry and
antidepressants and, 242
familial pure depressive disease (FPDD) and, 242, **244,** 251–252
shared brain circuitry and, **246,** 248–251, **250**
dopaminergic system and, 370–371, 372, **373**
glutamatergic afferent inputs from, 86
schizophrenia postmortem studies of
blood flow abnormalities in, 225
nucleus accumbens linked to, 227
serotonin transport uptake sites of, 65
SRIF concentrations in, 271
temporal lobe structure abnormalities and, 397
TRH concentrations and, 279
Anatomy of brain circuits. *See also* Biochemistry, of brain circuits; Brain circuits and function
ARNMD meeting presentations on, **11**
disease related to, xv, xvi

Angiotensin II, III, 62–63
Anorexia nervosa
CRF concentrations and, 265
SRIF concentrations and, 274, 275
Anterior cingulate region
corollary discharge and, 439–440
GABA receptor binding abnormalities in, 92–93, **94,** 98–102, **100–101**
glutamatergic dysfunction in, 85–92, **87, 88**
intrinsically cued behavior and, 437
major depression and, 253
in shared brain circuitry, **246,** 247–248
in systems level schizophrenia model, 98–102, **100–101**
Antidepressant action mechanism. *See also* Norepinephrine transporters; Serotonin transporters (SERT)
conclusions regarding, 328–329
dopamine function and
clinical studies of, 319
preclinical studies of, 319
summary regarding, 318
therapeutic studies of, 319
5-HT function and, 296, **297–298**
clinical studies of, 305–308, **306**
preclinical studies of
on behavioral sensitivity, 304–305
on electrophysiologic sensitivity, 303–304
on neurochemical sensitivity, 303
on receptor binding, 299–303, **300–301**
summary regarding, 308–309
therapeutic studies of, 308
norepinephrine function and
clinical studies of, 313–317, **314**
preclinical studies of
on α_2-adrenergic function, 313
on β-adrenergic function, 310–312
on norepinephrine uptake sites, 310
on tyrosine hydroxylase activity, 309–310, **311**
summary regarding, 317–318
other neurotransmitter systems and, excitatory amino acid systems: NMDA receptors and, 321–323
research directions regarding, 329–330
neuroanatomy of antidepressant action and, 333–334
postreceptor signal transduction and, 331–333
Antidepressants. *See also* Antidepressant action mechanism; Serotonin transporters (SERT)
amygdala and, 242
CRF concentrations and, 265–266
disorder prescribed for
bipolar disease, 5–6
major depression, 4
5-HT_2 receptor biding sites and, 205
neuropeptides and
CRF and, 262, 263–266, **264,** 269

Antidepressants *(continued)*
neuropeptides and
CRH and hypothalamic-pituitary-adrenal axis and
clinical studies of, 324–326, **325**
preclinical studies of, 323–324
therapeutic studies of, 326
neuropeptide Y and, 327
somatostatin and, 327–328
SRIF and, 272–275, **273,** 276, 280
TRH and, 279–282
norepinephrine function and, therapeutic studies of, 317
novel treatment approaches with for depressive illness, 334–336, **335**
other neurotransmitter systems and cholinergic function and, 321
$GABA_B$ receptor upregulation and, 320
platelet and brain targets for, 64–72, **66**
serotonin reuptake blocked by, 13, 72
Antipsychotics. *See also* Atypical antipsychotics
disorders prescribed for
autism, 7
bipolar disease, 6
schizophrenia, 224
neuroanatomical function of, 451–452
Apomorphine, 371, 378
Arginine-vasopressin (AVP)
ACTH secretion and, 18–19
brain stress response function of, 19–21
LHPA dysregulation in aged rats and, 32, 35–36
LHPA negative regulation and, 26–29
ARNMD. *See* Association for Research in Nervous and Mental Disease (ARNMD)
Asperger's syndrome, 131
Association for Research in Nervous and Mental Disease (ARNMD), 73rd meeting of, 1–2
purpose of, 1–2
research areas presented at, **11**
syndromes studied at, **11**
autism, 6–7, **8**
bipolar disease, 4–6, **5**
major depression, 3–4, **3–4**
schizophrenia, 6, **7**
timeliness of, xv
Associative memory
prefrontal cortex alterations and, 115–116
working memory and, 114
Atrial natriuretic peptide, 63
Atropine, 466
Atypical antipsychotics
clozapine and
activation of immediate to early genes by, 467–469
cholinergic system and, 465–467
dopaminergic system and, 451–456
limbic selectivity of, 455–456
low EPS incidence of, 453–455, 460, 463, 467, 472
vs. serotonergic affects, 457–464
effectiveness of, 452

glutamate role in the action of, 469–474
serotonin and, 456–464
conclusions regarding, 474–475
mesolimbic and mesocortical vs. nigrostriatal selectivity, 453–456
Auditory hallucinations, 441–442
Autism
diagnostic criteria for, **8**
overview of, 6–7
Autism Diagnostic Interview (ADI)
advantages of, 135
affected vs. unaffected vs. uncertain status measured by, 136, 140–141, 143–147, **144, 145, 146**
description of, 134
diagnoses from compared to referral diagnoses, 140–142, **141**
fragile X syndrome measured by, 132
Autism Diagnostic Observation Schedule (ADOS), 134–135
Autism. *See* Infantile autism
Autosomal inheritance, 132–133
AVP. *See* Arginine-vasopressin (AVP)

B

Basal ganglia
dopamine receptors in, 224, 225–226, 400
LSPT circuit and, 253
schizophrenia postmortem studies of, 225–227, **226**
D_2 receptors and, 225–226
Becker's muscular dystrophy, 131
Bed nucleus of the stria terminalis (BNST), 29
Benzodiazepine, 93
Beta-endorphin, 18
Beta-melanocyte-stimulating hormone. *See* β-MSH
Betaine, 57–58, **58**
Biochemistry
ARNMD meeting presentations on, **11**
of brain circuits, 10–13, **12**
disease related to, xvi
Bipolar disorder
diagnostic criteria for, **5**
LSPT circuit and, 253
overview of, 4–6
schizoaffective disorder and, 183
SRIF concentrations and, 274, 275
BNST. *See* Bed nucleus of the stria terminalis (BNST)
Brain circuits and function. *See also* Schizophrenic brain
in depressive subtypes, 253–254
in familial pure depressive disorder (FPDD), 242–244, **243, 244,** 251–252
imaging of
strategy of, 240–242
techniques of, 239–240
in LSPT circuit, 253–254
in self-induced dysphoria, **243,** 244–247, **244, 246**
shared circuits, **243, 244, 246,** 248–251, **250**
in verbal response selection, 247–248
Brain imaging. *See* Brain circuits and function
Brain stem
blood flow abnormalities in, 225
LHPA positive regulation and, 29–31
mRNA cloning in, 65–67, **66**

Brain stem *(continued)*
schizophrenia postmortem studies of, 225
suicide postmortem studies of
5-HT and 5-HIAA in, 199, **199,** 200, **213**
norepinephrine and metabolite concentrations in, 207–209, **207, 213**
Bulimia, SRIF concentrations and, 274, 275
Buspirone, 458

C

c-fos
clozapine and, 467–469
LHPA negative regulation and, 25
LHPA positive regulation and, 31
c-jun
LHPA negative regulation and, 24
LHPA positive regulation and, 31
cAMP. *See* Cyclic adenosine monophosphate (cAMP)
Canonical memory, 114
Capgras's syndrome, 443
Captopril, 63
Carbamazepine, 276, 276–277
Carbidopa, 223
CAT. *See* Computed axial tomographic (CAT) scan
Catatonic schizophrenia, 6
Catecholamines
norepinephrine transporters and, 59–60, 61
working memory and, 115
Caudal medulla, 30
Caudate nucleus
dopaminergic system and, 370–371, 372, **373, 374,** 400, 474
familial pure depressive disease (FPDD) and, 242
cDNA. *See* Complementary DNA (cDNA)
Cerebral cortex
dopamine receptors in, 224
SRIF in, 271
Cerebral cortical mechanisms dissolution
neuroleptics and, 120–122, 370–371
neuropathology of, 120–122
prefrontal cortex and, 113–114
associative memory function and, 115–116
blood flow studies of, 117
dopamine systems and, 120–122, **121**
functional organization, informational domains within, 117–119, **119**
internal representation through, 114–119, **119**
neuroleptics affecting, 120–122, 370–371
neuropathology of, 120–122
spatial working memory function and, 116–117
working memory function and, 114–117, 118–119, 397
Cerebral spinal fluid (CSF)
CRF concentrations in, 262, 263–265, **264**
dopaminergic system function and, 375–376
SRIF concentrations in, 272–275, **273**
Cerebral ventricular enlargement, 394–396, 406
Chlorpromazine
glutamatergic dysfunction and, 470
serotonergic system and, 462

Chlorprothixene, 458
Cholesterol, 17
Cholinergic system
  antidepressants and, 321
  clozapine and, 465–467
Chromosome 5, 178
Chromosome 22, 179
Cingulate cortex
  blood flow abnormalities in, 225
  dopaminergic system and, **373**
Circadian rhythm
  glucocorticoid and mineral-ocorticoid receptors negative feedback regulation and, 26, 29
  LHPA axis regulation of, 22–24
  LHPA dysregulation in aged rats and, 32, 36
Citalopram
  5-HT uptake and, 68
  prefrontal serotonin transporter biding sites and, 202
Clozapine. *See also* Atypical antipsychotics, clozapine and
  dopamine receptors affected by, 121, 224, 371
  for schizophrenia, 6, 224
Cocaine
  dopamine transport blocked by, 13
  norepinephrine and serotonin transporters and, 50, 59, 69
  uptake 1 inhibited by, 52–53
Cognitive processes. *See also* Frontotemporal abnormalities; Memory
  dopaminergic system and, 401
  "over-inclusiveness" of in schizophrenia, 92
  schizophrenia thought pathology and
    developmental maturation of, 495–497
    internal cerebral representations of the external world and, 497–500
    interspike interval (ISI) between action potentials and, 501–502
    loose associations and, 495–497
Complementary DNA (cDNA), 17–18
  cloning of hNET cDNA and, 55–56, **56,** 65–68, **66**
  cloning of SERT cDNA and, 65–67, **66,** 71, 72
  norepinephrine and serotonin transporter structure and, 53, **54,** 55–56, **56,** 71
Computed axial tomographic (CAT) scan
  introduction of, 223
  ventricular size abnormalities studied by, 224–225
Computerized tomography (CT)
  brain structure abnormalities studied by, 393–394
    anatomical asymmetries, 404
    lateral cerebral ventricular enlargement, 394–396
Concordance rates, of schizophrenic twins, 170
Corollary discharge modulation, 439–440
  auditory hallucinations and, 441–442
  delusional misinterpretations and, 442
  delusions of control and passivity experiences and, 443
  inappropriate affect and, 442–443

Corticolimbic system, of the schizophrenic brain, 98–102, **100–101**
Corticosteroids, 19–21, 24, 26–29
Corticosterone, 19, 24
  LHPA dysregulation in aged rats and, 32–36
Corticotropin-releasing factor (CRF), 18, 260–270, **264, 267, 268**
  ACTH and, 262–263, 269
  in cerebral spinal fluid (CSF) of depressed patients, 262, 263–266, **264,** 269
  future research issues on, 269–270
  HPA hyperactivity in major depression and, 262–263, 269–270
  locus ceruleus noradrenergic neurons and, 261–262
  other psychiatric disorders and, 265, 269
  pituitary and adrenal gland volumes and, 266–267, **268,** 269
  receptor downregulation of in suicide victims, 266, **267,** 269
  stress response behavior reactions of, 260–261, 269
Corticotropin-releasing hormone (CRH)
  ACTH secretion and, 18–19
    circadian rhythm function and, 22–24
  brain stress response function of, 19–21
  LHPA dysregulation in aged rats and, 32, 35–36
  LHPA negative regulation and, 26–29
  LHPA positive regulation and, 30–31
Cortisol, 19, 24
COS cells, 53, **54,** 55
Creatine, 57–58, **58**
CRF. *See* Corticotropin-releasing factor (CRF)
CRH. *See* Corticotropin-releasing hormone (CRH)
CSF. *See* Cerebral spinal fluid (CSF)
[^{3}H]Cyanoimipramine binding
  serotonin transporters and, 65
  in suicide victims, 201, **201,** 202
Cyclic adenosine monophosphate (cAMP), 63
Cystic fibrosis, 131
Cytogenetic testing, of autism, 139
Cytomegalovirus infection, 130

D

Delusional misidentification, 443
Delusional misinterpretations, 442
Delusions of control, 443
Dementia, SRIF concentrations and, 271, 272
Depolarization blockade, 371, 376, **377**
Depression. *See* Major depression
Desipramine
  CRF concentrations and, 266
  SRIF affected by, 276
  as uptake 1 antagonist, 52
N-Desmethylclozapine, 459
Dexamethasone
  adrenal volume and, 266–267, **267**
  SRIF concentrations and, 274–275
Diethylaminoethyl, **54**
Disorganized schizophrenia, 6
Disulfide bridge formation, **56,** 67

DNA. *See also* Complementary DNA (cDNA)
  restriction fragment length polymorphism (RFLP) marker of, 177–178
Dopamine, for Parkinson's disease, 223
Dopamine-β-hydroxylase
  anatomy of, 370–372
  brain stem noradrenergic neurons and, 209
Dopaminergic system. *See also* Antidepressant action mechanism, dopamine function and; Atypical antipsychotics; Schizophrenic brain, postmortem studies of
  cerebral cortical mechanisms and, 120–122, **121**
  clozapine and
    activation of immediate to early genes and, 467–469
    cholinergic system and, 465–467
    glutamatergic dysfunction and, 469–474
    serotonin system and, 456–464
  cocaine effects on, 13
  cognitive specificity and, 401
  conclusions regarding, 382–383
  decreased function of
    cortical function affected by, 379–380
    depolarization blockade and, 371, 376, **377**
    dopamine function affected by, 380–381
  hypothesis of in schizophrenia, 369–370
  increased function of
    homovanillic acid (HVA) and, 372, **373,** 375–379, **377, 378,** 400, 401
    peripheral measures of
      CSF studies, 375–376
      plasma studies, 376–379, **377, 378**
    PET studies of, 374–375
    postmortem studies of, 372–374, **373, 374**
  linking increased with decreased function within, 381–382
  neuroimaging studies of, 400–401
  proteins and, **12,** 13
  receptors of
    1 through 5, 13, 371–372
    2 through 4, **12,** 13, 115, 371–372
  reuptake substrate of for norepinephrine influx, 52
  suicide postmortem studies of, 198
  working memory affected by, 115
Dorsal raphe, 30
Dorsolateral prefrontal cortex. *See* Prefrontal cortex region, dorsolateral
DSM-III-R criteria
  for infantile autism, 135
  for schizophrenia, 169
  for schizotypal and schizoid personality disorder, 185
DSM-IV criteria
  for infantile autism, 135
  for schizoaffective disorder, 182
Duchenne's muscular dystrophy, 131
Dysphoria. *See* Self-induced dysphoria
Dysthymia, SRIF concentrations and, 274

E

Eigenimage, of frontotemporal activity pattern, 430–432, **431, 433, 435**
Electroconvulsive therapy
CRF concentrations and, 265
for major depression, 4
TRH concentrations and, 278
Entorhinal cortex
schizophrenia postmortem studies of
blood flow abnormalities in, 225
nucleus accumbens linked to, 227
structural deformities of, 225, 228, **229**
temporal lobe structure abnormalities and, 396
Environmental factors
in schizophrenia
as single vs. heterogeneous disorder, 179
twin studies of, 170–171, 176
Epilepsy
SRIF treatment of, 271
TRH treatment of, 279
Eticlopride, 470
Extrapyramidal symptoms (EPS)
of atypical antipsychotic drugs, 453–454
of clozapine, 453–455, 460, 463, 472
cholinergic system and, 465, 467

F

Familial pure depressive disorder (FPDD)
description of, 242–244, **243, 244**
LSPT circuit and, 253
shared brain circuitry and, 251–252
Family studies
of schizophrenia, 167–169
diagnosis of families, 185–186
of paranoid personality disorder, 184
pseudo-autosomal locus studies and, 179
of schizoid personality disorder, 184–185
of schizotypal personality disorder, 183, 185
Federal funding reduction, xvi
54-kilodalton (kDA) species in PC12 cells, norepinephrine transporter structure and, 53
Fluoxetine
CRF concentrations and, 265–266
5-HT uptake and, 68
Fluperlapine
cholinergic system and, 465
serotonergic system and, 462
Fluphenazine
atypical antipsychotics vs., 453
dopaminergic system and, 456
FMR-1 gene
autism linkage to, 150–151
fragile X syndrome linkage to, 147–149
southern blot typing of the CGG repeat of, 149–150
FPDD. *See* Familial pure depressive disorder (FPDD)
Fragile X syndrome, 132, 138, 139, 147–149
Frontal cortex. *See also* Frontotemporal abnormalities; Prefrontal cortex region

asymmetries of, 404
c-fos expression and, 468
GABA dysfunction in, 92–93, **94**
glutamatergic dysfunction and, 89–90, 469, 472
hypofunction and, 398
circumstances of, 399–400
medication affecting, 398–399
intrinsically cued behavior and, 436–439
Frontotemporal abnormalities
conclusions regarding, 444
data supporting
acquisition and preprocessing of, 424–425, **426**
subjects, 425–427
developmental cortical interactions and, 422
discussion of, 434–436
intrinsically and extrinsically cued behavior and, 436–439
neuronal basis of sensory representations and, 443–444
schizophrenia and frontotemporal integration, 440–441
delusional misinterpretations and, 442
delusions of control and passivity experiences and, 443
hallucinations and, 441–442
inappropriate affect and, 442–443
self-monitoring and corollary discharge and, 439–440
functional connectivity and
definition, explanation of, 423
differences in amount of (covariance matrix), 427–429, **429**
distributed activity patterns defined by, 429–432, **431, 433**
differences between, 432–434, **435**
psych fractionation and, 421–422
Functional brain imaging. *See* Brain circuits and function
Funding reduction, xvi

G

G proteins, 10
GABA. *See* γ-Aminobutyric acid (GABA)
GAT/NET gene family
cloning of, 50
norepinephrine transporter structure and, 57–61, **58,** 64
SERT cDNA cloning and, 65–67, **66,** 72
Gender differences
in infantile autism, 132, **142**
in major depression, 3
in schizophrenia, 166, 167
Genetic counseling, schizophrenia and, 187–188
Genetic heterogeneity, 131–132
Genetic marker definition, 177
Genetics. *See also* GAT/NET gene family; Genomic mechanism; Infantile autism; Schizophrenia, behavioral genetics of
ARNMD meeting presentations on, **11**
disease related to, xv, xvi
neurobiology paired with, xv

Genomic mechanism. *See also* GAT/NET gene family; Genomic mechanism; Infantile autism; Schizophrenia, behavioral genetics of
  brain stress response function and, 20–21
  clozapine and, 467–469
  glucocorticoid and mineralocorticoid receptors as negative feedback receptors and, 25
  LHPA positive regulation through, 31
Globus pallidus, 224
Glucocorticoid receptor (GR)
  LHPA dysregulation in aged rats and, 33–34
  LHPA negative feedback control by, 24–29
Glucocorticoids
  adrenal gland synthesis of, 17
  brain stress response function of, 16, 19–21
    circadian rhythm function and, 22–24
  LHPA dysregulation in aged rats and, 32–36
  perinatal development affected by, 95
Glutamatergic dysfunction, 84
  clozapine and, 469–474
  glutamate decarboxylase (GAD) activity dysfunction and, 92
  neuronal cell concentrations and, 85–89, **87, 88,** 122
  ontogenesis of and excitotoxicity, 97–98
  pre- and postnatal development abnormalities and, 95–97, 102
  receptor binding studies of, 89–92
    entorhinal cortex abnormalities and, 228
    frontal cortex receptor binding sites and, 90–91
    hippocampus receptor binding sites and, 89–91, 228
    phencyclidine (PCP) receptor binding activity, 90, 91–92
Glycine, 57–58, **58**
GR. *See* Glucocorticoid receptor (GR)
Grant funding reduction, xvi
Growth hormone-releasing factor, 270–271, 272

H

Haloperidol
  activation of immediate to early genes by, 467–469
  atypical antipsychotics vs., 453
  cholinergic system and, 465–466
  dopaminergic system affected by, 121, 378, 455–456
  EPS of, 460
  glutamatergic dysfunction and, 470–474
  prescribed for schizophrenia, 6
  serotonergic system and, 457, 463
Heterocyclic antidepressants, 69
5-HIAA
  serotonergic system of suicide victims and, 198–200, **199**
  SRIF concentrations and, 275
Hippocampus
  clozapine and
    glutamatergic system and, 472
    serotonergic system and, 458
  dopaminergic system and, 371
  GABA dysfunction in, 92, 98–102, **100–101**

glutamatergic system
abnormalities in, 89–91
clozapine and, 472
myelination changes and, 96–97
ontogenesis of and excitotoxicity, 97–98
postnatal development of, 96, 102
LHPA
dysregulation of in aged rats and, 32–36
negative regulation of, 26–29
mineralocorticoid receptor in, 24–26
psychological stress reaction of, 38
schizophrenia postmortem studies of, 228, **229**
blood flow abnormalities in, 225
nucleus accumbens linked to, 227
structural deformities of, 225, 228
serotonin transport uptake sites of, 65
SRIF concentrations in, 271
in systems level schizophrenia model, 98–102, **100–101**
temporal lobe structure abnormalities and, 396–397
TRH concentrations and, 279
Histidinemia, 132
Homovanillic acid (HVA)
cholinergic system and, 466
dopaminergic system and, 372, **373**
in CSF, 375–376, 381, 400, 401
in plasma (pHVA), 376–379, **377, 378**
5-HT. *See also* Antidepressant action mechanism, 5-HT function and; Serotonin; Serotonin transporters (SERT); Suicide postmortem studies
antidepressants and, 50, 59
clozapine and, 456–464
Na^+, Cl^-, K^- cotransport and, 52, **53**
SRIF affected by, 276
Huntington's disease
CRF concentrations and, 265
glutamatergic dysfunction and, 472
HVA. *See* Homovanillic acid (HVA)
5-Hydroxytryptamine. *See* 5-HT
Hypofrontality
conditions causing, 399–400
medication affecting, 398–399
neurodevelopment of schizophrenia and, 406
Hypothalamus. *See also* Limbic-hypothalamic-pituitary-adrenal axis (LHPA); Thyrotropin-releasing hormone (TRH)
ACTH secretion and, 18–19
CRF and, 262–263, 269–270
CRH in, 18
glucocorticoid and mineralocorticoid receptors in, 24–26
LHPA dysregulation in aged rats and, 35
medial parvicellular aspect of the paraventricular nucleus of (mpPVN), 18
brain stress response function of, 19–21
LHPA dysregulation in aged rats and, 35–36
LHPA positive regulation and, 29–31

Hypothalamus *(continued)*
serotonin transport uptake sites of, 65, 459
SRIF in, 271
ventricular enlargement and, 228, 394–396

I

ICD-10 system, infantile autism and, 135
Imaging techniques. *See also* Brain circuits and function; *specific techniques*
advancements in, 223–224, 239
application of, xvi
Imipramine, 52. *See also* [^{3}H]Cyanoimipramine binding; [^{3}H]Imipramine binding
[^{3}H]Imipramine binding
serotonin transporters and, 65
in suicide victims, 200–202, **201**
Inappropriate affect, 442–443. *See also* Affective disorders; Schizophrenia
Incidence rate, of schizophrenia, 165
Infantile autism
autosomal inheritance and, 132–133
causes of, 130–132
diagnostic accuracy and, 131–132
genetic etiology evidence and, 130
transmission modes and, 130
conclusions regarding, 151–154, **151, 152, 153**
$(CCG)_n$ amplification, 151
FMR-1 gene findings, 151–154
results, 157
testing for linkage to autosomal markers: genotyping, 154–155
testing of models and calculating lod scores, 155–156, **156**
on X linkage, 154
diagnostic accuracy and
allelic heterogeneity, 131–132
genetic heterogeneity, 131–132
locus heterogeneity, 131
genetic studies of
characteristics of unaffected siblings in autism multiplex families, 140–141, **141,** 143–145, **145**
characteristics of uncertain siblings in autism multiplex families, 136, 146–147, **146**
clinical characteristics of autism multiplex families, 142, **142**
clinical characteristics of autistic, unaffected, and uncertain groups, 140–141, 143, **144**
comparison of referral and ADI diagnoses and, 140–142, **141**
initial results of, 140
issues in
definition of affected status, 136, 140–141, **141**
definition of unaffected status, 136, 140–141, **141**
linkage analysis, 136–137
multiplex families, 134
selection of diagnostic instruments, 134–135

multiplex families recruitment and evaluation, 134, 136
blindness in diagnoses and, 139
diagnostic instruments and, 134, 138–139
fragile X syndrome and cytogenetic testing and, 139
initial screening procedures and, 138
recruitment methods and, 137–138
linkage studies of, 130
fragile X syndrome, 147–149
immortalizing lymphocytic cell lines, 147, 149
linkage to *FMR-1*: autism and, 150–151, **151, 152, 153**
linkage to *FMR-1*: fragile X syndrome and, 147–149
problems associated with, 130–131
southern blot typing of the CGG repeat in *FMR-1,* 149–150
X linkage, 147
phenocopies and, 130–131, 134
polygenic inheritance and, 131
statistics regarding, 129–130
X-linked inheritance and, 132
Insulin, norepinephrine transport and, 63
Interspike interval (ISI) between action potentials, 501–502
Intramolecular disulfide bridge, **56**
ISI. *See* Interspike interval (ISI) between action potentials

J

Jargon aphasia, 441–442

K

[^{3}H]Kainate binding, glutamatergic dysfunction and, 469
kDA. *See* 54-kilodalton (kDA) species
[^{3}H]Ketanserin binding
atypical antipsychotics and, 460
in suicide victims, 203–204

L

Latent structure analysis, 174
Lesch-Nyhan syndrome, 131
Levodopa
atypical antipsychotics and, 461
for Parkinson's disease, 223
LHPA. *See* Limbic-hypothalamic-pituitary-adrenal axis (LHPA)
Limbic-hypothalamic-pituitary-adrenal axis (LHPA)
aged rat as model of mild dysregulation of, 31–36
glucocorticoid and mineralocorticoid receptors and, 24–26
main elements of, 17–19
negative regulatory circuits, 26–29
neuronal control of
positive regulatory circuits, 29–31
physical stress and
psychological sequelae to, 15–16
unpredictable vs. predictable stressors and, 16
psychological stress reaction and, 36–39
receptors involved in negative feedback within, 24–26
regulation of
circadian rhythm and, 22–24
stress responsiveness and, 19–21

Linkage studies
of infantile autism, 130
fragile X syndrome and, 147–149
immortalizing lymphocytic cell lines and, 147, 149
linkage to *FMR-1*: autism and, 150–151, **151, 152, 153**
linkage to *FMR-1*: fragile X syndrome and, 147–149
problems associated with, 130–131
southern blot typing of the CGG repeat in *FMR-1* and, 149–150
X linkage and, 147
of schizophrenia
chromosome 5 studies, 178
chromosome 22 studies, 179
gametes formation, chromosome cross-over and, 176–177
genetic marker definition and, 177
phenotypic expressions of genotype issue of, 179–180
pseudo-autosomal locus studies and, 179
RFLP explanation, 177–178
sample size limitations of, 180–181
single vs. heterogeneous disorder issue of, 179
Lithium chloride
for bipolar disease, 5
SRIF affected by, 276
Locus ceruleus
CRF and, 261–262
LHPA positive regulation and, 30
norepinephrine and metabolites in, 209–210, 261–262
serotonin transport uptake sites of, 65
Locus heterogeneity, 131
Loxapine
glutamatergic dysfunction and, 472, 473
serotonergic system and, 462
Lymphocytic cell lines, autism and, 147, 149

M

Magnetic resonance imaging (MRI) scan
brain structure abnormalities studied by, 225, 228, 393–394
frontotemporal abnormalities studied by, 422
introduction of, 223
Major depression. *See also* Familial pure depressive disorder (FPDD); Self-induced dysphoria
diagnostic criteria for, **3–4**
dopaminergic activity and, 252
LHPA dysregulation and, 38–39
LSPT circuitry and, 252, 253–254
neuropeptides and
CRF concentrations and, 262–270, **264**
SRIF concentrations and, 271–276, **273,** 280
TRH concentrations and, 279–282
overview of, 3–4
SERT activity and, 72
suicide and, 197
Mania
CRF concentrations and, 265
SRIF concentrations and, 274
Manic syndrome, of bipolar disease, 4–5

Mathematical genetic transmission models
of schizophrenia
latent structure analysis and, 174
multifactorial polygenic (MFP) models, 175–176
oligogenic models, 175
single major locus (SML) models, 173–176
Mazindole, 52–53, 381
Melancholic depression diagnostic criteria, **4**
Melperone, 462
Memory
associative memory, 116
canonical memory, 114
nonspatial memory studies, 118
spatial working memory, 115, 116–117
working memory and, 114–119, 397
Mesoridazine, 457, 458
Messenger RNA (mRNA)
antidepressants' affect on, 13
brain stress response function of, 20–21
circadian rhythm function and, 22–24
c-fos expression and, 468
glutamatergic transmission dysfunction and, 89
in the hippocampus, 228
LHPA and
dysregulation of in aged rats, 33–36
negative regulation of, 26–29
neuron functioning and, 10, **12**
serotonin transport and, 65–68, **66**
[125I]Metaiodobenzylguanidine (MIBG), 55
3-Methoxy-4-hydroxyphenylglycol (MHPG), in cerebrospinal fluid, 208–209
[3H]*N*-Methylspiperone (NMSP), atypical antipsychotics and, 461
MFP. *See* Multifactorial polygenic (MFP) genetic transmission models
MHPG. *See* 3-Methoxy-4-hydroxyphenylglycol (MHPG)
Mianserin, 463
MIBG. *See* [125I]Metaiodobenzyl-guanidine (MIBG)
Michaelis-Menten saturation kinetics, 61
Mineralocorticoid receptor (MR)
LHPA dysregulation in aged rats and, 33–34
LHPA negative feedback control by, 24–29
Molecular genetics, **11**
Molindone, 457, 458
Monoamine transporters. *See also* Antidepressant action mechanism; Antidepressants; Norepinephrine (NE)
mood disorder etiology, treatment and, 9
Mood disorders. *See also* Affective disorders; Bipolar disorder; Major depression
general issues in the study of, 8–10
LHPA dysregulation and, 38–39
overview of, 2–8, **3**, **5**, **7–8**
mpPVN. *See* Hypothalamus, medial parvicellular aspect of the paraventricular nucleus of (mpPVN)
MR. *See* Mineralocorticoid receptor (MR)

MRI. *See* Magnetic resonance imaging (MRI) scan
mRNA. *See* Messenger RNA (mRNA)
β-MSH, 18
γ-MSH, ACTH derivation and, 18
Mucopolysaccharidosis, type II, 132
Multifactorial polygenic (MFP) genetic transmission models, of schizophrenia, 175–176
Multiple sclerosis, SRIF concentrations and, 272
Multiplex families. *See* Infantile autism

N

N-linked glycosylation sites, 56–57, **56,** 67
National Institutes of Health, xvi
Negative regulatory circuits, of LHPA axis, 26–29
NET. *See* Norepinephrine transporters (NET)
Neurobiological advances, 10
Neurodevelopment model of brain pathology, 405–406
Neurofibromatosis, 138
Neuroimaging. *See also specific techniques*
  ARNMD meeting presentations on, **11**
  brain structure abnormalities studied by, 393–394
Neuroleptic drugs
  cerebral cortical mechanisms dissolution and, 120–122, 370–371
  dopaminergic system affected by, 120–122, 369–371, 376, 400
  frontal lobe hypofunction and, 398–399
  for schizophrenia, 121–122
Neuropeptides. *See also* Antidepressants, neuropeptides and
  affective disorders and
    advancement in knowledge of, 259–260
    mood disorder etiology, treatment and, 9
    research directions on, 282–284
    suicide postmortem studies of, 198
  corticotropin-releasing factor (CRF)
    ACTH and, 262–263, 269
    affective disorders and, 260–270, **264, 267, 268**
    in cerebral spinal fluid (CSF) of depressed patients, 262, 263–266, **264,** 269
    future research issues on, 269–270
    HPA hyperactivity in major depression and, 262–263, 269–270
    locus ceruleus noradrenergic neurons and, 261–262
    other psychiatric disorders and, 265, 269, 275–276
    pituitary and adrenal gland volumes and, 266–267, **268,** 269
    receptor downregulation of in suicide victims, 266, **267,** 269
    stress response behavior reactions of, 260–261, 269

somatotropin release-inhibiting factor (SRIF)
  affective disorders and, 270–277, **273**
  behavioral and physiological effects of, 272
  distribution of throughout CNS, 271
  effects of in neuropsychiatric disorders, 272
  excitatory and inhibitory actions of, 271–272
  growth hormone secretion and, 270
  neurotransmitters and, 270–271, 276–277
  postmortem studies of, 276
  receptor subtypes of in CNS, 271
  role of in major depression, 272–275, **273**, 276, 280
thyrotropin-releasing hormone (TRH)
  affective disorders and, 277–282
  antidepressant effects of, 278
  HPT axis function of, 277–278, 279–281
  hypothalamic and extrahypothalamic distribution of, 278
  physiological and behavioral effects of, 278–279, 281–282
  role of in depression, 279–282
  seizure disorders treatment and, 278–279
  TSH and, 278–282

Neuropharmacology. *See also* Antipsychotics; Atypical antipsychotics; Neuroleptic drugs; Pharmacology; *specific substances*
  biochemically known neurons and, 13
Neurotransmitter. *See also* Antidepressants; Suicide postmortem studies; *specific substances*
  release and clearance of, 50, **51**
Nigrostriatal system, atypical antipsychotic drugs and, 453–456
Nisoxetine, 52–53
[^{3}H]Nitroquipazine binding, serotonin transporters and, 65
NMSP. *See* [^{3}H]*N*-Methylspiperone (NMSP)
Nomifensine, 52–53
Noradrenergic system. *See* Corticotropin-releasing factor (CRF); Norepinephrine transporters (NET); Suicide postmortem studies
Norepinephrine (NE). *See also* Norepinephrine transporters (NET)
  for major depression, 4
  production of research, 13
Norepinephrine transporters (NET). *See also* Antidepressant action mechanism, norepinephrine function and
  catecholamine substrates and, 59–60
  mechanism, structure, control of, 50, **51**

Norepinephrine transporters (NET) *(continued)*
molecular basis of uptake 1, 52–64, **53, 54, 56, 58**
angiotensin II/III and, 62–63
atrial natriuretic peptide and, 63
catecholamine biosynthesis and, 61
cloning of hNET cDNA and, 55–56, **56**
cocaine, amphetamine, tricyclic antidepressants and, 59
conclusions regarding, 73–74
cyclic adenosine monophosphate (cAMP) and, 63
dopamine influx substrate and, 52
endogenous mechanisms of, 61–64
GAT/NET gene family relationships and, 57–59, **58,** 64
genomic locus for, 60–61
insulin and, 63
ion-cotransport and, 52, **53,** 69–70
phenylethylamine substrates for, 52–53
protein phosphorylation and, 56–57, **56,** 63
SK-N-SH cells and, 60–61
transmembrane domain (TMD) structure of, 55–57, **56,** 59–60
SRIF and, 271
Norrie's disease, 132, 138
Nortriptyline, 52
Nucleus accumbens
c-fos expression and, 467–469
clozapine and
cholinergic system and, 466
dopaminergic system and, 454–455
glutamatergic dysfunction and, 470–471, 474
serotonergic system and, 457–458, 459
depression and, 252
dopaminergic system and, 370–371, 372, **373**
haloperidol and, 456
GABA concentration abnormalities in, 92
schizophrenia postmortem studies of, 225–227
blood flow abnormalities in, 225
D_2 receptors and, 224, 225–226, **226,** 227
SRIF in, 271
Nucleus of the solitary tract, LHPA positive regulation and, 30

O

Obsessive-compulsive disorder, SRIF concentrations and, 276
Occipital lobe asymmetries, 404
Olanzapine, 453
c-fos expression and, 469
glutamatergic dysfunction and, 470, 471
low EPS incidence of, 453–454
serotonergic system and, 457, 459
Olfactory tubercle, dopaminergic system and, 370–371
Oligogenic genetic transmission models, of schizophrenia, 175
Oxytocin, ACTH secretion and, 18

P

Pallidum
familial pure depressive disease (FPDD) and, **244,** 251–252
shared brain circuitry and, 252
Panic disorder, 265
Paranoid personality disorder, 183
Paranoid schizophrenia, 6
Paraventricular nucleus (PVN) of the hypothalamus
LHPA negative regulation by, 26–29
medial parvicellular aspect of (mpPVN), 18, 19–21, 29–31, 35–36
Parkinson's disease
anticholinergic drugs and, 465
clozapine and, 453
dopamine replacement treatment for, 223
psychomotor retardation in, 437
SRIF concentrations and, 272
Paroxetine, 68
[^{3}H]Paroxetine binding
serotonin transporters and, 65
in suicide victims, 201–202, **201**
Passivity experiences, 443
Pasteur, Louis, 494
Pathophysiology of schizophrenia
conclusions regarding, 407
functional abnormalities, 397–398
brain neurochemistry and, 400–401
frontal lobe hypofunction, 398–399
hypofrontality, 399–400
hypofrontality and, 398–399, 406
medication affecting, 398–399
neurodevelopment abnormalities
in limbic cortices, 406
model for, 405–406
structural abnormalities
lateral cerebral ventricular enlargement, 394–396, 406
medial temporal lobe abnormalities, 396–397
structural-functional interactions, 401
asymmetry of pathology vs. pathology of asymmetry, 403–404
role of functional networks in psychosis, 402–403
PCR. *See* Polymerase chain reaction (PCR) analysis
Peptides. *See* Corticotropin-releasing factor (CRF); Neuropeptides; Somatotropin release-inhibiting factor (SRIF); Thyrotropin-releasing hormone (TRH)
Perinatal development vulnerability, 95
Perphenazine, 455
Personality disorders, suicide and, 197
PET. *See* Positron-emission tomography (PET)
Pharmacology. *See also* Antipsychotics; Atypical antipsychotics; Neuroleptic drugs; Neuropharmacology; *specific substances*
application of, xvi
ARNMD meeting presentations on, **11**
Phencyclidine (PCP), 469
receptor sites of, 90, 91–92

Phenocopies, infantile autism and, 130–131, 134
Phenylketonuria, 131, 132, 138
pHVA. *See* Homovanillic acid (HVA)
Pilocarpine, 473
Pituitary gland. *See also* Limbic-hypothalamic-pituitary-adrenal axis (LHPA)
  ACTH derived from, 17–18
  brain stress response function of, 20–21
  SRIF and, 272
  volume of in affective disorder patients, 266–267, **268**
Plasma studies, of dopaminergic system, 376–379, **377, 378**
Polymerase chain reaction (PCR) analysis, autism and, 147
POMC. *See* Proopiomelanocortin (POMC)
Positive regulatory circuits of LHPA axis, 26–29
Positron-emission tomography (PET)
  application of, 240–241
    to familial pure depressive disease (FPDD), 242–244, **243**
    to self-induced dysphoria, 245–247, **246**
    to verbal response selection, **243, 246,** 247–248
  brain structure abnormalities studied by, 393–394, 400
    asymmetries, 404
    hypofrontality, 398–399
  clozapine effectiveness measured by, 452
  dopamine function measured by, 226, 374–375, 379–380, 400
  frontotemporal abnormalities studied by, 423, 424
  functional networks studied by, 402–403
  introduction of, 223, 239
Postmortem studies
  of dopaminergic system, 372–374, **373, 374**
  multiple disciplines in, xvi
Postnatal development, glutamatergic development dysfunction during, 95–97, 102
Posttraumatic stress disorder
  ACTH and, 262–263
  CRF and, 262–263
Prefrontal cortex region. *See also* Frontal cortex; Frontotemporal abnormalities
  blood flow abnormalities in, 225
  brain circuitry and
    familial pure depressive disease (FPDD) and, 242–244, **243, 244,** 251–252
    LSPT circuit and, 253
    self-induced dysphoria and, **243,** 245–247
    shared brain circuits and, **246,** 248–252, **250**
    in verbal response selection, **246,** 247–248
  c-fos expression and, 467–469
  cerebral cortical mechanisms dissolution and, 113–114
    associative memory function and, 115–116
    blood flow studies of, 117
    functional organization, informational domains within, 117–119, **119,** 402
    internal representation and, 114–119, **119**

spatial working memory function and, 116–117
working memory function and, 114–119, 397
dopaminergic system and, 120–122, **121,** 370, 372, **373**
atypical antipsychotics and, 456, 466
cerebrospinal fluid HVA concentrations and, 372, **373,** 375–379, **377, 378,** 381, 400, 401
cognitive specificity of, 401
decreased function and, 379–381
linking increased and decreased function of, 381–382
neuroimaging studies, 400–401
executive function defects and, 397–398
GABA receptor binding abnormalities in, 92–93, **94**
glutamatergic dysfunction and, 471
intrinsically cued behavior and, 436–439
modulating corollary discharge and, 439
neuroleptics affecting, 120–122, 370–371
neuropathology of, 120–122
serotonin transporter binding sites in, 202
suicide postmortem studies of
adrenergic receptors in, **208, 209,** 210–212, 212–214, **213**
CRF receptor binding and, 266, **267**
5-HT and 5-HIAA receptors in, 199, **199,** 200, **213**
5-HT_{1A} receptors in, 205, **206, 213**
5-HT_2 receptors in, 203–205, **204, 213**
norepinephrine and metabolites in, 207–208, **213**
in systems level schizophrenia model, 98–102, **100–101**
Prenatal development
glutamatergic development dysfunction during, 95–97, 102
myelination changes and, 96–97
Preoptic area, SRIF in, 271
Prevalence rate, of schizophrenia, 164–165
Proline, 57–58, **58**
Proopiomelanocortin (POMC)
brain stress response function of, 19–21
cloning of, 17–18
Prosopagnosia, 443–444
Protein kinase C, SERT phosphorylation sites and, 71
Pseudo-autosomal locus studies, schizophrenia linkage studies and, 179
Psychological stress. *See also* Limbic-hypothalamic-pituitary-adrenal axis (LHPA)
LHPA dysregulation and, 37–39
Psychopharmacology. *See* Antipsychotics; Atypical antipsychotics; Neuroleptic drugs; Neuropharmacology; Pharmacology; *specific substance*
Psychosis not otherwise specified, schizophrenia spectrum disorder and, 182–183

Psychotic spectrum disorders, 182–183
Putamen, 370, **373, 374**
PVN. *See* Paraventricular nucleus (PVN) of the hypothalamus

R

Raphe magnus, LHPA positive regulation and, 30
Raphe nuclei
  mRNA cloning in, 65, **66**
  serotonin transport uptake sites of, 65
Raven's Matrices, 400
Reafference copy, 439
Receptor binding studies, of glutamatergic dysfunction in schizophrenia, 89–92
Remoxipride
  c-fos expression and, 469
  low EPS of, 453
  prefrontal cortex dopamine receptors affected by, 121
Residual schizophrenia, 6
Restriction fragment length polymorphism (RFLP) analysis
  autism and, 147
    testing for linkage to autosomal markers: genotyping, 154–155
  description, explanation of, 177–178
RFLP. *See* Restriction fragment length polymorphism (RFLP) analysis
Risk factors
  of schizophrenia, 166–167
    lifetime risk, 166
Risperidone, 453
  c-fos expression and, 469
  glutamatergic dysfunction and, 470, 471
  low EPS incidence of, 453–454, 463
  serotonergic system and, 457, 459, 463–464
Ritanserin
  dopaminergic system and, 455
  serotonergic system and, 459, 463
Rubella, autism and, 130

S

Schizoaffective disorder, 182–183
Schizoid personality disorder, 183, 184–185
Schizophrenia. *See also* Cerebral cortical mechanisms dissolution; Frontotemporal abnormalities; Pathophysiology of schizophrenia; Schizophrenic brain
  basic science and, 493–494
  behavioral genetics of
    adoption studies of, 171–172, 183, 184
    family studies of, 167–169, 179, 183–184
    linkage analysis and, 176–181
    mathematical models of genetic transmission and, 173–176
    multifactorial polygenic model of, 175–176
    oligogenic genetic transmission model of, 175
    single major locus model of, 173–176
    twin studies of, 169–171, 175–176, 183
  cerebral lateralization hypothesis of, 403–404

clinical implications of
diagnosis, 185–186
genetic counseling, 187–188
treatment, 186–187
clinical problems research base for, 494
diagnostic criteria for, **7**
dopaminergic system and
decreased function of
cortical function, 379–380
dopamine function, 380–381
hypothesis of in schizophrenia, 369–370
increased function of
anatomy of, 370–372
cerebrospinal fluid studies of, 375–376
PET studies of, 374–375
plasma studies of, 376–379, **377, 378**
postmortem studies of, 372–374, **373, 374**
linking increased with decreased function of, 381–382
conclusions regarding, 382–383
epidemiology of
gender differences, 166, 167
incidence rate, 165
lifetime risk factor, 166
overview of, 163–164
prevalence rate, 164–165
risk factors, 166–167
socioeconomic factors and, 167
general issues in the study of, 8–10
overview of, 6
role of functional networks in, 402–403
spectrum disorders of
psychotic spectrum disorders, 182–183
schizotypal personality disorder, 183–185
SRIF concentrations and, 274
subtypes of, 6
suicide and, 197
symptoms of
auditory hallucinations, 441–442
delusional misinterpretations, 442
delusions of control and passivity experiences, 443
gender differences in, 167
inappropriate affect, 442–443
"over-inclusiveness" of cognitive processing, 92
thought pathology in
developmental maturation of, 495–497
internal cerebral representations of the external world and, 497–500
interspike interval (ISI) between action potentials and, 501–502
loose associations and, 495–497
Schizophrenic brain
conclusions regarding, 102–103
GABA system dysfunction in, 84, 92–93, **94**
anterior cingulate, prefrontal cortex abnormalities and, 92–93, **94**
benzodiazepine binding site abnormalities and, 93
frontal cortex abnormalities and, 92–93

Schizophrenic brain *(continued)*
GABA system dysfunction in
glutamate decarboxylase (GAD) activity dysfunction and, 92
in layer II of anterior cingulate region and, 93–95
systems level schizophrenia model and, 98–102, **100–101**
glutamatergic dysfunction in, 84
anatomical findings regarding, 85–89, **87, 88**
neuronal cell concentrations and, 85–89, **87, 88,** 122
pre- and postnatal development abnormalities and, 95–97, 102
receptor binding studies of, 89–92
frontal cortex receptor binding sites and, 90–91
hippocampus receptor binding sites and, 89–91
phencyclidine (PCP) receptor binding activity and, 90, 91–92
neuronal degeneration of
causative mechanisms in, 83–84
ontogeny-excitotoxicity relationship and
glutamatergic transmission role in, 84, 97–98
layer II findings regarding, 93–95
pre- and postnatal development of glutamatergic transmission and, 95–97, 102
postmortem studies of
antipsychotic dopamine receptor blockage and, 224
of basal ganglia, 225–227, **226**
conclusions regarding, 230–231
of the dorsolateral prefrontal cortex, 229–230
of entorhinal cortex, 227–228, **229**
genetic factors and, 224
of the hippocampus, 228, **229**
of the nucleus accumbens, 225–227
structural abnormalities and, 224–225
technology advances in, 223
systems level approach to, 98–102, **100–101**
Schizotypal personality disorder, 183–185
Scopolamine, 466
Self-induced dysphoria, **243,** 244–247, **244, 246**
Serine-threonine phosphorylation sites, norepinephrine transport and, **56,** 63, 67
Seroquel, 453
5-HT_{2A} and, 455
low EPS incidence of, 453–454
Serotonin. *See also* 5-HT; Serotonin reuptake inhibitors (SRIs); Serotonin transporters (SERT); Suicide postmortem studies
clozapine and, 456–464
neurons producing, 13
Serotonin receptors. *See* Serotonin transporters (SERT); Suicide postmortem studies

Serotonin reuptake inhibitors (SRIs). *See also* 5-HT
for major depression, 4
SRIF affected by, 276
Serotonin transporters (SERT). *See also* Antidepressant action mechanism; Suicide postmortem studies
molecular basis of
mechanism, structure of, 50, **53**
proposed transmembrane topology and structural features of, 55–56, **56**
platelet and brain targets for antidepressants and, 64–72, **66**
antidepressant 5-HT uptake inhibitors and, 72
cloning of cDNA, mRNA and, 65–68, **66**
CNS uptake sites and, 64–65
conclusions regarding, 73–74
GAT/NET gene family and, **58,** 67–68, 72
ion-cotransport and, **53,** 70–71
phosphorylation sites and, 71
structural transport features and, 68–69
transporter cDNAs and, 71, 72
SRIF and, 271
SERT. *See* Serotonin transporters (SERT)
Sertindole, 453
5-HT_{2A} and, 455
low EPS incidence of, 453–454
Sertraline, 202
Setoperone, 462
Short-term memory. *See* Working memory
Single major locus (SML) genetic transmission models, of schizophrenia, 173–176
Single photon emission computed tomography (SPECT)
brain blood flow measured by, 230
brain structure abnormalities studied by, 393–394, 400
hypofrontality, 398–399
frontal cortex dopamine function measured by, 379, 400
introduction of, 223
Single-gene metabolic disease, 132–133
SK-N-SH
cDNA and, 55
norepinephrine transporters and, 60–61
SML. *See* Single major locus (SML) genetic transmission models
Smooth-pursuit eye movement dysfunction, schizophrenia and, 174
Somatization disorder, 265
Somatotropin release-inhibiting factor (SRIF), 270–277, **273**
affective disorders and, 270–277, **273**
behavioral and physiological effects of, 272
distribution of throughout CNS, 271
effects of in neuropsychiatric disorders, 272
excitatory and inhibitory actions of, 271–272
growth hormone secretion and, 270
neurotransmitters and, 270–271, 276–277
postmortem studies of, 276
receptor subtypes of in CNS, 271

Spatial working memory, 115, 116–117
SPECT. *See* Single photon emission computed tomography (SPECT)
[^{3}H]Spiroperidol binding
atypical antipsychotics and, 450
to D_1 receptors, 371
to 5-HT_2 receptors in suicide victims, 203
SRIF. *See* Somatotropin release-inhibiting factor (SRIF)
SRIs. *See* Serotonin reuptake inhibitors (SRIs)
Stress axis, system. *See also* Limbic-hypothalamic-pituitary-adrenal axis (LHPA)
mood disorder etiology, treatment and, 9
psychological stress response and, 37–39
Striatum
c-fos expression and, 467–469
clozapine and
anticholinergic drugs and, 465–467
dopaminergic system and, 454–455
glutamatergic dysfunction and, 470, 471–474
serotonergic system and, 457–459, 461, 462
D_2, D_4 receptors and, 227
dopaminergic system and, 224, 370–371, 372–374, **374**
D_2 receptor density and, 374–375, 455–456
haloperidol and, 378, 455–456
linking increased and decreased function of, 381–382
neostriatum and, 370
shared brain circuitry and, 252
familial pure depressive disease (FPDD) and, **244**
psychomotor deficiencies and, 437–438
Substance abuse suicide, 197
Substantia nigra
cDNA cloning in, 65
c-fos expression and, 468
dopaminergic system and
anatomy of, 370–371
dopamine-producing cells of, **12,** 13
receptors in, 224
shared brain circuitry and, 252
Parkinson's disease and, 224
serotonergic system and, 65, 459
Suicide postmortem studies
of CRF concentrations, 264–265, **264**
of noradrenergic system, 206–207
adrenergic receptors in
α-adrenergic receptors, 211–212
β-adrenergic receptors, 210–211
conclusions regarding, 212–214, **213**
norepinephrine and metabolites, 207–210, **207, 208, 209**
predisposition factors and, 197–198
of serotonergic system
conclusions regarding, 212–214, **213**
serotonin (5-HT) and 5-hydroxyindoleacetic acid (5-HIAA) and, 198–200, **199**

serotonin receptors and
5-HT_{1A} serotonin receptors, 205, **206**
5-HT_2 serotonin receptors, 203–205, **204**
other receptor subtypes, 206
transporter binding site, 200–202, **201**
SERT density and, 72
Sulpiride
glutamatergic dysfunction and, 470–471
serotonergic system and, 457
Superior colliculus, corollary discharge and, 439
Sylvian-insular cortices, 248

T

Tardive dyskinesia, 465, 466
Taurine, 57–58, **58**
Tegmental area, dopaminergic system and, 370–371
Tegretol, 5
Temporal cortex region. *See also* Frontotemporal abnormalities
asymmetries of, 404
dopaminergic system and, **373**
structure abnormalities of, 225, 396–397
suicide postmortem studies of
adrenergic receptors in, **209,** 210–211, **210**
norepinephrine and metabolites in, 207
Thalamus
blood flow abnormalities in, 225
brain circuitry and
familial pure depressive disease (FPDD) and, 242, **244,** 251–252
shared brain circuitry and, **246,** 248–251, **250**
dopaminergic system and, 371
GABA concentration abnormalities in, 92
glutamatergic system and, 86, 471–472
major depression and, 253
serotonin transport uptake sites of, 65
Thioridazine
anticholinergic effect of, 465, 466–467
dopaminergic system and, 456
low EPS of, 453, 467
serotonergic system and, 457, 458
Thiothixene, 453
Thyroid-stimulating hormone (TSH)
SRIF and, 272
TRH and, 278–282
Thyrotropin-releasing hormone (TRH), 277–282
affective disorders and, 277–282
antidepressant effects of, 278
depression and, 279–282
HPT axis function of, 277–278, 279–281
hypothalamic and extrahypothalamic distribution of, 278
physiological and behavioral effects of, 278–279, 281–282
seizure disorders treatment and, 278–279
TSH and, 278–282
Tiospirone
5-HT_{2A} and, 455
low EPS incidence of, 453–454
serotonergic system and, 462
TMD. *See* Transmembrane domain (TMD)
Tower of London task, 380

Transmembrane domain (TMD)
GAT/NET gene family relationships and, 58–59, 67
norepinephrine and serotonin transporter structure and, 55–57, **56,** 59–60, 67
TRH. *See* Thyrotropin-releasing hormone (TRH)
Tricyclic antidepressants
norepinephrine and serotonin transporters and, 59, 69
norepinephrine transmission inhibition by, 50
Trihexyphenidyl, 465
Tuberous sclerosis, 132, 138
Twin studies
of autism
concordance rate of, 130
monozygotic autistic twins and, 138, **142**
of hypofrontality, 399
of schizophrenia, 169–171
multifactorial polygenic (MFP) vs. single major locus (SML) genetic transmission models and, 175–176
monozygotic vs. dizygotic, 169–170, 175–176
schizotypal personality disorder and, 183
ventricular enlargement and, 228, 396
Tyrosine hydroxylase, **12,** 13
activity of in noradrenergic system, 207
brain stem noradrenergic neurons and, 209

U

Undifferentiated schizophrenia, 6

V

Vaccinia-T7 expression system, norepinephrine transporter studies and, 55
Valproic acid, for bipolar disease, 5
Ventricular enlargement, 406
CAT study of, 224–225
lateral cerebral enlargement and, 394–396
schizophrenia type I/type II dichotomization and, 395
twin studies of, 228, 396
Verbal response selection, 247–248
Visuospatial working memory, 115, 116–117

W

Wisconsin Card Sorting Test
dorsal lateral prefrontal cortex function in, 229–230
frontal lobe function and, 379, 381, 399, 401
working memory and, 114–115, 118, **119**
Working memory
prefrontal cortex mechanisms and, 114–119
blood flow studies of, 117
dopamine systems and, 120–122, **121**
functional organization, informational domains of, 117–119, **119**
human studies of, 116–117
neuroleptics affecting, 120–122
rhesus monkey studies of, 114–116
temporal lobe structure abnormalities and, 397

X

X-linked inheritance
  autism and, 132, 147–149
  fragile X syndrome and, 132, 138, 139, 147–149
  Norrie's disease and, 132, 138

Z

zif-268, LHPA positive regulation and, 31
Zimelidine, 276
Ziprasidone, 453
Zotepine, 462